Clinical Haematology

Clinical Haematology

Seventh Edition

R. D. Eastham
MD (Cantab) FRCP (Lond) FRCPath FRCPsych
DCP Dipl Path
*Honorary Consultant Pathologist to the Frenchay Group of
Hospitals, Bristol; Honorary University Lecturer, Bristol University*

R. R. Slade
BSc MB BS MRCP MRCPath
*Consultant Haematologist, Southmead
Hospital, Bristol; Clinical Dean, Southmead Hospital, Bristol*

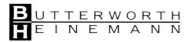

Butterworth-Heinemann Ltd
Linacre House, Jordan Hill, Oxford OX2 8DP

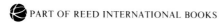 PART OF REED INTERNATIONAL BOOKS

OXFORD LONDON BOSTON
MUNICH NEW DELHI SINGAPORE SYDNEY
TOKYO TORONTO WELLINGTON

First published 1961
Reprinted 1962
Second edition 1966
Reprinted 1968
Third edition 1970
Fourth edition 1974
Fifth edition 1977
Sixth edition 1984
Seventh edition 1992

British Library Cataloguing in Publication Data
Eastham, R. D.
  Clinical haematology. – 7th ed.
  I. Title II. Slade, R.
  616.1

ISBN 0 7506 1339 4

Library of Congress Cataloguing in Publication Data
Eastham, R. D.
  Clinical haematology/R. D. Eastham, R. R. Slade. – 7th ed.
  p. cm.
  Includes bibliographical references and index.
  ISBN 0 7506 1339 4
  1. Hematology.   I. Slade, R. R.   II. Title.
  [DNLM: 1. Blood.   QY 400 E13c]
  RB145.E33
  616.1'5075–dc20
  DNLM/DLC
  for Library of Congress   91–26656
                                                CIP

Typeset by STM Typesetting Limited, Amesbury, Wilts
Printed and bound in Great Britain by Bath Press, Avon

Contents

Preface to the Seventh Edition

The seventh edition of *Clinical Haematology* has been extensively revised, brought up-to-date, and produced in a new format. With Dr Slade joining Dr Eastham, more information on clinical practice has been added to the interpretation of laboratory results. The contents of the first three chapters have been rearranged by Dr Slade, who has written the sections on the haemoglobinopathies and thalassaemias in Chapter 3, bone marrow malignancies, aplastic anaemia and AIDS in Chapter 5, and blood transfusion at the end of Chapter 6. Chapter 6 has been rewritten and rearranged, and now includes details about the early stages of clotting, natural anticoagulant factors, and the mechanisms whereby clot integrity is sustained without generalized thrombosis ensuing. Advances have necessitated extensive rewriting of the sections dealing with platelets, fibrinolysis and anticoagulant therapy. There is a large index to ensure easy reference.

R. D. E.
R. R. S.

Preface to the First Edition

This book is similar in design and intent to *Biochemical Values in Clinical Medicine* in that I have attempted to provide an accurate summary of the ways in which various clinical conditions can be related to haematological results.

Since clinical haematology is a different discipline from clinical biochemistry, it was not considered adequate merely to list the various laboratory tests and the significance of their results. Accordingly, the book falls into the following sections:

1. Haemoglobins and associated pigments.
2. Red blood cells.
3. Anaemia.
4. Peripheral white blood cells.
5. Bone marrow.
6. Bleeding, clotting and transfusion.

The relevant laboratory tests are included in each section. Individual coagulation factors (e.g. Factors V, VII, etc.) are considered in detail. Where known, their physical characters are listed. In this respect the recently agreed International Nomenclature for the various factors has been used (e.g. Factors I, II, III, IV, V, VII, VIII, IX, X).

The aetiology of certain clinical conditions (e.g. pancytopenia, purpura in children, macrocytic anaemia) have been considered. Because the rate of expansion of knowledge in Haematology, as in Clinical Biochemistry, is very great at the present time, many new tests which are not, as yet, performed in routine laboratories have been described. This extension of recent knowledge has also been used as an excuse for giving details, for example, of such conditions as von Willebrand's disease, which, although rare, has a very interesting relationship with haemophilia and other conditions with reduced plasma antihaemophiliac globulin content. (The name von Willebrand has been used in connection with four syndromes.)

It is hoped that this book, which is not intended to replace standard haematology textbooks, will encourage more discussion of haematological cases and problems between clinicians and clinical haematologists. It is also hoped that it will be of some assistance to junior medical hospital staff in their requests for tests, and interpretation of results of these tests.

I am grateful to Dr A. B. Raper, Consultant Haematologist, Bristol United Hospitals, for reading the manuscript, and to Mr K. W. Denson FIML, for helpful advice, criticism, and much valuable information relating to coagulation problems.

R.D.E.

Abbreviations

ABO	Landsteiner blood groups
ACTH	adrenocorticotrophin
[AD]	autosomal dominant
ADA	adenosine deaminase
ADP	adenosine diphosphate
AHG	factor VIII
AICAR	5-amino-4-imidazole carboxamide ribotide
AIDS	acquired immune deficiency syndrome
ALL	acute lymphoblastic leukaemia
AML	acute myeloid leukaemia
AMP	adenosine monophosphate
cAMP	cyclic adenosine monophosphate
APTT	activated partial thromboplastin time
[AR]	autosomal recessive
AS	heterozygote sickle-cell disease
ATP	adenosine triphosphate
AT-III	antithrombin III
BCR	British comparative ratio (prothrombin ratio)
BFU	burst-forming cell
CFU	colony-forming unit
CGL	chronic granulocytic (myeloid) leukaemia
CML	chronic myeloid leukaemia
CSA	colony-stimulating activity
CSF	colony-stimulating factor
DDAVP	synthetic analogue of vasopressin
$DF^{32}P$	di-isopropylfluorophosphate (labelled)
DIC	disseminated intravascular coagulopathy
DNA	deoxyribonucleic acid
2,3-DPG	2,3-diphosphoglycerate
dU	deoxyuridine
E-B Virus	Epstein–Barr virus
EDTA	ethylenediamine tetraacetic acid, sequestrene
EP	endogenous pyrogens
ER	endoplasmic reticulin
ESR	erythrocyte sedimentation rate
Fc	the constant portion of the heavy chain of an immunoglobulin
FDP	fibrin/fibrinogen degradation products
FEP	free erythrocyte protoporphyrin

FIGLU	formiminoglutamic acid
FPA	fibrinopeptide A
FPB	fibrinopeptide B
G	glucose
GC	glutamyl-cysteine
Gd^A, Gd^B etc.	different forms of glucose-6-phosphate dehydrogenase
GVHD	graft versus host disease
HDL	high-density lipoprotein
HEMPAS	hereditary erythroblastic multinuclearity associated with a positive acidified serum test
HETE	12-L-hydroxy-5,8,10,14-eicosatetraenoic acid
HGH	human growth factor
HIV	human immunodeficiency virus
HL-A	human leucocyte antigen
HMWK	high-molecular-weight kininogen
HPPF	human plasma protein fraction
HRGP	histidine-rich glycoprotein
HS	hereditary spherocytic haemolytic disease
5-HT	5-hydroxytryptamine, serotonin
HTLV	a retrovirus
ICR	international comparative ratio (prothrombin ratio)
IF	intrinsic factor
IgG, IgA, IgM, IgD, IgE	immunoglobulins
IMP	inosine monophosphate
INR	international normalized ratio
IQ	intelligence quotient
ISC	irreversibly sickled cells
ITP	idiopathic thrombocytopenic purpura
K_x	antigen necessary for the proper expression of Kell in red cells
LASS	labile aggregation stimulating substance
LAV	lymphadenopathy virus
LDH	lactate dehydrogenase
LDL	low-density lipoprotein
LE	lupus erythematosus
LEM	leucocyte endogenous mediator
LMWK	low-molecular-weight kininogen
L1, L2, L3	used in classification of acute lymphatic leukaemia
M1, M2, M3, ..., M6	system of classification of acute myeloblastic leukaemia
MAF	macrophage activating factor
MCAT	mean cell average thickness
MCF	mean corpuscular fragility (i.e. strength of saline to produce 50% haemolysis)
MCF	macrophage chemotactic factor
MCH	mean corpuscular haemoglobin
MCHC	mean corpuscular haemoglobin concentration
MCT	mean cell thickness
MCV	mean cell volume
MHC	major histocompatibility complex
MIF	migration inhibition factor
MIT	total marrow iron turnover
MLC	mixed lymphocyte culture
MMA	methylmalonic acid
MPV	mean platelet volume
NADH	nicotinamide adenine dinucleotide – coenzyme I
NADPH	nicotinamide adenine dinucleotide phosphate – coenzyme II

NBT	nitroblue tetrazolium test
OPSI	overwhelming postsplenectomy infection
PCV	packed cell volume
PDGF	platelet-derived growth factor
PF3	platelet factor 3
PF4	platelet factor 4
PG	prostaglandin (e.g. PCE_1 etc.)
Ph	Philadelphia chromosome
pH	reciprocal of $logarithm_{10}$ of hydrogen ion concentration
Pi	inorganic phosphate
PIVKA	protein-induced vitamin K absence or antagonist
PNH	paroxysmal nocturnal haemoglobinuria
PNP	purine nucleoside phosphorylase
P_{O_2}	oxygen partial pressure
$P_{50}O_2$	oxygen partial pressure corresponding to 50% saturation of haemoglobin
PPD	purified protein derivative
PSC	pluripotent haemopoietic stem cell
PTH	parathyroid hormone
[R]	rare disorder
RAEB	refractory anaemia with excess blasts
RBC	erythrocyte, red blood cell
Rh	rhesus factor
RNA	ribonucleic acid
SAM	S-adenosyl methionine
SH-	sulphydryl groups
S-phase	Cells in DNA-synthesis phase of cycle
SS	homozygote sickle-cell disease
TCI, TCII, TCIII	transcobalamins I, II and III
^{99m}Tc	technetium, radioactive
TdT	terminal deoxynucleotidyl transferase
THF	tetrahydrofolate
THFA	tetrahydrofolic acid
TIBC	total iron-binding capacity
TTP	thrombotic thrombocytopenic purpura
TxA_2	thromboxane A_2
UIBC	unsaturated iron-binding capacity
WDLL	well-differentiated lymphatic leukaemia

Chapter 1

Red cell physiology and pathology

Blood volume

Normal range

Total blood volume

Full term infant $\simeq$ 85 ml/kg body weight.
Pre-term infant $\simeq$ 108 ml/kg body weight.

(At birth, delayed clamping of the cord is equivalent to a transfusion of about 150 ml of whole blood in a 3.5-kg infant.)

1. 72–100 ml/kg body weight.
2. 2500–4000 ml/m^2 body surface area.

Total plasma volume

1. For 49–59 ml/kg body weight.
   Infants $\simeq$ 41.3 ml/kg body weight.
   Adult males $\simeq$ 46 ml/kg body weight.
   Adult females $\simeq$ 45 ml/kg body weight.
2. For 1400–2500 ml/m^2 body surface area.

(The plasma volume is variable and difficult to measure accurately. It cannot be used to deduce the red cell volume.)

Total red cell volume

Newborn infant $\simeq$ 29 ml/kg body weight.
Adult males $\simeq$ 30 ml/kg body weight (25–35 ml/kg $\pm$ 2 s.d.).
Adult females $\simeq$ 25 ml/kg body weight (20–30 ml/kg $\pm$ 2 s.d.).

Red cell volume increased in:

1. Primary polycythaemia vera.
2. Secondary erythraemia:
   (a) anoxia;
   (b) renal.

Red cell volume normal, but plasma volume decreased, in 'stress' erythraemia. This condition should not be treated as though it were primary polycythaemia vera. PCV may exceed 55% with haemoglobin exceeding 17 g/dl but red cell volume within normal range.

The *interstitial fluid volume* is three times as great as the plasma volume, and protects the plasma volume from marked change following loss.

In anaemia (other than immediately after haemorrhage) the normal blood volume is maintained by a compensatory increase in the plasma volume.

Increased blood volume

Physiological

1. Normal pregnancy

The total blood volume increases by up to 45% maximal by the thirty-second week. The total plasma volume increase by 25–55%, more than the 20–40% increase in the red cell mass, resulting in the apparent anaemia of normal pregnancy with the haemoglobin concentration remaining above 10 g/dl.

2. Vigorous and prolonged exercise

As in regular marathon training, this type of exercise results in increase in plasma volume greater than the increase in red cell mass, with a fall in the haemoglobin concentration. At the same time, red cell 2,3-DPG increases, improving oxygen delivery to the tissues.

References
Eichner, E. R. (1985) *Am. J. Med.* **78**, 321.
Wardrop, C. A. J. (1987) *Brit. Med. J.* **295**, 455.

Pathological

1. Overtransfusion with saline, blood, plasma, glucose solution, dextran etc., especially if the patient is hypothermic.
2. Polycythaemia vera (red cell mass increased).
3. Occasionally in congestive cardiac failure.

Decreased blood volume

Pathological

1. Acute haemorrhage

The plasma volume is rapidly restored from fluid in the interstitial fluid space.

2. Dehydration

This is following water deprivation, persistent vomiting, diarrhoea, loss of fluid from surgical drains, etc.

Packed cell volume or haematocrit

This is the volume of red blood cell per 100 ml of whole blood. SI units conversion factor = 0.01 i.e. 44–62% becomes 0.44–0.62.

Normal range
- Infant (full term, cord blood)   0.44–0.62
- Infant (3 months)   0.32–0.44
- Child (1 year old, mean)   0.36–0.44
- Child (10 years old, mean)   0.37–0.44
- Adult males   0.40–0.54
- Adult females   0.36–0.47

The haematocrit can be measured by: centrifugation (with error due to trapping of plasma, especially in polycythaemia and conditions with variation of red cell size and shape); conductivity (with error due to any pathological proteins in the plasma); electronic counter (accurate if instrument calibration accurate).

Decrease
- *Absolute* – any case of anaemia, from whatever cause.
- *Relative* – normal pregnancy. The plasma volume increases by a maximum of +55%, and the red cell mass increases by up to +30%, by about 60 days before normal delivery.

Increase
- *Absolute* – normal newborn, transient; living at high altitude; primary polycythaemia (see p. 123); some renal disorders, including carcinoma, sarcoma, nephroblastoma, benign renal tumour, hydronephrosis, and polycystic kidneys; arterial hypoxia – congenital and acquired heart disease, chronic lung disease; benign familial erythrocytosis (R).
- *Relative* – conditions with reduced plasma volume, including dehydration, stress erythrocytosis associated with alcohol and smoking.

Factors affecting blood flow
- Red cell rouleaux formation and aggregation
- Erythrocyte sedimentation rate (ESR)
- Plasma viscosity
- Relationship between the ESR and the plasma viscosity
- Serum viscosity
- Red cell deformability
- Whole blood viscosity

Red cell rouleaux formation and aggregation

When whole blood ceases to move, red cells tend to aggregate, reducing the surface tension of the system. Aggregates of red cells lying face to face (rouleaux) can be seen in anticoagulated whole blood after it has been standing for a few minutes. The half-time for red cell aggregation has been reported in normal blood as 5.6 seconds, falling to 3.3 seconds by week 37 of normal pregnancy.

Aggregation, and the formation of rouleaux, are greatly increased by increases in hydrophilic colloids, such as fibrinogen, α_2-globulin, immunoglobulin IgM, and by increase in the concentration of red cells. It can be increased artificially by other hydrophilic colloids, such as large-molecule dextran and gum acacia (both used as plasma substitutes), and it is inhibited by increasing albumin concentration. Red cell aggregation is responsible for an increase in whole blood viscosity at lower shear rates. On standing in vitro for up to 8 hours this tendency of red cells to aggregate in anticoagulated blood decreases markedly with changes in the red cell membrane, affecting erythrocyte sedimentation rate (ESR) readings.

Reference
Huisman, A., Aarnoudse, J. G., Krans, M., *et al.* (1988) *Br. J. Haematol.* **68**, 121.

Erythrocyte sedimentation rate (ESR)

The ESR is a qualitative test of changes in the plasma proteins, and is also affected by the haematocrit. When anticoagulated blood stands in a column, the red cells aggregate and sediment, leaving clear plasma above. The larger the aggregates, the faster the sedimentation, because the rate of fall depends on the square of the radius of the aggregates. Paradoxically, although a single particle falls more slowly with increasing viscosity, the plasma proteins causing greatest aggregation are also the most viscous and therefore slow the rate of fall – fibrinogen, acute phase proteins and immunoglobulins. Albumin reduces red cell aggregation, and therefore reduces the ESR.

Westergren method

Four parts of blood are diluted with one part of sodium citrate solution (109 mmol/l). The estimation must be carried out within 6 h of collection, otherwise the deterioration in the red cell membrane reduces the ESR to 'normal'.

Normal range
- *Men* – up to 5 mm/h.
- *Women* – up to 7 mm/h (Up to 20 mm/h in normal pregnancy).
- *Newborn* – there is no justification for taking the volume of blood needed for this crude qualitative test.

- *Normal pregnancy* – the normal increase in plasma fibrinogen plus the normal fall in the haematocrit results in an increased normal upper limit. Underlying inflammatory disease can be detected by C-reactive protein estimation.
- *Old age* – it has been claimed that a proportion of otherwise normal old people have abnormally raised ESR values. If the haematocrit is normal, and the plasma proteins are normal, then the ESR will be normal. An unsuspected decrease in plasma albumin, which has been found in some old people who are malnourished, results in a relative increase in plasma fibrinogen and globulin (both within normal absolute values). This, in turn, results in an increased ESR, since the albumin, which would reduce red cell aggregation, is low. These blood samples will have a normal or low–normal plasma viscosity, with a raised ESR in an apparently normal old subject.

References
Harris, C. J. (1972) *J. Med. Lab. Technol.* **29**, 405.
Crawford, J., Eye-Boland, M. K. and Cohen, H. J. (1987) *Am. J. Med.* **82**, 239.

Pathological

1. Increase in ESR
- Increase in plasma fibrinogen and/or globulin.
- Decreased plasma albumin concentration.
- Decreased haematocrit, even though the plasma proteins are normal.
- Any combination of the above.
- Cold agglutinins active at room temperature.

2. Normal ESR in the presence of active inflammatory disease
- Haematocrit more than 0.5, regardless of any changes in the plasma proteins.
- Abnormal red cells with faulty aggregation – including spherocytes, and sickle cells.
- Very high concentrations of plasma immunoglobulins, when the plasma is so viscous that sedimentation is obstructed, e.g. macroglobulinaemia and some cases of myeloma.

(A normal ESR does not exclude organic disease.)

Plasma viscosity

Normal values (British population)

Newborn

Values are 0.98 – 1.25 mPa s at 37°C. For each 1°C below 37°C, the plasma viscosity increases by + 2.4%.

Adult values

These are reached by the third year of life: 1.16 – 1.33 mPa s at 37°C (1.50 – 1.72 mPa s at 25°C, rising to 1.80 mPa s in normal pregnancy). There is a slow normal increase in plasma fibrinogen after late middle age, with an increase in plasma viscosity. The coefficient of variation for the estimation is less than 1%; the estimation, which takes less than 1 min to perform, can be carried out 24 h after collection, and the method has now been automated.

References
Cooke, B. M. and Stuart, J. (1988) *J. Clin. Pathol.* **41**, 1213
ICSH (1984) *J. Clin. Pathol.* **37**, 1147 (recommendations for method)

Pathological

Any condition, which changes plasma fibrinogen, globulins and/or albumin concentrations, results in change in the plasma viscosity. There is a direct correlation between plasma fibrinogen and globulin concentrations with the plasma viscosity.

Increase
- Both acute and chronic inflammatory disease.
- Paraproteinaemia.
- Down's syndrome patients with increasing age. Also to a lesser degree in institutionalized patients with mental handicap.

Decrease
- Severe inanition with low plasma protein concentration, e.g. terminal tuberculosis.
- Therapeutic defibrination with ancrod (snake venom).

Relationship between the ESR and the plasma viscosity

The plasma viscosity and the ESR are directly related until the plasma is so viscous that even very large red cell aggregates only sediment very slowly. There is a direct correlation between plasma fibrinogen, α- and γ-globulin, and both the ESR and plasma viscosity. Plasma albumin concentration is also directly correlated to the plasma viscosity, but inversely correlated to the ESR (as albumin inhibits red cell aggregation). Changes in the haematocrit dramatically affect the ESR, but have no effect on the plasma viscosity. Both tests are non-specific methods for detecting changes in the plasma proteins. Whilst the plasma viscosity can be measured using stored plasma, the ESR must be measured within 6 h of blood collection.

Reference
Hutchinson, R. M. and Eastham, R. D. (1973) *J. Clin. Pathol.* **30**, 345

Serum viscosity

This estimation detects changes in serum globulin and albumin only, and has no advantages over plasma viscosity, but has the disadvantage that any tags of fibrin in serum are liable to block the apparatus.

It has been found that increased serum hyaluronic acid concentrations found in Wilms' tumour cause the serum viscosity to be significantly increased.

Reference
Wu, A. H. B., Parker, O. S. and Ford, L. (1984) *Clin. Chem.* **30**, 914

Red cell deformability

Reticulocytes deform to pass from the marrow sinusoids into the circulation. Following this, red cells have to pass regularly through the splenic filters and the very small peripheral capillaries; they deform without damage to half their diameter in the process, the red cell membrane rotating round the contained haemoglobin like the tread of a tank. The spleen sieves off cells which are no longer flexible, including spherocytes, rigid cells, cells with inclusion bodies and cells which have undergone excessive surface remodelling. Red cell deformability increases with rising temperature, until at 48°C the red cells become elongated and irregularly deformed by small shear stress. This can happen acutely to cells in the area of a burn or scald.

Reference
Stuart, J. (1985) *J. Clin. Pathol.* **38**, 965 (review and methods)

Decrease
- With increasing normal red cell age, the cells become more viscous.
- Membrane defects in hereditary spherocytic anaemia, elliptocytosis and pyropoikilocytosis. Also a rare haemolytic anaemia with high membrane phosphatidyl choline content.

Reference
Yawata, Y., Sugihara, T., Mori, M., *et al.* (1984) *Blood* **64**, 1129
- Malarial infections with parasites in the red cells.
- Sickle-cell disease: haemoglobin S becomes excessively viscous when deoxygenated.
- Abnormal spectrin in the red cell membrane in Duchenne muscular dystrophy.

Reference
Nagano, Y., Wong, P. and Rosen, A. D. (1980) *Clin. Chim. Acta* **108**, 469
- Smokers.
- Diabetes mellitus: both a decrease in red cell deformability in insulin-dependent diabetes and no difference from normal controls have been reported.

References
Williamson, J. R., Gardner, R. A., Boylan, C. W., *et al.* (1985) *Blood* **65**, 283
Bryszewska, M., Watula, C. and Torzecka, W. (1986) *Br. J. Haematol.* **62**, 111

Increase

After a high fatty fish diet, or intake of eicosapentaenoic acid ($C_{20:5}$) and docosahexaenoic acid ($C_{22:6}$), with incorporation of these fatty acids into red cell membrane over 6 weeks, red cell deformability is increased, with a corresponding decrease in whole blood viscosity but no change in plasma viscosity.

Whole blood viscosity

Whole blood is viscous and thixotropic (i.e. high viscosity at low shear, with low viscosity at increased flow velocity, or velocity gradient). At low shear rates ($< 1/s$), whole blood viscosity varies with the plasma concentration of large molecule proteins with a high frictional ratio (e.g. fibrinogen). At high shear rates ($> 100/s$) whole blood viscosity reflects erythrocyte deformability.

When whole blood viscosity is measured in relation to the radius of the capillary through which it is flowing, there is a sudden great increase when the radius falls below $5-7$ μm, when red cells have to deform as they pass along the capillary. This increase in whole blood viscosity therefore has its greatest effect in the arterioles and capillaries, the vessels which carry oxygen to the tissues.

Within the normal range, there is a linear relation between the PCV and the logarithm of the whole blood viscosity, but it is difficult to use regression lines to correct to a standard PCV. Normal blood results may not be applicable to blood from patients. Unfortunately, measurement of whole blood viscosity suffers from poor sensitivity and specificity, with overdependence on the packed cell volume, which limit its clinical usefulness. Measurement of red cell deformability and plasma viscosity is clinically more valuable. The efficiency of the circulation of erythrocytes is proportional to the ratio of the haematocrit to the whole blood viscosity. Maximum efficiency values are found at a haematocrit value of about 0.42. This has implications both for the transfusion of blood in anaemia and for the treatment of polycythaemia. Whole blood viscosity at both high and low shear is significantly reduced when the haematocrit is reduced to 0.4 by venesection, with development of microcytosis, in patients with a high risk of stroke. Microcytosis is not important if venesection is to reduce whole blood viscosity. Controlled low-dose iron therapy with frequent venesection is necessary in secondary polycythaemia due to hypoxic lung disease or cyanotic congenital heart disease, as both the oxygen saturation and the oxygen-carrying capacity fall with the development of microcytic hypochromic red cells. Relieving the microcytosis reduces whole blood viscosity and also improves oxygen delivery to the tissues.

Increase in whole blood viscosity

- Increase in haematocrit: when the haematocrit increases above 0.5, the work of the heart at rest is greatly increased.
- At a constant haemoglobin concentration, whole blood viscosity increases with decrease in MCV, from whatever cause.
- Rigid cells which do not deform normally – sickle-cell disease, spherocytes, target cells.
- Increased plasma viscosity – increased plasma fibrinogen, IgM, cryoglobulin.
- Post splenectomy: whole blood viscosity is increased, as the less deformable red cells are not removed from the circulation.

References
Challoner, T., Briggs, C., Rampling, M. W. and Thomas, D. J. (1986) *Br. J. Haematol* **62**, 671
Milligan, D. W., MacNamee, R., Roberts, B. E., *et al.* (1982) *Br. J. Haematol.* **50**, 467
Nicol, C. G., Harkness, J. and Whittington, R. B. (1982) *Clin. Phys. Physiol. Meas.* **3**, 303
Pearson, T. C., Guthrie, D. L., Slater, N. G. P., *et al.* (1982) *Br. J. Haematol* **52**, 166
van de Pette, J. E. W., Guthrie, D. L. and Pearson, T. C. (1986) *Br. J. Haematol* **63**, 369

Sensorineural hearing impairment affects about 12% of adults in Britain, and ischaemia is a possible cause. The effects of difficulties in the flow of whole blood through very small vessels are demonstrated by the finding that such hearing impairment is directly proportional to high shear rate blood viscosity and red cell rigidity, and inversely proportional to the plasma viscosity.

Reference
Browning, G. G., Gatehouse, S. and Lowe, G. D. O. (1986) *Lancet* **i**, 121

The effects of exercise on the blood

Neutrophilia occurs, especially in untrained subjects. Vigorous and prolonged regular exercise, e.g. marathon training, results in an increased total blood volume, the plasma volume increase being greater than the red cell mass increase, resulting in a lower circulating haemoglobin concentration. At the same time the red cell 2,3-DPG increases, increasing the oxygen availability per unit volume of blood. The plasma viscosity falls and red cell deformability increases in regular joggers, again facilitating oxygen delivery to the tissues. Haemolysis resulting from the pounding

of blood in the feet is associated with a moderate increase in plasma free haemoglobin, a loss of iron in the urine and an increase in the MCV due to reticulocytosis. There is also a slight increase in faecal blood loss, and this may also contribute to the fall in the haemoglobin concentration in 'runner's macrocytosis'. Some athletes have attempted to raise their haemoglobin levels before big events by receiving the erythrocytes from two units of their own blood, taken earlier and frozen, to be reinfused after their haemoglobin levels have recovered. The extra haemoglobin results in an increase in maximal oxygen uptake, but this increase is related to the individual's initial aerobic fitness.

References
Eichner, E. R. (1985) *Am. J. Med.* **78**, 321
Ernst, E. (1985) *J. Am. Med. Assoc.* **253**, 2962
McCarthy, D. A., Perry, J. D., Melsom, R. D. and Dale, M. M. (1987) *Br. Med. J.* **295**, 636
Sawka, M. N., Young, A. J., Muza, S. R., *et al.* (1987) *J. Am. Med. Assoc.* **257**, 1496
Wardrop, C. A. J. (1987) *Br. Med. J.* **295**, 455

Red blood cell count

(SI units conversion factor $= 10^6$, i.e. $4000000/mm^3$ becomes $4 \times 10^{12}/l$.)

Normal range

- Infant
  (full term, cord blood) $4.0 \times 10^{12} - 5.6 \times 10^{12}/l$
- Infant (3 months) $3.2 \times 10^{12} - 4.5 \times 10^{12}/l$
- Infant (1 year old, mean) $3.6 \times 10^{12} - 5.0 \times 10^{12}/l$
- Children
  (10 years old, mean) $4.2 \times 10^{12} - 5.2 \times 10^{12}/l$
- Adult males $4.5 \times 10^{12} - 6.5 \times 10^{12}/l$
- Adult females $3.9 \times 10^{12} - 5.6 \times 10^{12}/l$

Reference
Dacie, J. V. and Lewis, S. M. (1968) *Practical Haematology*, 4th ed., London, Churchill.

Physiological

There is a moderate fluctuation during the 24 h of about $\pm 4\%$, probably related to exercise, meals and fluid intake etc.

Strong emotions such as fear, anger, excitement, cause a temporary increase in the red cell count; a similar increase follows abdominal massage, cold showers etc. Probably red cells sequestered in the spleen are released into the circulation.

Pathological

Increased count

- Primary polycythaemia vera.
- Secondary polycythaemia.
- *See* packed cell volume p. 2

Note: Any reduction in the oxygen tension in the blood results in an increase in the red cell count above normal, e.g. (1) high altitudes, and (2) severe congenital heart disease.

Decreased count

This occurs in anaemia—*See* Classification of anaemia, p. 15.

The red cell count is more severely reduced in anaemias due to deficiencies other than iron, e.g. pernicious anaemia. The red cell count in some cases of fairly severe iron deficiency anaemia may be nearly normal.

It is found that, in normal animals of different species, the red cell count and the mean red cell volume are inversely related.

Whole blood haemoglobin

(SI units = g/dl; conversion factor from g/100 ml = 1.0)

Normal range

• Infant (full term, cord blood)	13.6 – 19.6 g/dl
• Infant (3 months)	9.5 – 12.5 g/dl
• Infant (1 year old)	11.0 – 13.0 g/dl
• Children (10 years old)	11.5 – 14.8 g/dl
• Adults (ignoring sex difference, mean)	14.8 g/dl
• Adult males	13.5 – 18.0 g/dl
• Adult females	11.5 – 16.4 g/dl
• Elderly males (65 – 85 years + mean)	13.62 g/dl
• Elderly females (65 – 85 years + mean value)	13.11 g/dl

References
Dacie, J. V. and Lewis, S. M. (1975) *Practical Haematology*, 5th edn. London, Churchill
Myers, M., Saunders, C. and Chalmers, D. C. (1968) *Lancet* ii, 261

Mean corpuscular haemoglobin (MCH)

(SI units—no change)

Normal range

• Infants (3 months)	24 – 34 pg
• Infants (1 year)	23 – 31 pg
• Children (10–12 years)	24 – 30 pg
• Adults	27 – 32 pg

Pathological

Increase

Macrocytosis (up to 50 pg).

Decrease

This occurs in microcytosis, associated with iron deficiency (down to 15 pg).

Note: When the packed cell volume (PCV) is estimated by centrifugation of whole blood, trapping of plasma between red cells inevitably occurs, with consequent overestimation of red cell size, especially if there is anisocytosis of the red cells. In these circumstances, the mean corpuscular haemoglobin concentration (MCHC) is a better measure of hypochromia.

When the PCV is automatically calculated from measurements of the mean red cell volume (MCV) and the red cell count, trapping errors are eliminated (e.g. Coulter 'S' counter), and an MCH of less than 27 pg indicates hypochromia, the MCHC only falling with very gross hypochromia.

Mean corpuscular haemoglobin concentration (MCHC)

(SI units—no change).

The MCHC is the amount of haemoglobin in 100 ml of red blood cells, and this concentration is remarkably constant throughout the mammals, in spite of variations in red cell size and count. Using electrical impedance, red cell volume measurement (e.g. Coulter 'S-plus'), the results of MCV and MCH are linear between 27 and 35 g/dl, with a flat response above 35 g/dl, due to inaccurate measurement of abnormal cells with altered shapes, deformability properties and conductivity. Light-scattering methods of MCV measurement are accurate between 30 and 120 fl, and results for the MCHC are linear between 27 and 45 g/dl. The normal range is accepted as 30–35 g/dl of red cells, but, with the availability of MCV and MCH measurements, it is no longer clinically useful.

Increased values (above 36 g/dl)

These occur with severe prolonged dehydration, hereditary spherocytosis, cold agglutinin disease, xerocytosis and intravascular haemolysis with much free haemoglobin in the plasma.

Decreased values (less than 30 g/dl)

These occur with iron anaemia, excessive rapid overhydration, thalassaemia and sideroblastic anaemia.

Reference
Mohandas, N., Kim, Y. R., Tycko, D. H., *et al.* (1986) *Blood* **68**, 506

Mean cell volume (MCV)

Normal range

• Adult 76–96 fl (mean = 90 fl).

The MCV in normal infants is 75–85 fl, increasing in childhood to reach adult values by 20 years. There is a small slow increase in red cell volume up to old age.

The inaccurate measurement by electronic counters of pathological red cells with altered shapes and deformability has been greatly improved by a new method.

References
Kelly, A. and Munan, L. (1977) Br. J. Haematol. **35**, 153
Mohandas, N., Kim, Y. R., Tycko, D. H., et al. (1986) Blood **68**, 506

Increase

Physiological

- Normal pregnancy, with an increase of + 5 fl; also the contraceptive pill.
- Small increase after the menopause.

Pathological

- Vitamin B_{12} and/or folate deficiency.
- Reticulocytosis.
- Aplastic anaemia and pure red cell aplasia.
- Primary acquired sideroblastic anaemia.
- Myelodysplastic anaemia; preleukaemia (diagnosed in retrospect!).
- Alcohol, with or without folate deficiency – a useful screening test for suspected drinkers.
- Long-term anticonvulsant therapy, with or without folate deficiency.
- Cytotoxic drugs, including cyclophosphamide, azathioprine and vidarabine.
- Chronic obstructive airway disease, with falling Po_2 and rising Pco_2.
- Severe hyperglycaemia – some electronic counters may over-estimate the MCV.
- Liver disease – 'thin macrocytes'.
- Down's syndrome.

Reference
Eastham, R. D. and Jancar, J. (1983) Br. J. Psychiatr. **143**, 203

- Hypothyroidism and myxoedema.
- Lesch–Nyhan disease [R], in some cases.

Decrease

Pathological

- Iron deficiency – the MCH falls below 25 pg and the MCV falls in parallel.
  A microcytic (predominant) and a normocytic (minority) population of red cells may occur in some cases.
- Thalassaemia.
- Anaemia of chronic disease – in chronic infection, uraemia, malignancy and autoimmune disease (e.g. rheumatoid arthritis).
- Haemoglobin E disease – found in Burma, South-East Asia and in the Veddas in Sri Lanka, otherwise rare.

- Sideroblastic anaemia.
- Lead poisoning rarely presents with microcytic anaemia.
- Hyperthyroidism – within the normal range for the MCV, it is low, rising by about 6 fl following thyroid treatment.
- Pyropoikilocytosis.

Discriminating factors

To distinguish between iron deficiency anaemia and thalassaemia trait:

- Computer-devised formula: MCV – RBC – (5 × Hb) – 8.4. A negative result is given with thalassaemia, a positive result with iron deficiency.
- MCV/RBC > 13 in iron deficiency, < 13 in thalassaemia trait.
- MCH/RBC > 3.8 in iron deficiency, < 3.8 in thalassaemia trait.

A false diagnosis of thalassaemia trait using the above formulae may occur in pregnancy with microcytic anaemia, polycythaemia vera venesected to iron deficiency, and iron deficiency anaemia treated with iron.

Results suggesting iron deficiency may be found in mild classic heterozygous α-thalassaemia and in some heterozygotes for β-thalassaemia.

Red cell distribution width (RDW)

The RDW is a mechanical number calculation to express the size distribution curve of the red cell population of a sample.

Raised RDW with normal haemoglobin concentration

High reticulocyte count, as may be found in a haemoglobinopathy.

Raised RDW with anaemia

In decreasing order of magnitude of RDW: sickle-cell disease, sickle-cell – β-thalassaemia, sickle-cell trait, β-thalassaemia trait, iron deficiency.

Raised RDW with microcytosis

Iron deficiency and, in nearly 50% of heterozygous thalassaemia. The two conditions can be distinguished.

References
Flynn, M. M., Reppur, T. S. and Bhagavan, N. (1986) Am. J. Clin. Pathol. **85**, 445
Roberts, G. T. and El Bedawi, S. B. (1985) Am. J. Clin. Pathol. **83**, 222
Cesana, B. M., Maiolo, Anna T., Gidiuli, Nosa et al. (1991) Clin. Lab. Haematol. **13**, 141

Erythrocyte mean cell diameter (MCD) and mean cell thickness (MCT or MCAT)

MCD

Normal range 6.7–7.7 μm (mean = 7.2 μm). With the availability of rapid accurate measurements of MCV, MCH and RDW, this measurement is now obsolute.

MCT

Normal range 1.7–2.5μm (mean = 2.1μm). This measurement is now obsolete.

Reticulocytes

Reticulocytes are non-nucleated red cells, 7–10 μm in diameter, which contain RNA, small mitochondria and ribosomes. These ribosomes are mainly polyribosomes, which give polychromatic staining with Romanowsky dyes, and a reticular appearance with new methylene blue. The reticulocyte can deform, is motile and has an irregular cell margin. Denucleation of late polychromatic erythroblasts within the marrow parenchyma is followed by migration of the reticulocytes, stimulated by erythropoietin, through channels which develop across the endothelial cells. As the cell matures, reticulum becomes more scanty until only a few granules remain, this maturation taking 1–2 days in the marrow followed by 24 hours in the circulation.

Normal range

- 3-month fetus: 90% of circulating red cells.
- 6-month fetus: 15–30%.
- Full term newborn infant for first 3 days: 2–7%, falling after 3 days to <1% at the end of the first week, reflecting greater availability of oxygen after birth.
- Children and adults: 0.5–1.5% (absolute count $25 \times 10^9 - 85 \times 10^9$/l).
- In normal pregnancy there is an early decrease in maternal iron stores with an increase in the reticulocyte count until week 28, not dependent on increased erythropoietin.

Reference
Howells, M. R., Jones, S. E., Napier, J. A. F., *et al.* (1986) *Br. J. Haematol.* **64**, 595

Increase

- After specific treatment for deficiency anaemia (e.g. iron, vitamin B_{12}, folic acid).
- Following haemorrhage or haemolysis.
- Myelosclerosis–the count may be increased in the presence of reduced red cell production.
- Very high reticulocyte counts found in acute erythraemic myelosis.
- Other forms of leucoerythroblastic anaemia.

Decrease

When the absolute count is less than 40×10^9/l, this indicates reduced erythropoiesis, e.g. aplastic and hypoplastic anaemia.

Correction for reticulocyte maturation times

Premature release of 'shift' or 'stress' reticulocytes from the bone marrow into the circulation results in the reticulocytes spending up to 3 days in the circulation before complete maturation with loss of reticulum. Since the maturation time is proportional to the severity of the anaemia, corrections can be made (Table 1.1).

Reference
Callender, S. T. E. and Pippard, M. J. (1982) In: *Blood and its Disorders*, 2nd edn, p. 1462, Hardisty, R. M. and Weatherall, D. J., Eds. Oxford: Blackwell Scientific

Red cell ageing

The normal red cell lifespan in humans is about 120 days. It contains no nucleus or messenger RNA (mRNA) and at first, as a reticulocyte, has high enzyme concentrations which fall with increasing red cell age. Potassium and water are lost progressively, the MCV falls and the MCHC rises, with a loss of 25% of its haemoglobin during its life, and increasing resistance to hypotonic saline.

The red cell membrane is remodelled and reduced, with increasing viscosity and decreasing deformability, making splenic retention of effete red cells easier. As

Table 1.1   Corrections

PCV (%)	Reticulocyte maturation in circulation (days)
45	1.0
35	1.5
25	2.0
15	2.5

$$\text{Reticulocyte Index} = \frac{\text{Reticulocyte}(\%) \text{ observed} \times \text{Observed PCV} \times \text{Maturation coefficient}}{45}$$

haemoglobin begins to denature, it forms hemichromes that cross-link the major membrane-spanning proteins (band 3), into clusters. These clusters provide recognition sites for IgG antibodies directed against senescent cells, which bind to aged cells and trigger their removal from the circulation.

References
Beutler, E. (1985) *Br. J. Haematol.* **61**, 377
Low, P. S., Waugh, S. M., Zinke, K. *et al.* (1985) *Science* **227**, 531
Sutera, S. P., Gardner, R. A., Boylan, C. W. *et al.* (1985) *Blood* **65**, 275
Snyder, L. M., Garver, F., Liu, S. C. *et al.* (1986) *Br. J. Haematol.* **61**, 415
Van der Vegt, S. G. L., Ruben, A. M. Th., Werre, J. M. *et al.* (1986) *Br. J. Haematol.* **61**, 393

Nucleated red cells in the peripheral blood

The presence of nucleated red cells in the peripheral blood may indicate some disturbance in red cell maturation. Nucleated red cells are found in the peripheral blood in:

1. Leucoerythroblastic anaemia.
2. Untreated megaloblastic anaemia, especially if anaemia fairly severe and patient mobile.
3. Leukaemia: circulating nucleated red cells are more common in acute leukaemias and chronic myeloid leukaemia, than in chronic lymphatic leukaemia.
4. Erythraemic myelosis:
   (a) acute erythraemic myelosis: basophilic normoblasts appear in large numbers;
   (b) chronic erythraemic myelosis: orthochromic pyknotic normoblasts are predominant.

Severe oxygen lack may result in release of nucleated red cells into the peripheral blood:

5. Congestive cardiac failure.
6. Severe pulmonary disease.

Reference
Ward, H. P. and Holman, J. (1967) *Ann. Intern. Med.* **67**, 1190

Circulating nucleated red cells in infants with associated jaundice and splenomegaly
- Erythroblastosis fetalis (Rh or ABO incompatibility).
- Acholuric jaundice.
- Obliteration of the bile ducts.
- Congenital syphilis.

Red cell structure

The normal red cell has to maintain its discoidal shape and also be able to undergo frequent extensive reversible deformability. It has also to maintain osmotic equilibrium with the surrounding plasma, in spite of the osmotic effect of high haemoglobin concentration and cation differences with the plasma. Cell membrane sodium pump activity, which keeps the intracellular sodium concentration low and potassium concentration high relative to the plasma, depends on adequate ATP. ATP is generated in the cell during glycolysis. The red cell membrane contains magnesium-dependent, calcium-dependent and low calcium concentration-dependent ATPases. Normal intracellular glycolysis produces adequate NADH, NADPH and ATP. Glutathione is synthesized and maintained as reduced glutathione in the cell membrane. Normal haemoglobin is synthesized in the normal immature red cell. Finally, the negative charge on the red cell surface is maintained.

Red cell membrane proteins

The proteins of the red cell membrane can be separated into distinct bands on specialized gels. Spectrin (bands 1 and 2) consists of two polypeptide chains, α and β, and exists as tetramers $(\alpha_2\beta_2)$, 100 nm as rods in the membrane. These are bound by ankyrin (bands 2.1, 2.2, 2.3 and 2.6) and by protein band 3 (the anion channels that bridge the lipid layer) to form a network. Spectrin is kept dephosphorylated to maintain the discoid shape, because, on phosphorylation, the red cell tends to become spheroidal. Short actin filaments and protein band 4.1 bind to the ends of the spectrin tetramers, cross-linking adjacent spectrin molecules.

Red cell membrane lipids

Seventy per cent of the total lipid consists of phospholipids, 30% consists of cholesterol, with a small amount of glycolipid and fatty acids.

Red cell membrane carbohydrates

These make up 8% of the dry weight of the red cell membrane, and are attached to membrane proteins and specific lipids (glycolipids). Sialoglycoproteins α, β, γ' and δ, occur in the red cell membrane. α-Sialoglycoproteins carry the blood group M or N activity, and cells with no α-sialoglycoprotein are refractory to invasion by malarial parasites. Both β- and γ-sialoglycoproteins are associated with the maintenance of the discoid red cell shape. Sialic acid is lost progressively from the red cell surface as it ages in the circulation.

References
Agre, P., Orringer, E. P. and Bennett, V. (1982) *N. Engl. J. Med.* **306**, 1155
Anstee, D. J. and Tanner, M. J. A. (1986) *Br. J. Haematol.* **64**, 211
Goodman, S. R., Shiffer, K. A., Casoria, L. A. *et al.* (1982) *Blood* **60**, 772
Schrier, S. L., Hardy, B., Junga, I. *et al.* (1981) *Blood* **58**, 953

Red cell shape

Irregular shape distortion (poikilocytosis)

A great variety of irregularly shaped red cells of various sizes is found in untreated megaloblastic anaemia, severe iron deficiency anaemia, severe lead poisoning, acute haemolytic anaemia due to substances, including acetylphenylhydrazine and naphthalene, and some cases of myelosclerosis.

Crenated red cells

1. Abetalipoproteinaemia

This is associated with retinitis pigmentosa and damage to the central nervous system in severely affected homozygotes.

2. Artificially produced

These are produced artificially by suspension of red cells in hypertonic saline. Red cells may crenate in the extracorporeal circulation during coronary artery bypass surgery. This may be prevented by the addition of albumin to the extracorporeal blood.

References
Bassen, F. A. and Kornzweig, A. L. (1950) *Blood* **5**, 381
Kamada, T., McMillan, D. E., Sternlieb, J. J. *et al.* (1987) *Lancet* **ii**, 818

Schistocytes

These are fragmented red blood cells of less than 3 μm diameter, which stain pink with Romanowsky stains.

1. These fragmented red cells may appear in the peripheral blood during the first few hours after a severe burn. They are then rapidly cleared from the circulation.
2. Disseminated intravascular coagulopathy.
3. Other cases of microangiopathic haemolytic anaemia.
   (a) haemolytic uraemic anaemia (intravascular haemolysis).
   (b) thrombotic thrombocytopenic purpura;
   (c) malignant hypertension;
   (d) calcified aortic valve stenosis;
   (e) early synthetic aortic and mitral valve replacements;
   (f) Kasabach–Merritt syndrome;
   (g) arteriovenous malformation.
4. Severe sepsis.
5. Severe megaloblastic anaemia.
6. Myelofibrosis.
7. Falciparum malaria.
8. Hypersplenism.
9. Occasionally in sideroblastic anaemia.
10. Acute leukaemia.
11. β-Thalassaemia–haemoglobin E disease.

Acanthocytes ('Burr' cells)

Red cells develop spiny projections in certain conditions:

1. Abetalipoproteinaemia, hereditary acanthocytosis associated with retinitis and neurological lesions.
2. Uraemia: schistocytes may also occur.
3. Microangiopathic haemolytic anaemia.
4. Thrombotic thrombocytopenic purpura.
5. Pyruvate kinase deficiency haemolytic anaemia.
6. Hypothyroidism.
7. Some cases of carcinoma.
8. Some cases of cirrhosis: in severe liver disease 'spur cells' develop. Following acquisition of cholesterol to the red cell surface, there is splenic remodelling of the red cell surface. Splenectomy ameliorates the condition.

Reference
Cooper, R. A., Kimball, K. B. and Durocher, J. R. (1974) *N. Engl. J. Med.* **290**, 1279

9. Found in one case showing progressive neurological disease.
10. Possibly may be found in some cases of haemolytic anaemia.
11. 'Burr' cells may occur in thrombotic thrombocytopenic purpura.
12. Severe burns. Echinocytes with slightly reduced erythrocyte lipid and reduced plasma lipoproteins found in severe burns. The cells are flat and spiculated.

Reference
Harlan, W. R., Shaw, W. A. and Zelkowitz, M. (1974) *Arch. Intern. Med.* **136**, 71

Echinocytes

The red cell biconcave discocyte with its large surface area relative to its volume is in an equilibrium state between the echinocyte and the stomatocyte. The echinocyte has a tendency towards membrane externalization, whilst the stomatocyte has a tendency towards membrane internalization. Echinocytes increase the whole blood viscosity, whilst stomatocytes impair blood flow through the microcirculation. Echinocytes may be found in blood films in: pyruvate kinase deficiency, phosphoglycerate kinase deficiency, after intralipid infusion, cardiac bypass with increased plasma fatty acids and after extensive burns.

References
Chabanel, A., Reinhart, W. and Chien, S. (1987) *Blood* **69**, 739
Hsu, R. C., Kanofsky, J. R. and Yachnin, S. (1980) *Blood* **56**, 109
Reinhart, W. H. and Chien, S. (1986) *Blood* **67**, 1110
Siegel, I., Liu, T. L., Zaret, P. *et al.* (1984) *J. Am. Med. Assoc.* **251**, 1574

Pyropoikilocytes [R]

In pyropoikilocytosis with haemolytic anaemia, the MCV averages 25 fl, the red cell calcium is abnormally high and saline osmotic fragility is abnormally increased. Spectrin in the red cell membrane is abnormal or absent, and has an increased propensity to undergo aggregation in the cell membrane, producing membrane instability. The condition is related to congenital spherocytosis and elliptocytosis, and the severity of the condition varies from mild non-haemolytic to poikilocytic haemolytic anaemia, depending on the quantity of affected spectrin in the membrane. These cells fragment at a lower temperature than normal (45°C instead of 49°C).

References
Coetzer, T. L. and Palek, J. (1986) *Blood* **67**, 919
Marchesi, S. L., Knowles, W. J., Morrow, J. S. *et al.* (1986) *Blood* **67**, 141

Regular shape distortion

Spherocytes

● Hereditary spherocytosis

The reticulocytes appear to be normal, but develop into spherocytes with no central depression, a smaller MCD and larger MCT than normal, a reduced tendency to form rouleaux and pseudoagglutinations, and increased saline osmotic fragility. Haemolysis is rare in vitro in collected blood samples (compare acquired spherocytosis). Various forms have been described:

1. Autosomal hereditary spherocytosis [AD]–the most common haemolytic anaemia in people of northern European descent.
   (a) mild–without anaemia; 25% of this group; haemolysis occurs during attacks of illness causing splenomegaly;
   (b) moderate, with mild-to-moderate anaemia (66%);
   (c) severe, transfusion dependent, with aplastic anaemia associated with virus infection.
2. [AD] with moderate numbers of acanthocytes [R].
3. [AR] severe [R].
4. Severe atypical hereditary spherocytosis.

These various varieties are associated with defects in spectrin, protein band 4.1, and ankyrin in the red cell membrane.

References
Becker, P. S. and Lux, S. E. (1985) In: *Clinics in Haematology*, Schrier, S. L., Ed. vol. 14, p. 15, London, W. B. Saunders
Coetzer, T. L., Lawler, J., Liu, S-C. *et al.* (1988) *N. Engl. J. Med.* **318**, 230
Smedley, J. C. and Bellingham, A. J. (1991) *J. Clin. Pathol.* **44**, 441

● Acquired spherocytosis

Damage to the red cell membrane or loss following partial phagocytosis of red cells coated with immunoglobulin results in spherocyte formation.

1. Acquired warm antibody-type autoimmune haemolytic anaemia.
2. Haemolytic disease of the newborn due to ABO incompatibility.
3. Following thermal injury.
4. Following storage of blood, spherocytes develop.
5. Osmotic spherocytosis, e.g. red cells suspended in hypotonic saline.

Elliptocytes (ovalocytes)

The red cells are normally oval in camels. Up to 1% of red cells are oval in normal people.

● Hereditary elliptocytosis

Heterogeneous, due to various defects in the structure and linkages of spectrin, ankyrin (protein band 2.1) and protein band 3. Ovalocytosis in one of these conditions has been found to protect children between 2 and 4 years of age, when they are most vulnerable, against both *Plasmodium falciparum* and *P. vivax* in Papua New Guinea.

1. Common hereditary elliptocytoses:
   (a) non-haemolytic hereditary elliptocytosis;
   (b) mild hereditary elliptocytosis;
   (c) hereditary elliptocytosis with infantile poikilocytosis;
   (d) common hereditary elliptocytosis with sporadic haemolysis;
   (e) severe haemolytic elliptocytosis;
   (f) hereditary pyropoikilocytosis;
   (g) elliptocytosis with dyserythropoiesis.
2. Spherocytic elliptocytosis.
3. Stomatocytic elliptocytosis – common in Melanesians and protecting against malaria.

References
Marchesi, S. L., Knowles, W. J., Morrow, J. S. *et al.* (1986) *Blood* **67**, 141
Palek, J. (1985) In: *Clinics in Haematology*, Schrier, S. L., Ed. vol 14 p. 45, London, W. B. Saunders
Schrier, S. L. (Ed.) (1985) *Clinics in Haematology*, vol 14, p. 1, London, W. B. Saunders

● Acquired elliptocytosis

1. Pernicious anaemia and other macrocytic anaemia.
2. Severe iron-deficiency anaemia.
3. Thalassaemia.
4. Severe anaemia associated with:
   (a) severe infections;
   (b) carcinomatosis;
   (c) leukaemia.
5. Occasionally associated with hereditary spherocytosis.
6. Pseudothalassaemia.

Leptocytes (target cells, Mexican hat cells)

The red cells are thinner than normal, with a greater surface area relative to cell volume. There is no bridge joining the central spot and the peripheral ring of haemoglobin. Polychromatic cells are excluded. They are more resistant to the saline osmotic fragility test than normal, since they can accommodate more saline before becoming spherical and eventually haemolysing. Normal controls contain up to 3.3% of red cells as target cells (up to 2.5% in normal pregnancy), i.e. less than 1 target cell per high-power field.

Hereditary

* Thalassaemia major and minor.
* Sickle-cell disease.
* Sickle-cell haemoglobin C disease.
* Haemoglobin C–thalassaemia.
* Plasma lecithin–cholesteryl acyl transferase deficiency.
* Haemoglobin C disease.

Acquired

* Hypochromic anaemia.
* Postsplenectomy.
* Liver disease – hepatitis, obstructive jaundice and cirrhosis.

Normal red cells transfused into these cases develop into target cells, and target cells from these patients, when suspended in normal plasma, revert to their normal discoid shape.

* Occasionally in sideroblastic anaemia.
* Prolonged severe dehydration.

Stomatocytes

The red cells have a slit in place of a central concavity.

Hereditary

* Hereditary stomatocytosis [R]

In this hereditary haemolytic anaemia, stomatocytosis occurs with reticulocytosis of up to 40%, a reduced red cell life and increased red cell osmotic fragility. The red cells have an abnormally high sodium content ($\times$ 9 normal) and increased water content, with red cell potassium reduced by half.

* Hydrocytosis [AD] [R]

This is a congenital haemolytic anaemia with a permeability defect in the red cell membrane allowing excess water to enter the cell, causing red cell swelling and stomatocyte formation. The red cell osmotic fragility is increased. Splenectomy increases the red cell life from 3.7 to 9.2 days.

* Xerocytosis [AD] [R]

This is a congenital haemolytic anaemia with abnormal red cell membrane permeability leading to cellular dehydration. The MCHC is raised and red cell osmotic fragility is reduced. As the red cells age, they undergo progressive dehydration with loss of deformability. Blood films contain stomatocytes and target cells.

Reference
Lande, W. M. and Mentzer, W. C. (1985) In: *Clinics in Haematology*, Schrier, S. L., Ed., vol 14, p. 89, London, W. B. Saunders

Acquired stomatocytosis

Small numbers of stomatocytes are found in: acute alcoholism, alcoholic cirrhosis, infectious mononucleosis (some cases), glutathione-peroxidase deficiency, lead poisoning, thalassaemia minor and some cases of malignant disease.

Red blood cell inclusion bodies

Nuclear or cytoplasmic remnants

Howell–Jolly bodies

These spherical intracellular eccentrically placed 1 μm granules contain DNA, and are left during accelerated pyknosis, abnormal karyorrhexis, or are pinched-off bleb formations along the nuclear membrane surface. They occur in megaloblastic anaemia, disorders of the spleen, including congenital absence of the spleen, functional asplenism in sickle-cell disease, splenic atrophy and post splenectomy, haemolytic anaemia in crisis and in some cases of leukaemia.

Isaac's bodies

These are non-nuclear intracellular bodies.

Reticular material (punctate basophilia)

This results from ribosomal abnormalities, and is found in lead poisoning, following acute haemorrhage and in pernicious anaemia.

Stippled cells

Seen in β-thalassaemia major – excess α-chains stain with crystal violet. Also in pyrimidine-5′-nucleotidase deficiency and with unstable haemoglobins.

Iron-containing inclusion bodies

Siderocytes

These are erythrocytes which contain stainable iron – normal = 0.4–0.6% of red cells. They are found in the normal and pre-term newborn infant, chronic haemolytic anaemia, lead poisoning, megaloblastic anaemia, infections, severe burns and haemochromatosis.

Sideroblasts

* These are normoblasts with stainable iron in their cytoplasm, representing an intracellular depot of

iron available for haem formation. They are increased in number in haemolytic anaemia, megaloblastic anaemia, haemochromatosis and haemosiderosis.

- Abnormal sideroblasts of increased size but normal distribution, with increased numbers of abnormally large, iron-staining granules are found in thalassaemia, and in other conditions with defective globin synthesis.

'Ring' sideroblasts

These have a perinuclear halo or crescent of iron-staining granules (i.e. mitochondria containing excess iron) and are found in:

- Hereditary sex-linked hypochromic anaemia.
- Primary acquired refractory sideroblastic anaemia.
- Secondary sideroblastic anaemia associated with the antituberculous drugs cycloserine, p-aminosalicylate (PAS), isoniazid, lead poisoning, chloramphenicol in some cases, acute alcohol poisoning, some cases of thalassaemia, di Guglielmo's erythraemia and polycythaemia vera during the development of leukaemia.

Pappenheimer bodies

These are Feulgen-negative, iron-containing granules probably related to siderocytes, which appear basophilic when stained with Romanowsky stains. They appear after splenectomy in hereditary spherocytosis, in other haemolytic anaemias including erythroblastosis fetalis and Blackwater fever and in some cases of carcinoma.

Heinz bodies

These are of denatured haemoglobin, occurring as 1:20, iron-containing inclusion bodies in fully developed red cells, which are Prussian blue negative. They appear as blue-black particles when stained with methyl violet or cresyl blue in saline, and are decolorized by methyl alcohol. Red cells containing Heinz bodies are less deformable than normal, and are more susceptible to mechanical haemolysis and removal by the spleen. The attachment of denatured haemoglobin to red cell membrane reduced-glutathione groups deplete membrane-available reduced SH groups.

- Heinz bodies in otherwise normal red cells

Oxidizing drugs include: acetanilide, aniline, chlorates, diaminophenyl sulphone, erythrol trinitrate, naphthalene, large doses of phenacetin, phenothiazine, phenylhydrazine and acetyl phenylhydrazine, pyridine, resorcinol, salicylazosulphapyridine, sulphanilamide, sulphapyridine, trinitrotoluene. The effect of these drugs is enhanced by splenectomy.

As glutathione peroxidase is a selenium-containing enzyme, selenium deficiency in cattle is associated with anaemia with Heinz bodies in the red cells.

Reference
Morris, J. G., Gripe, W. S., Chapman, H. C. Jr. *et al.* (1984) *Science* **223**, 491

- Heinz bodies in defective red cells

1. Glucose-6-phosphate dehydrogenase deficiency:
   (a) drug-induced haemolytic anaemia (primaquine, pamaquin and Negroes);
   (b) favism;
   (c) non-immune haemolytic anaemia of the newborn. In the newborn infant, and especially in pre-term infants, the red cell glucose-6-phosphate dehydrogenase activity is low, rendering the cells susceptible to the action of drugs (e.g. vitamin K analogues, naphthalene etc.);
   (d) non-spherocytic congenital haemolytic anaemia due to glucose-6-phosphate dehydrogenase deficiency.
2. Stomatocytosis.
3. Pyruvate kinase deficiency.
4. Triose-phosphate isomerase deficiency.
5. 2,3-Diphosphoglyceryl mutase deficiency.
6. Glutathione reductase deficiency.
7. Glutathione peroxidase deficiency.
8. Reduced glutathione deficiency.

(Absence of catalase activity is not associated with Heinz body formation.)
9. Haemolytic anaemia with many Heinz bodies associated with burns and antibiotic therapy.

References
Sevitt, S., Jackson, D., Stone, P. *et al.* (1973) *Lancet* **ii**, 471

- Heinz bodies associated with haemoglobinopathies

1. α-Thalassaemia: excess tetramers of β-chains (haemoglobin H) precipitate both in vitro and in vivo to form both fine disperse precipitates in cells and also Heinz bodies.
2. Haemoglobin Zurich, haemoglobin Köln, haemoglobin Ube I, Haemoglobin Seattle etc., are associated with the formation of Heinz bodies, especially after splenectomy and following the action of the drugs listed above. The haemoglobins manifest heat lability.

   In unstable haemoglobinopathies, haem loss from mutant β-chain is an early step in Heinz body formation. Haem-depleted compound results in β-chain precipitate (the bulk of the Heinz body molecule).

Reference
Jacob, H. S. and Winterhalter, K. H. (1970) *J. Clin. Invest.* **49**, 2008

Protozoa and bacteria

Malaria

Plasmodium vivax (benign tertian), *P. falciparum* (malignant tertian) and *P. malariae* (quartan) all invade human red cells during the life cycle. The red cells containing maturing *P. falciparum* become distorted with knob-like protuberances on their surfaces and also become less deformable; there is therefore a greater uptake of parasitized cells from the circulation. The spleen 'pits' malarial parasites from the cells. Sequestration of parasitized red cells in small blood vessels may play a part in both the encephalopathy of cerebral malaria and bone marrow dysfunction in severe malaria. Red cells parasitized with *P. falciparum* activate platelets, encouraging local microthrombi.

Sickle-cell haemoglobin (HbS), glucose-6-phosphatase deficiency and possibly ovalocytosis give some protection from the more severe effects of malaria.

References

Cranston, H. A., Boylan, C. W., Carroll, G. L. *et al.* (1984) *Science* **223**, 400

Inyang, A. L., Sodeinde, O., Okpako, D. T. *et al.* (1987) *Br. J. Haematol.* **66**, 375

Schmitzer, B., Soderman, T., Mead, M. L. *et al.* (1972) *Science* **177**, 175

Wickramasinghe, S. N., Phillips, R. E., Looareesuwan, S. *et al.* (1987) *Br. J. Haematol.* **66**, 295

- Maurer's dots

These are coarse violet dots, varying considerably in size, which appear in parasitized red blood cells during heavy infestation with *Plasmodium falciparum* (malignant tertian malaria).

- Schuffner's dots

In the course of benign tertian malaria (*P. vivax*) fine reddish dots may appear in any red blood cell containing a young ring form of the parasite or an older form.

Bacteria

Bartonella basilliformis: babesia

Human babesiosis:

- Europe – *B. divergens* and *B. bovis* from cattle can be fatal in splenectomized subjects.
- USA – *B. microti*. Infection from deer tick via deer mouse and meadow vole. Relatively avirulent in patients with spleens, in islands off the New England coast.

Reference

Anderson, A. L., Cassaday, P. B. and Healy, G. R. (1974) *Am. J. Clin. Pathol.* **62**, 612

Artefacts

Cabot's rings, thread-like rings and convolutions sometimes seen in red cells, are thought to be artefacts, and cannot be seen when using a phase-contrast microscope. Obviously, unclean slides and unfiltered dyes can result in apparent red cell inclusion bodies.

Chapter 2

Anaemia

Classification of anaemia

The concentration of haemoglobin in the peripheral blood is reduced below the normal range in anaemia.

Impaired formation

Deficiency of substances essential for erythropoiesis

- Iron deficiency.
- Megaloblastic anaemias (vitamin B_{12}, folic acid).
- Protein deficiency.
- Vitamin C deficiency.
- Copper deficiency.

Disturbance of bone marrow function

- Thalassaemia.
- Haemoglobinopathies.
- Sideroblastic anaemia.
- Congenital dyserythropoietic anaemia.
- Aplastic anaemia.

Secondary to other conditions

1. Infection.
2. Kidney disease.
3. Liver disease.
4. Malignancy.
5. Some autoimmune diseases (e.g. rheumatoid arthritis).
6. Some endocrine deficiencies.
7. Burns. Immediate blood loss followed by depressed erythropoiesis.

Red cell loss

- Bleeding
- Haemolysis

Total red cell volume

Red cells from the patient are labelled with ^{51}Cr or ^{99m}Tc and reinjected.

Normal adult males – 30 ml/kg body weight (2 s.d. ± 5 ml).

Normal adult females – 25 ml/kg body weight (2 s.d. ± 5 ml).

Plasma volume

Measured using ^{125}I-labelled albumin. The volume varies during the day in normal individuals. Normal (both men and women) = 40–50 ml/kg body weight.

Hypersplenism

Red cells are labelled with ^{51}Cr or ^{99m}Tc at 49.5°C (i.e. thermal damage without haemolysis of the red cells) for 20 min. The damaged red cells are injected and the splenic uptake is measured. The splenic blood volume can also be measured using undamaged tagged red cells, followed by surface counting over the spleen. Surface counting over the body following the injection of ^{51}Cr can be used to determine the site of red cell destruction.

Tests of absorption

1. Radiolabelled iron has been used to determine iron absorption.

2. *Schilling test*

Using ^{57}Co or ^{58}Co, absorption of tagged vitamin B_{12} in the absence or presence of added intrinsic factor is used in anaemia due to vitamin B_{12} deficiency.

Dicopac test

Free cyanocobalamin is labelled with ^{58}Co and cyanocobalamin which is bound to intrinsic factor (human gastric juice) is labelled with ^{57}Co. As in the Schilling test, a relatively large dose of non-radioactive cyanocobalamin (the 'flushing' dose) is given at the same time. The 24-h urine sample is then tested.

Normal
$^{57}Co = 21\%$ (12–30%).
$^{58}Co = 20\%$ (11–28%) excreted in urine.

Intrinsic factor deficiency etc.
$^{57}Co = 10\%$ (5–14%).
$^{58}Co = 2\%$ (0.5–5%) excreted in urine.

Generalized malabsorption not caused by lack of intrinsic factor

^{57}Co = less than 4%.
^{58}Co = less then 4%.

Renal dysfunction depresses the results.

References
Pathy, M. S., Kirkman, S. and Molloy, S. J. (1979) *J. Clin. Pathol.* **32**, 244
Wahner, H. W. and Phyliky, R. L. (1983) *Mayo Clin. Proc.* **58**, 541

3. *Folic acid absorption test*

[^{3}H] Folic acid 200 μg is given orally after intramuscular injection of 15 mg non-labelled folic acid.

- Normal

Of the oral dose 30–54% appears in the subsequent 24 h urine sample. This test is claimed to be better than xylose absorption in assessment of upper small intestinal function.

Reference
Elsborg, L. (1981) *Acta Med. Scand.* **209**, 323

Anaemia due to nutritional deficiencies, other than iron deficiency

Pyridoxine deficiency

- Very rare when occurring naturally.
- Sideroblastic anaemia in patients receiving pyridoxine antagonists (e.g. cycloserine, pyrazinamide).

Riboflavine deficiency

This 'never' occurs.

Vitamin C deficiency

Erythropoiesis is usually normoblastic. Vitamin C-deficient diets are almost invariably also deficient in folic acid and other nutrients. Haemorrhage in severe cases of scurvy may cause iron deficiency.

Vitamin E deficiency [R]

This occurs in pre-term infants given iron supplements and a diet rich in linoleic acid. Anaemia, reticulocytosis, abnormal red cell morphology, increased platelet count and oedema, develop at about 6 weeks.

Copper deficiency

This is with anaemia, neutropenia, low serum copper and ceruloplasmin.

- Extensive bowel resection.
- Pre-term babies on a copper-poor milk diet.
- Infants and children with severe malnutrition and chronic diarrhoea.

Calorie deficiency

This may result in mild normochromic anaemia with acanthocytosis in severe anorexia nervosa.

Protein–energy malnutrition

This occurs in children under 5 years old in poorer communities in the less developed countries. Concomitant infectious diseases and parasitic infestation, plus malabsorption, aggravate nutritional deficiency.

Reference
Wickramasinghe, S. N. (1988) *Clin. Lab. Haematol.* **10**, 117

Iron metabolism

Reference
Jacobs, A. and Worwood, M. (Eds.) (1974, 1980) *Iron in Biochemistry and Medicine*, vol. I and vol. II London, Academic Press

Dietary sources

These include liver, meat, eggs and dried fruits.

Increased iron absorption following iron fortification of food is effective only if the diet contains animal protein.

Iron absorption

Normally about 10% of the iron in a normal diet is absorbed. Iron absorption is proportional to the rate of erythropoiesis and inversely proportional to the body iron stores. Ferrous iron is absorbed more readily than ferric iron, and the rate of absorption of iron is improved at low pH because the formation of iron phosphates, which are not absorbed, is reduced. Non-haem iron absorption in subjects with hypochlorhydria is satisfactory, unless it is severe and sustained.

Reference
Skikne, B. S., Lynch, S. R. and Cook, J. D. (1981) *Gastroenterology* **81**, 1068

It has been postulated that the intestinal mucosa secretes apotransferrin into the gut lumen, where it combines with iron, to be reabsorbed, and it is thought that the effects of ferritin, lactoferrin and albumin on iron absorption are minimal. Iron deficiency, pregnancy and hypoxia all induce duodenal, brush border, glycoprotein iron carriers, and the initial entry of iron into the enterocyte is the major regulatory step in the control of iron absorption, and is a rate-limiting process.

References
Cox, T. M. and Peters, T. J. (1980) *Br. J. Haematol* **44**, 75
Cox, T. M., O'Donnall, M. W., Voyles, C. R. *et al.* (1981) *Gut* **22**, A867, T21
Huebers, H. A., Huebers, E., Csiba, E. *et al.* (1983) *Blood* **61**, 283

Increased

PHYSIOLOGICAL

Iron absorption is increased in:

- Anoxia.
- Iron deficiency.
- Increased erythropoiesis.
- Increased sucrose content of diet.

Large quantities of ascorbic iron enhance iron absorption by converting ferric iron to ferrous iron in the food.

Up to 5 mg of iron can be absorbed from the diet each day during pregnancy, and this does not increase in the presence of hypochromic iron-deficient anaemia.

Iron requirements are normally increased:
- In women, who require more iron than men, to replace iron lost during menstruation and to the fetus during pregnancy. There is a rapid mobilization of iron from tissue stores with an early fall in serum ferritin during the first trimester, and with a modest increase in serum erythropoietin in late pregnancy. By 6–8 weeks postpartum most of the iron has returned to the body iron stores.

Reference
Howells, M. R., Jones, S. E., Napier, J. A. F. *et al.* (1986) *Br. J. Haematol.* **64**, 595

- In infants, and especially pre-term infants – the body iron stores are used by 6 months and 200 mg of iron are required to expand the red cell mass (500 ml of blood contains about 250 mg of iron).
- Growing children – 200–300 mg iron are required at adolescence.

PATHOLOGICAL

Increased

In haemochromatosis iron is continuously absorbed, even though the body stores become excessive. Absorption continues at the rate of 3–5 mg/day or 1000 mg/year. It is thought that the initial rate-limiting entry of iron into the enterocyte is not controlled.

Decreased

Iron absorption is reduced by:
- Low iron content of diet.
- Alkalis in antacids raising the duodenal pH.
- Phytates and phosphates in the diet block iron absorption.
- Tannin in tea.

Decreased demand for iron is caused by:
- Decreased erythropoiesis.
- Acute and chronic disease.

- Pyrexia.
- Iron overload.

A high calcium content in a diet containing marginal amounts of iron is associated with reduced iron absorption, i.e. iron deficiency is more frequent in babies fed cows' milk than human milk.

Atrophy of the gastric mucosa with increasing age is associated with iron deficiency, from poor iron absorption.

Intestinal malabsorption also causes decreased iron absorption.

Reference
Barton, J. C., Conrad, M. E. and Parmley, R. T. (1983) *Gastroenterology* **84**, 90

Body iron

Total body iron: 4–5 g. This total is made up of the following:

1. *Circulating red cell mass*

This is 2.7 g (60% of total).

2. *Ferritin + haemosiderin stores*

There are stores in liver and bone-marrow (1.2–1.5 g) (30% of total). The body ferritin pool includes:

- An anabolic fraction accepting iron from transferrin; the take-up from labelled transferrin is rapid.
- a catabolic fraction accepting iron from degraded haemoglobin, and from any ineffective erythropoiesis. Compared with the anabolic fraction there is a 6 h lag before uptake. There is a rapid uptake of labelled iron from damaged labelled reticulocytes.

Reference
Shepp, M., Toff, H., Yamada, H. *et al.* (1972) *Br. J. Haematol.* **22**, 377

3. *Myoglobin (in muscles)*

This is 0.14 g (3–5% of total).

4. *Haem enzymes*

cytochrome oxidase	
cytochromes $b + c$	<1% of total.
peroxidases	
catalase	

5. *Plasma iron*

This is <0.1% of total.

The labile intracellular muscle iron pool is in equilibrium with the serum iron, which accounts for a significant proportion of the daily plasma iron turnover.

Note: Whilst cytochrome *c* activity is depressed in iron deficiency, catalase activity is not diminished.

The normal infant's body contains about 400 mg of iron. Therefore 3–4 g of iron are accumulated during growth over the subsequent 20 years. In the first few months, iron intake from a milk diet is negligible. By the eighth month 0.3–0.4 mg iron is needed daily. From 4 to 12 years 0.4–1 mg is needed daily. The adolescent male requires 1 mg daily, and the adult male requires about 0.6 mg iron daily.

The importance of adequate iron in the body is shown by the findings in iron-deficiency anaemia:

- Reduced skin reaction to candida antigen.
- Reduced skin reaction to purified protein derivative (PPD) injection.
- Impairment of lymphocyte transformation.

Reference
Joynson, D. H. M., Jacobs, A., Walker, D. M. *et al.* (1972) *Lancet* ii, 1058

- Low urine hydroxyproline excretion, increased following iron therapy.

Reference
Ganzoni, A. M. and Fumagelli, I. A. C. (1970) *Acta Haematol.* **44**, 200

6. *Brain non-haem iron*

Severe iron deficiency in children is associated with:

- Inattention.
- Poor motivation.
- Hyperactivity.
- Lower IQ than normal.

The iron concentration in the brain increases normally during infancy and childhood, over the first 20 years, to adult values, with the highest concentration in the phylogenetically oldest parts of the brain. Falling iron stores in the infant are associated with glial proliferation, myelinization and dendrite arborization at this period.

Reference
Leibel, R., Greenfield, D. and Pollitt, E. (1979) *Br. J. Haematol.* **41**, 145

When total dose, iron–dextran infusion is given to mothers during pregnancy, the saturation of transferrin and the concentration of ferritin in the infant's cord blood at birth are higher than in babies born in untreated mothers, i.e. the fetal iron stores are increased.

Reference
Bingham, D., Khalaf, M. M., Walters, G. *et al.* (1983) *J. Clin. Pathol.* **36**, 907

7. The iron content of the nails reflects the body iron status.

Normal

The iron content is 6–26 μg/g nail (male and female).

Iron deficiency

Less than 4 μg/g nail.

Reference
Sobolewski, S., Laurence, A. C. K. and Bagshaw, P. (1978) *J. Clin. Pathol.* **31**, 1068

Iron turnover

Normal red blood cell life = 120 days. To maintain the normal haemoglobin level the red cell iron turnover = 0.25–0.5 mg/day per kg body weight = 22 mg/day = 6.58 g haemoglobin replaced daily (in a 70-kg man) resulting in the excretion of 193–234 mg urobilinogen daily.

The total daily plasma iron turnover = 20–40 mg/day, i.e. 3–4 mg iron in serum turns over 12 times each day (30 mg/day = 0.5 millimoles/day); 90% of the red cell iron is recycled.

Increased rate of iron turnover

- Iron-deficiency anaemia, even though the serum iron concentration may be low.
- Haemolytic anaemia.
- Polycythaemia vera (compare secondary polycythaemia).
- Megaloblastic anaemia (associated with the short life and rapid destruction of the abnormal red cells).
- Possibly some cases of leukaemia.

Note: The maximum rate of haemoglobin synthesis is about 6–8 times the normal rate, i.e. up to 50 g haemoglobin daily. As soon as the rate of blood loss exceeds the rate of blood formation, the whole blood haemoglobin level falls below normal, and a new equilibrium may then result.

Decreased rate of iron turnover

- Hypoplastic anaemia.
- Infection (*or* possibly shorter cell life, with increased turnover).

Iron loss from the body

Adult males

Iron = 0.5–1.5 mg may be lost each day in sweat, urine etc.

Adult females

Menstrual loss

Iron loss = 1.0–2.5 mg/day (mean, for whole month); the mean menstrual loss = 10.3 mg/period.

Reference
Elwood, P. C., Rees, G. and Thomas, J. D. R. (1968) *Br. J. Prev. Soc. Med.* **22**, 127

Pregnancy

- Fetus   400 mg ⎫
- Placenta   150 mg ⎬ = average 2.7 mg/day
- Blood loss 175 mg ⎭

i.e. allowing for 40 weeks of amenorrhoea, an extra 400 mg of iron are needed per pregnancy.

- Lactation 0.5 mg/day

Thus women do not develop haemochromatosis before the menopause.

Blood donation

In both sexes donation of 2 pints of blood per year requires absorption of an extra 1 mg of iron per day.

Urine iron

Increased output

- Paroxysmal nocturnal haemoglobinuria, and any other form of haemoglobinuria.
- After intravenous iron therapy there may be increased urine iron for a short time.

Serum iron

SI units conversion factor = 0.179, i.e. 70–180 μg/100 ml becomes 13–32 μmol.l.

Normal range

Cord blood serum iron: 72–237 μg/100 ml.

Reference
Weippl, G., Pantlitschko, M., Bauer, P. *et al.* (1973) *Clin. Chim. Acta.* **44**, 147

Adult males: 19.5–50 μmol/l; adult females: 1–32 μmol/l. Serum iron exists in the ferric state and is attached to the serum β-globulin transferrin (two atoms of iron per molecule of protein). The normal adult body contains about 4–5 g of iron, of which up to 3 g are present in the red blood cells; thus specimens of serum for analysis must be free from any haemolysis for some methods of serum iron estimation.

Physiological

1. Normal diurnal variation

The serum iron is higher in the early morning and lower in the afternoon due to fluctuating release of iron from reticuloendothelial cells.

Reference
Uchida, T., Akitsuki, T., Kimura H. *et al.* (1983) *Blood* **61**, 799

It is recommended that all specimens be collected between 9 and 10 a.m. Sleep deprivation results in low serum iron levels with loss of diurnal variation until sleep occurs. Iron released following the destruction of senile red cells is processed by reticuloendothelial cells into: (1) quick-release iron with a half-survival

time of 34 min; (2) slow-release iron with a half-survival time of 7 days; the two types are normally in equal amounts. The diurnal fluctuation in serum iron reflects the variable partitioning between early and late release phases. In acute inflammation there is a marked prompt increase in iron storage (late phase). Following depletion of iron stores there is a marked increase in early release iron.

References
Fillet, G., Crook, J. D. and Finch, C. A. (1974) *J. Clin. Invest.* **53**, 1527
Kuhn, E., Brodann, V., Brodanova, M. *et al.*, (1967) *Cas. Lek. Cesk.* **106**, 1342

2. Normal pregnancy

There is a progressive fall in the maternal serum iron from mid-term onwards, with a rising total iron-binding capacity.

3. Menstrual cycle

The serum iron falls just before menstruation.

4. Infancy

The normal serum iron at birth is 27–36 μmol/l, with a low total serum iron-binding capacity. Within a few hours of birth the serum iron falls to less than 18 μmol/l, eventually reaching adult levels by 3–7 years of age. Diurnal variation is absent at birth and the adult pattern is developed by 1–3 years of age.

5. Saturation with vitamin C

This results in an increase in serum iron levels.

Reference
Schwarz, E. and Baehner, R. L. (1968) *Acta Paediatr. Scand.* **57**, 433

Pathological

INCREASE

- Excessive iron intake

1. Excessive intravenous or intramuscular iron therapy.
2. Repeated blood transfusions: each pint of citrated blood contains more than 0.2 g of iron (i.e. transfusions in aplastic anaemia, where there is a falling haemoglobin level, but no external blood loss).
3. Haemochromatosis: in this condition there is excessive absorption of iron from the alimentary tract.
4. Acute poisoning, e.g. ingestion of ferrous sulphate tablets by very young children. Serum iron levels of more than 180 μmol/l may rapidly develop, and death may occur within 6 h.
5. Pancreatic disease: iron absorption is increased.
6. Allopurinol (xanthine oxidase inhibitor) increases iron absorption.

Note: There is no mechanism for excretion of excess iron. Women regularly lose 10–40 mg of iron at each menstrual period. Paradoxically, this loss may be greater in the presence of iron-deficiency anaemia.

During pregnancy the fetus obtains 400–500 mg of iron from the maternal circulation.

- Increased rate of blood destruction

As in haemolytic anaemias.

- Liver disease

In both acute hepatitis and in active portal cirrhosis the serum iron level is increased, presumably due to the liberation of stored iron from the necrosing liver cells. Circulating ferritin has been identified. A high incidence of abnormal liver function tests was found in apparently healthy blood donors with abnormally high serum iron values.

Reference
Crosby, W. H., Likhite, V. V. and O'Brien, J. E. (1974) *JAMA* **227**, 310

- Nephritis
- Refractory anaemia

Iron absorption is normal, but iron is not being used because haemoglobin synthesis is slowed.

- Oral contraceptives
- Primary inherited sex-linked sideroblastic anaemia
- Primary acquired sideroblastic anaemia

Some cases.

- Acute leukaemia
- Congenital hypochromic microcytic anaemia with iron overload

Reference
Stavem, P., Saltvedt, E. Elgjo, K. *et al.* (1973) *Scand. J. Haematol.* **10**, 153

- Thalassaemia minor
- Active porphyria cutanea tarda

DECREASE

Erythropoiesis is decreased if the serum iron persists below 12.5 μmol/l.

- Iron-deficiency anaemia

See 'Iron-deficiency anaemia'.

Post-surgery

Falling to low levels on first postoperative day and remaining low for 6 days.

- Remission in pernicious anaemia

Rapid blood regeneration uses up available iron.

- Acute and chronic infections

A low serum iron level frequently develops within 24 h of onset.

Carcinoma

Normal quantities of storage iron and increased red blood cell turnover.

- Nephrosis

Probably related to loss of specific iron-binding serum globulin in urine.

- Acth or adrenocortical extract therapy

The serum iron level falls, lowest level being reached after 8 h.

- Kwashiorkor
- Congenital atransferrinaemia

References
Reissmann, K. R. and Dietrich, M. R. (1956) *J. Clin. Invest.* **35**, 588
Trinder, P. (1956) *J. Clin. Pathol.* **9**, 170

Serum iron-binding capacity

The total serum iron-binding capacity is a measure of the serum concentration of transferrin, the specific iron-carrying protein. Transferrin is present in the serum at a concentration of 1.8–2.6 g/l and has a half-life of 8–11 days. Direct measurement of transferrin is difficult and only performed in research laboratories. At least 21 distinct transferrins have been isolated. Their distribution is:

1% Caucasians = C + B$_2$.
10% US Negroes = C + B$_2$.
Majority = C homozygotes.

Serum transferrin

Transferrin has a molecular weight of 76 000–80 000 and consists of a single polypeptide chain, with two metabolic iron-binding sites. Two molecular forms of transferrin-iron exist and the two binding sites do not share equal properties of iron exchange with cells. For each Fe^{3+} atom, bicarbonate (or less commonly oxalate) is attached to the molecule. This probably regulates the transfer of ingested iron from the labile intestinal epithelial pool to plasma. (It has been suggested that in the haemochromatosis there is failure to synthesize adequate ferritin in epithelial cells of the intestine, resulting in excess formation of plasma transferrin and hence excessive iron absorption.) Reticulocytes remove the bicarbonate iron from the transferrin molecule and iron becomes free for ingestion into the cell. Bound in this way iron cannot even be removed by chelating agents. Free iron atoms cannot enter developing red blood cells. Transferrin attaches to the cell membrane and the iron is chelated by cell acceptors. Similarly reticuloendothelial cells transfer iron derived from senescent red cells to developing red blood cells.

Reference:
Huebers, H. A. and Finch, C. A. (1984) *Blood* **64**, 763 (Review)

The serum iron-binding capacity consists of the following.

Total serum iron-binding capacity (TIBC)

Normal adult range: 45–72 μmol/l of iron per 100 ml serum.

Serum unsaturated iron-binding capacity (UIBC)

Normally about 35% of the serum transferrin is bound with iron, i.e. UIBC = TIBC minus serum iron.

SI unit conversion factor = 0.17, i.e. 250–400 μg/ 100 ml becomes 45–72 μmol/l.

The iron-binding protein appears to be active in bacteriostasis, unless it is fully saturated with iron by making iron unavailable to invading bacteria. Falling serum iron levels in infection appear to inhibit bacterial growth. Transferrin saturation with iron:

- <30%; unsatisfactory release of iron to marrow cells.
- 30–60%; satisfactory release of iron to marrow cells.
- >60%; iron deposited in tissue stores.

Reference
Bullen, J. T., Rogers, H. J. and Griffiths, E. (1972) *Br. J. Haematol.* **23**, 389

Note: When iron salts are injected intravenously, toxic symptoms develop as soon as the iron-binding capacity is exceeded.

Physiological

In normal pregnancy the TIBC rises to an average of 80.5 μmol/l, unrelated to either serum iron or haemoglobin levels, whilst the serum iron tends to fall, i.e. high UIBC.

In infants, the TIBC falls after birth, and subsequently rises to about 72 μmol/l by 2 years. Later, adult levels are attained.

Pathological

Raised serum iron-binding capacity (total)

WITH RAISED SERUM IRON CONCENTRATION

The total transferrin concentration is increased, but the unsaturated iron-binding capacity is reduced:

- Liver damage, e.g. acute hepatitis and active portal cirrhosis.
- Increased blood destruction, e.g. haemolytic anaemia.
- Excessive iron intake, e.g. (1) prolonged parenteral iron therapy, (2) repeated blood transfusions in refractory anaemia, (3) haemochromatosis and (4) high iron diet with low phosphate content (Bantus using iron cooking pots).
- Primary inherited sex-linked sideroblastic anaemia.
- Oral contraceptives.
- Idiopathic neonatal iron storage disease [R]: serum iron, total iron-binding capacity and tissue iron are all increased, accumulating during life in utero. Death occurs by 4 months.

Reference
Blisard, K. S. and Barstow, S. A. (1986) *Human Pathol.* **17**, 376

WITH LOW SERUM IRON CONCENTRATION

High UIBC:

- Acute and chronic blood loss: The available iron is used for blood regeneration.
- Some cases of iron deficiency.
- Polycythaemia vera.

LOW SERUM IRON-BINDING CAPACITY (TOTAL)

UIBC is normal or low.

- Acute and chronic infections and inflammation

The serum iron falls proportionally more than the transferrin content.

Reference
Hershko, C., Cook, J. D. and Finch, C. A. (1974) *Br. J. Haematol.* **28**, 67

- Falls to lowest levels

These occur by third day after surgical operation.

- Pernicious anaemia in relapse
- Uraemia
- Carcinomatosis
- Nephrotic syndrome

Excessive loss of protein bound iron in the urine.

- Kwashiorkor

Serum transferrin is reduced more than other serum proteins in proportion to the clinical severity.

Hypochromia develops when the transferrin saturation persists below 16%.

Reference
McFarlane, H., Ogbeide, M. I., Reddy S. *et al.* (1969) *Lancet* **i**, 392

- Scurvy
- Haemolytic anaemia

High serum iron with slightly reduced TIBC.

- Rheumatoid arthritis

The low TIBC rises with effective steroid therapy.

- Congenital atransferrinaemia [R]

Early childhood hypochromic anaemia, with very low serum transferrin, systemic iron overload, and virtually no iron stored in the liver.

Reference
Goya, N., Miyazaki, S., Kodate, S. *et al.* (1972) *Blood* **40**, 239

Stainable iron present in urine deposits

- Paroxysmal nocturnal haemoglobinuria.
- Thalassaemia major.
- Pernicious anaemia, if severe.
- Hereditary absence of haptoglobin.

Urine iron excretion after desferrioxamine

Normal adult males

800 μg iron excreted in the urine in 24 h.

- Cases of iron overload

More than 2200 μg iron excreted in the urine in 24 h.

- Cases of iron deficiency with depleted iron stores

Less than 600 μg iron excreted in the urine in 24 h. When the test is preceded by a small dose of an oral iron preparation, less than 150 μg iron are excreted in the urine in 24 h. (Evidence of ineffective erythropoiesis in iron deficiency.)

Reference
Harker, L. A., Funk, D. D. and Finch, C. A. (1968) *Am. J. Med.* **45**, 105.

Ferritin

Ferritin is the major iron storage protein, with a family of closely related isoferritins, occurring in liver, spleen, bone marrow, kidney, heart, pancreas, intestine and placenta. The iron-free apoferritin consists of a spherical protein shell with a molecular weight of 450 000, built up of 24 chemically identical subunits, with a core of ferric oxide phosphate. Ferritin synthesis is stimulated by iron, and the serum ferritin in normal subjects is proportional to the mobilizable iron stores of the body. Each ferritin molecule can accumulate 4000 iron atoms and, when fully saturated, 20% of its weight is iron.

The human ferritin gene is assigned to chromosome 19, whereas the genetic fault in haemochromatosis is due to a defect on chromosome 6.

Reference
Caskey, J. H., Jones, C., Miller, E. *et al.* (1983) *Proc. Natl. Acad. Sci. USA* **80**, 482

Serum ferritin

Circulating ferritin is probably secreted by the reticuloendothelial cells. Absorption of ferrous iron in males is inversely proportional to the logarithm of the serum ferritin concentration. There is a normal circadian rhythm, with a morning peak and evening trough. Stainable iron in the bone marrow only crudely measures available iron stores.

References
Magnusson, B., Bjorn-Rasmussen, E., Hallberg, L. *et al.* (1981) *Scand. J. Haematol.* **27**, 201
Worwood, M. (1982) In: Jacobs, A. (ed.) *Clinics in Haematology*, Vol. II, pp. 275–307. Philadelphia: Saunders

NORMAL VALUES

There is correlation between maternal serum ferritin and cord serum ferritin.

- From 6 months until puberty, serum ferritin values are low.
- Adults (males and females) 15–300 μg/l.

PHYSIOLOGICAL

Serum ferritin levels fall in pregnancy, especially after 35 weeks if no iron supplements are given.

After severe prolonged physical exercise in young men, serum ferritin is increased for 2 days afterwards, with greatest increases in those with the lowest initial values, ?synthesis of ferritin stimulated rapidly by iron release from damaged red cells, as ferritin increase correlated with decrease in haemoglobin and increase in serum bilirubin.

Reference
Vidnes, O. and Opstad, P. K. (1981) *Scand. J. Haematol.* **27**, 165

In blood donors, using serum ferritin estimations, it was shown that males and non-menstruating females could make up to five donations per year without depleting their body iron stores. Menstruating females could also make the same number of donations if they received iron supplements. The iron loss per donation was 250 mg.

Reference
Simon, T. L., Garry, P. J. and Hooper E. M. (1981) *JAMA* **245**, 2038

PATHOLOGICAL

Increase

1. Iron overload: serum ferritin levels are related to the volume of blood transfused in transfusion haemosiderosis.
2. Haemochromatosis: serum ferritin levels correlate with the amount of iron mobilized by venesection, but fluctuate widely during courses of venesection, and also if the patient is taking alcohol.

   In males serum ferritin levels may exceed 500 μg/l, being lower in female homozygotes. There is a significant difference between serum ferritin values in male control subjects and male heterozygotes.

   Serum ferritin levels rise to two to eight times the pre-venesection value shortly after venesection.

Reference
Leyland, M. J., Brown, P. J., Walker, R. J. *et al.* (1977) *Lancet* **ii**, 1030

3. Malignancy: increased in:
   (a) Hodgkin's disease;
   (b) non-Hodgkin's lymphoma;
   (c) other malignancy, including acute myeloblastic and lymphoblastic leukaemia.

Reference
Jakobsen, E., Engerset, A., Sandstal, B. *et al.* (1982) *Scand. J. Haematol.* **28**, 264

4. Transient increase with peak on third day after surgical operation (cf. serum iron and TIBC).
5. Alcoholics in proportion to liver damage.
6. Liver damage.

7. Infection. Serum ferritin levels can persist for up to 5 weeks after an infection with a fall in serum iron.

References
Birgegård, G. Hällgren, R., Killander, A. *et al.* (1978) *Scand. J. Haematol.* **21**, 333
Elin, R. J., Wolff, S. M. and Finch, C. A. (1977) *Blood* **49**, 147

8. Rheumatoid arthritis, in active synovitis, falling with remission.
9. Upper limit of normal in megaloblastic anaemia, falling during specific treatment.

Reference
Hussein, S., Laulicht, M. and Hoffbrand, A. V. (1978) *Scand. J. Haematol.* **20**, 241

10. Sickle-cell crisis due to vascular occlusion and tissue damage.

Reference
Brownell, A., Lowson, S. and Brozovic, M. (1986) *J. Clin. Pathol.* **39**, 253

11. Increase in pregnant carriers of β-thalassaemia.

Reference
White, J. M., Richards, R., Jelenski, G. *et al.* (1986) *J. Clin. Pathol.* **39** 256

Decrease

- Iron-deficiency anaemia: serum ferritin less than 10 µg/l. Serum ferritin is a reliable index of maternal iron stores, if sampled 1 month after total dose infusion of iron dextran, but is unreliable if tested earlier after the dose.

  Serum ferritin detects iron deficiency, when it is missed by serum iron and TIBC estimations. The correlation between serum ferritin, and serum iron and TIBC is satisfactory if the TIBC level is normal, but not otherwise.

Reference
Peter, F. and Wang, S. (1981) *Clin. Chem.* **27**, 276

- Vitamin C deficiency: serum ferritin rises again with vitamin C therapy.

Urine ferritin

Normal value = 2.2 µg/l (3% of serum value). Increased in intravascular haemolysis and in haematological malignancies.

Reference
Lipschitz, D. A., Allegre, A. and Cook, J. D. (1980) *Blood* **55**, 261

Free erythrocyte protoporphyrin (FEP)

The free red cell protoporphyrin increases in inverse proportion to the availability of ferrous iron to the erythroid marrow.

Normal values

Males: less than 30 µg/dl
Females: less than 40 µg/dl

Physiological

Increase

Increases by week 37 of pregnancy. This increase is much smaller when iron supplements are given during pregnancy.

Pathological

1. Iron deficiency (with low serum ferritin). Protoporphyrin is slowly lost from circulating red cells, and raised FEP levels persist even after iron therapy has been started.
2. Anaemia of chronic disease.
3. In thalassaemia and haemoglobin disease the FEP is normal.

References
Bothwell, T. H., Charlton, R. W., Cook, J. D. *et al.* (1979) *Iron Metabolism in Man*, pp. 44–81, Oxford: Blackwell
Marsh, W. C. Jr., Nelson, D. P. and Koenig, H. M. (1983) *Am. J. Clin. Pathol.* **79**, 655, 661

Measurement of available body iron stores

- Eventually the whole blood haemoglobin concentration cannot be maintained when available iron stores have been depleted by the weekly removal of up to 1 litre of blood. This method can only be used in cases of haemochromatosis.
- Liver biopsy: stainable iron is found mainly in the reticuloendothelial cells in normal subjects. Stainable iron may be increased in parenchymal cells in haemochromatosis.
- Bone marrow-stainable iron gives variable results.
- Using chelating agents, the excretion of chelatable iron in the urine varies, and this method for the estimation of body iron stores is inaccurate.
- Considerable variations from hour to hour, and from day to day, occur in the serum iron, total iron-binding capacity and percentage saturation of transferrin in normal subjects. Infections, inflammation and malignancy all depress transferrin saturation. High transferrin saturation results are found in iron overload, hypoplastic anaemia, haemolytic anaemia and acute leukaemia. Increased serum iron and transferrin saturation results are found in homozygotes for haemochromatosis before serum ferritin levels rise above normal.
- Erythrocyte protoporphyrin values increase from 35 ± 13 µg/l red cells to about 200 µg/l red cells in severe iron deficiency.

- Serum ferritin: this measurement is very useful for routine assessments of iron stores. Low serum ferritin (< 15 μg/l) reflects a depletion of body iron stores. Raised serum ferritin levels occur in iron overload, but also in liver disease, infection, inflammation or malignant disease.

Red cell ferritin

Normal

Normal value = 3–40 ag/cell (1 ag = 10^{-18}g). Red cell ferritin is a residue of erythroblast ferritin. Most of the iron taken up from plasma transferrin by immature red cells is for haemoglobin synthesis. The excess is stored as red cell ferritin.

Increase

1. Iron overload:
   (a) idiopathic haemochromatosis – persists after phlebotomy;
   (b) alcoholic liver disease – falls after phlebotomy.
2. Thalassaemia.
3. Sideroblastic anaemia.
4. Megaloblastic anaemia.

Decrease

1. Iron deficiency.
2. Inflammation – with normal or raised serum ferritin.
3. Rheumatoid arthritis – patients with microcytic anaemia and low red cell ferritin respond to iron therapy with a rise in haemoglobin.

Reference
Cazzola, M. and Ascari, E. (1986) *Br. J. Haematol.* **62**, 209

Hypochromic microcytic anaemia

Iron deficiency

The earliest laboratory signs of iron deficiency, with a normal haemoglobin concentration, are increasing anisocytosis with increasing numbers of microcytic red cells, and falling saturation of serum transferrin below 32%.

Later, the MCH and MCV fall, with haemoglobin concentration subnormal but greater than 9 g/dl, and transferrin saturation less than 16%.

Severe iron deficiency results in the haemoglobin concentration falling below 9 g/dl, and the MCHC falls below normal (when measured by Coulter counter). Serum ferritin levels fall below 10 μg/dl and red cell free protoporphyrin increases.

Perhaps 30% of the world population are anaemic, and at least half of these, 500–600 million, are suffering from iron deficiency anaemia. Iron deficiency reduces work performance, but also impairs attention span and cognitive development in late infancy, pre-school and school-age children.

References
Cook, J. D. and Lynch, S. R. (1986) *Blood* **68**, 803
England, J. M., Ward, S. M. and Down, M. C. (1976) *Br. J. Haematol.* **34**, 589

Inadequate iron intake

1. Poor diet
- Low iron content.
- Available iron absorption blocked, e.g., high phytate and/or phosphate content.

2. Impaired iron absorption
- Gastric lesions: low gastric hydrochloric acid results in lower iron absorption.
- Gastric surgery followed by abnormally rapid emptying of gastric contents into duodenum is associated with impaired iron absorption, with rapid intestinal passage. Iron is normally maximally absorbed in the duodenum.
- Malabsorption syndrome.

Iron loss exceeding intake

1. Bleeding
- Replacement by bone marrow of blood lost following an acute haemorrhage.
- Chronic blood loss, e.g. bleeding from haemorrhoids.

2. Haematuria

In paroxysmal nocturnal haemoglobinuria, the loss of iron in the urine as haemoglobin and haemosiderin often results in hypochromic/microcytic anaemia. Iron-deficient anaemia is present in up to 50% of joggers and competition runners. The plasma haemoglobin is significantly raised after a 25-km run, with low plasma haptoglobin and iron concentrations, and raised TIBC.

Reference
Hunding, A., Jordel, R. and Paulev, P-E. (1981) *Acta. Med. Scand.* **209**, 315

Hypochromic anaemia without iron deficiency

Failure of release of iron from the reticuloendothelial system

Even though stainable iron may be present in the bone marrow, iron-deficiency anaemia persists:

- Infection.
- Chronic inflammatory disorders, e.g. rheumatoid arthritis.
- Uraemia.
- Malignancy.

Atransferrinaemia [R]

This must be a lethal condition.

Thalassaemia

Sideroblastic anaemia

Iron overload

Primary haemochromatosis

Loss of feedback control of iron entry via the enterocyte, related to genetic defect on chromosome 6, results in continued daily iron absorption throughout life, regardless of increasing iron stores.

Reference
Cox, T. M. and Peters, T. J. (1980) *Q. J. Med.* **49**, 249

Secondary haemosiderosis

Anaemia with ineffective erythropoiesis

- Transfusion-dependent thalassaemia.
- Sideroblastic anaemia requiring repeated transfusion.
- Hypoplastic or aplastic anaemia requiring repeated blood transfusions.

Liver disease

- Alcoholic cirrhosis.
- After portacaval anastomosis.

Excessive oral iron intake

- Prolonged excessive iron medication.
- Excessive iron absorption associated with heavy drinking of corn beer brewed with high iron content (South Africa).

Laboratory tests

- TIBC tending to saturation with raised serum iron.
- Serum ferritin levels high.
- Liver biopsy reveals excessive stainable iron, and iron concentration is abnormally high.
- Following quantitative phlebotomy – subjects with normal body iron stores become iron deficient when a total of 2 g of iron have been removed by weekly 500 ml phlebotomies.
- Chelation with desferrioxamine results in abnormally increased urine iron excretion.
- Patients suffering from iron overload and who are also vitamin C deficient, tend to have low serum ferritin levels. If they are given large doses of vitamin C, oxidant tissue damage may occur.
- Plasma iron, not bound to transferrin in chronic iron overload, is taken up by the myocardium. This results in increased peroxidation, which causes abnormalities in both rhythm and contractility of the heart muscle.

References
Finch, C. A. and Huebers, H. (1982) *N. Engl. J. Med.* **306**, 1520
Hershko, C. and Peto, T. E. (1987) *Br. J. Haematol.* **66**, 149

Macrocytic anaemia

There is a mean red cell volume greater than 94 fl, due to: (1) disruption of mitotic sequence in the bone marrow, or (2) increased erythropoietic stimulation in the presence of adequate iron supplies, leading to premature release of reticulocytes. There are two types: megaloblastic anaemia and macrocytic/normoblastic anaemia.

Macrocytic/normoblastic anaemia

1. Any case with reticulocytosis: reticulocytes are normally larger than normal adult red cells.
2. Occasionally during the course of:
   (a) Hodgkin's disease;
   (b) myeloma;
   (c) carcinomatosis;
   (d) leukaemia (very occasionally cells resembling megaloblasts may be seen in the marrow);
   (e) lymphoma;
   (f) hepatitis and liver disease (in cirrhosis, an occasional case may be megaloblastic);
   (g) pellagra;
   (h) myxoedema and hypothyroidism;
   (i) malaria;
   (j) aplastic anaemia;
   (k) lead poisoning;
   (l) hypopituitarism;
   (m) protein malnutrition, e.g. kwashiorkor;
   (n) cardiorespiratory disorders;
   (o) uraemia;
   (p) chronic alcoholism: combination of folate deficiency and/or direct toxic action of alcohol on erythropoietic developments;
   (q) azathioprine: macrocytosis is dose related. When the MCV exceeds 115 fl there is a risk of marrow hypoplasia.

Vitamin B_{12}

Occurrence and daily requirement

Vitamin B_{12} is present in meats, eggs and, to a lesser extent, milk. Plants do not contain the vitamin. It is synthesized, with other analogues which cannot be utilized but are included in some estimations, in the human intestines by organisms, including *Pseudomonas* sp. and *Klebsiella* sp. The daily intake on a normal diet is about 5 μg, and the daily requirement is less than 1 μg.

Absorption

Dietary cobalamin is hydrolysed from its peptide links with dietary protein, and two molecules bind to two molecules of gastric *intrinsic factor* (IF). IF is a mucoprotein, a dimer with a molecular weight of 114 000, secreted by the gastric parietal cells. Production and secretion of IF are stimulated by histamine, gastrin, gastrin analogues and insulin. Only about 1% of the normal daily production of IF is required for absorption of the daily 1 μg of vitamin B_{12}, 1 mg of IF binding 25 μg of the vitamin.

Vitamin B_{12} also binds to R-binder, present in saliva, gastric juice, bile and intestinal juices, especially at low pH. Pancreatic protease splits R-binders releasing vitamin B_{12}, which then binds to IF. Ileal receptors, which occur in the distal three-fifths of the small intestine, with the highest concentration just before the terminal ileum, bind to the IF–cobalamin complex. It then takes several hours for cobalamin to transfer across the ileal cells, to become bound to *transcobalamin II* in the portal circulation. IF is not absorbed. Less than 1% of oral vitamin B_{12} can be absorbed passively.

Transport in plasma

The total serum vitamin B_{12} binding capacity is 1194–2322 ng/l. Following absorption by the ileal mucosal cells, vitamin B_{12} is carried in the plasma by *transcobalamin I (TC-I)*. TC-I is an α-globulin with a molecular weight of 121 000, and is probably derived from granulocytes and other tissues. It has a total binding capacity of 700–800 ng/l, and carries about 470 pg of vitamin B_{12} per ml of plasma, mostly as methylcobalamin, as a circulating reserve store. The other carrier protein is transcobalamin II (TC-II).

Transcobalamin II

TC-II is a single polypeptide chain β-globulin with a molecular weight of 38 000. It is synthesized in the bone marrow, liver and ileal enterocytes, and has a short half-life. This protein is essential for transport of vitamin B_{12} to the cells, and plays a part in normal gastrointestinal absorption of the vitamin. It is only 10–20% saturated with cobalamin in the plasma.

Vitamin B_{12} enters the cells bound to TC-II via specific receptors on the cell surface. Endocytosis of this complex is followed by degradation of the binding protein by lysosomal protease, releasing free vitamin B_{12} into the cell cytoplasm.

Methylcobalamin is the main plasma transport form (60–70% of plasma, 20–30% of intracellular vitamin B_{12}), whereas 5'-deoxyadenosylcobalamin is the main intracellular form (20–25% of plasma, 70–80% of intracellular vitamin B_{12}).

References
Porck, H. J., Fräter-Schröder, M., Frants, R. R. *et al.* (1983) *Blood* **62**, 234
Rosenblatt, D. S., Hosack, A., Matiaszuk, N. V. *et al.* (1985) *Science* **228**, 1319
Seligman, P. A., LaDonna, L., Steiner, B. S. *et al.* (1980) *N. Engl. J. Med.* **303**, 1209

Functions of vitamin B_{12}

Two forms of the vitamin provide prosthetic groups to two classes of enzymes: 5'-deoxyadenosylcobalamin and methylcobalamin.

5'-Deoxyadenosylcobalamin

The oxidation of fatty acids with odd numbers of carbon atoms, and of the oxo-acids derived from the branched-chain amino-acids, isoleucine and valine, produces propionyl-CoA. Vitamin B_{12} is the cofactor and hydrogen donor to the isomerase, methylmalonyl-CoA mutase, which is one of three enzymes involved in the conversion of propionyl-CoA to succinyl-CoA, enabling its entry into the tricarboxylic acid cycle (citric acid cycle).

Methylcobalamin

Methylcobalamin is the cofactor, and methyl donor, for the enzyme tetrahydropteroylglutamate methyl transferase which generates methionine from homocysteine, receiving a methyl-group from N^5-methyltetrahydrofolate, producing tetrahydrofolate (THF). This is a main pathway in the metabolism of sulphur-containing amino acids.

Methionine is required for methyl transfer to choline in the formation of phospholipids and sphingomyelin. THF is converted to its pentaglutamate form in the cell, and is essential for the synthesis of 5,10-methylene-THF, required for thymidylate synthesis (an essential component of DNA).

Vitamin B_{12} values

1. Serum vitamin B_{12}

- Using various organisms, including *Euglena gracilis* and *Lactobacillus leishmanii*: 160–925 ng/l.
- Using isotope dilution methods: 200–1000 ng/l.

(Some cobalamin analogues will be measured which cannot be utilized by the human body.)

There is no decline in serum vitamin B_{12} with age, and no difference between males and females in good health.

Reference
Hitzhusen, J. C., Taplin, M. E., Stephenson, W. P. *et al.* (1986) *Am. J. Clin. Pathol.* **85**, 32

There is a specific radio-immunoassay of 5'-deoxyadenosylcobalamin in serum.

Reference
Quadros, E. V., Sheldon, P., Rothenberg, S. P. and Polu, S. (1988) *Br. J. Haematol.* **69**, 551

2. Red cell vitamin B_{12}

Values are 72–512 ng/l packed cells (varying with the method).

3. White cell vitamin B_{12}

Approximately 7500 ng/l packed cells (varying with the method).

4. Cerebrospinal fluid vitamin B_{12}

Values are 8–36 ng/l (mean = 17.8 ng/l). There is no direct correlation between serum and CSF vitamin B_{12}. CSF vitamin B_{12} levels fall in pernicious anaemia, and following long-term anticonvulsant therapy.

5. Body stores

About 1000–2000 μg (mainly in the liver).

6. Biological half-life of vitamin B_{12}

Thought to be about 365 days. When vitamin B_{12} treatment is interrupted in pernicious anaemia, there is a mean interval of 64 months (21–123 months) when macrocytosis develops, followed by anaemia.

Reference
Savage, D. and Lindenbaum, J. (1983) *Am. J. Med.* **74**, 765

Pathological

Increase in serum vitamin B_{12}

1. Pharmacological doses of vitamin B_{12}.
2. Myeloproliferative disorders:
   (a) chronic myeloid leukaemia, before treatment;
   (b) acute myeloblastic leukaemia;
   (c) acute promyelocytic leukaemia–levels may reach 2000–16 000 ng/l;
   (d) some cases of myelosclerosis;
   (e) some cases of erythraemic myelosis;
   (f) in about 33% of cases of chronic lymphatic leukemia;
   (g) some cases of monocytic leukaemia;
   (h) polycythaemia vera.
3. Some cases of carcinomatosis, especially with liver secondary deposits.
4. Liver disease, including acute hepatitis, cirrhosis, chronic liver disease and hepatic coma, with release of vitamin B_{12} from liver stores.

Decrease in serum vitamin B_{12}

1. Diet

A diet deficient in vitamin B_{12}, for example the vegetarian diet of strict vegans. A low maternal vitamin B_{12} is depleted in pregnancy, as there is preferential transfer of the vitamin to the fetus.

2. Lack of availability of dietary vitamin B_{12}

- Fish tapeworm anaemia: *Diphyllobothrium latum* selectively absorbs vitamin B_{12} from the diet, especially if the worm is lodged high up in the jejunum.
- Blind loop syndrome, tropical sprue, post-polygastrectomy: there is bacterial overgrowth with competition for vitamin B_{12}, with a relative increase in biologically inactive analogues of vitamin B_{12} produced by intestinal organisms. These enter the plasma and may produce 'normal' serum vitamin B_{12} results.

Reference
Murphy, M. F., Sourial, N. A., Burman, J. F. *et al.* (1986) *Br. J. Haematol.* **62**, 7

3. Defective absorption of vitamin B_{12} due to gastric lesions

INTRINSIC FACTOR

- Absence of IF following total surgical gastrectomy with vitamin B_{12} deficiency and iron deficiency developing in 5–10 years. After partial gastrectomy, 50% develop iron deficiency and 5–6% develop vitamin B_{12} deficiency. Destruction of gastric mucosa may be caused by corrosives or radiation. Carcinoma of the stomach usually progresses too rapidly for vitamin B_{12} deficiency to have time to develop.
- Parietal cell atrophy, as in pernicious anaemia.
- Gastritis.
- Intrinsic factor antibodies: type I IF antibodies, IgG immunoglobulins, inhibit the complexing of vitamin B_{12} with IF. They are present in the sera of 50–60% of patients with pernicious anaemia (with false negative test results for a few days after a dose of vitamin B_{12}). They are also present in the gastric juice of 80% of pernicious anaemia cases. Achlorhydria favours antigen–antibody complex formation, increasing vitamin B_{12} malabsorption. Type II antibody binds to the IF–vitamin B_{12} complex and prevents its absorption by the ileal mucosa. It occurs in 35% of cases of pernicious anaemia, and its presence is not diagnostic.

Reference
Fairbanks, V. F., Lennon, V. A., Kokmen, E. *et al.* (1983) *Mayo Clin. Proc.* **58**, 203

- Primary hypothyroidism: 40–50% have achlorhydria with intrinsic factor failure and low serum vitamin B_{12} levels, although megaloblastic anaemia is rare.
- Congenital intrinsic factor deficiency [R].

- Biologically inert intrinsic factor. The binding site for vitamin B_{12} is distinct from the ileal receptor binding site.

PARIETAL CELL ANTIBODIES

Ninty per cent of adult patients with pernicious anaemia have parietal cell antibodies in their sera and gastric juice. Complement-dependent cytotoxic antibodies to gastric parietal cells may contribute to loss of these cells in pernicious anaemia.

About 16% of women over 60 years of age and without pernicious anaemia also have parietal cell antibodies in their sera. These antibodies also occur in some cases of atrophic gastritis, chronic active rheumatoid arthritis and iron-deficiency anaemia.

Reference
de Aizpurua, H. J., Cosgrove, L. J., Ungar, B. *et al.* (1983) *N. Engl. J. Med.* **309**, 625

4. Ileal malabsorption of vitamin B_{12}

INTESTINAL MALABSORPTION

This includes idiopathic steatorrhoea, coeliac disease, sprue, regional ileitis, diverticulitis and diverticulosis, intestinal fistulae, strictures and resection. Broad-spectrum antibiotic therapy may cause clinical remission with improved vitamin B_{12} absorption.

Reference
Hughes, S. and Marsh, N. M. (1981) *Postgrad. Med. J.* **59**, 536

INHIBITION OF ILEAL ABSORPTION

PAS used in antituberculous treatment inhibits ileal absorption of vitamin B_{12}.

THE IMERSLUND–GRÄSBECK SYNDROME

In this syndrome, ileal receptors for vitamin B_{12} are normal at birth, but decline in numbers or functional quality, leading to selective malabsorption of vitamin B_{12} and the development of megaloblastic vitamin B_{12} deficiency.

References
Burman, J. F., Jenkins, W. J., Walker-Smith, J. A. *et al.* (1985) *Gut* **26**, 311
Mackenzie, I. L., Donaldson, R. M. Jr., Trier, J. S. *et al.* (1972) *N. Engl. J. Med.* **286**, 1021

5. Faults in plasma transport of vitamin B_{12}

- Congenital lack of TC-I and TC-III [R] has been described. Although serum vitamin B_{12} levels were abnormally low, no abnormal clinical signs or symptoms occurred, because TC-II was normal.
- Congenital lack of TC-I [R] is inherited, and is associated with severe megaloblastic anaemia in neonates. Affected infants and children can only survive if given daily injections of 1000 μg vitamin

B_{12} for life. Such massive doses allow passive diffusion of vitamin B_{12} into the body cells in adequate amounts.

Reference
Zeitlin, H. C., Sheppard, K., Baum, J. D. *et al.* (1985) *Blood* **66**, 1022

- Biologically ineffective, immunologically normal TC-II, with absence of thymidylate synthase before treatment. One case has been reported, which responded to massive parenteral doses of vitamin B_{12} or oral folic acid.

Reference
Harauni, F. I., Hall, C. A. and Rubin, R. (1979) *J. Clin. Invest.* **64**, 1253

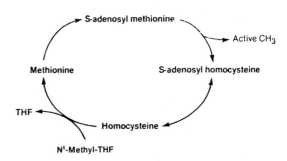

Activated methyl cycle. Shortage of methylcobalamin results in accumulation of N^5-methyl-THF, leading to shortage of 5,10-methylene-THF, and hence reduced synthesis of dTMP (folate trap).

Abnormalities of vitamin B_{12} metabolism

1. *Nitrous oxide anaesthesia and marrow dysfunction*

Continuous exposure to 50% nitrous oxide and 50% oxygen results in bone marrow aplasia in 5–7 days. Intermittent use of nitrous oxide (Entonox) anaesthesia over a 3-month period has resulted in myeloneuropathy with loss of myelinated nerve fibres.

Exposure to nitrous oxide eventually results in megaloblastic haemopoiesis before the marrow is damaged more severely, and such changes are seen in 5–24 h of exposure. Circulating vitamin B_{12} in its active form is oxidized to methylcob(II)alamin and methylcob(III)alamin, inactive precursor forms of the vitamin and in consequence, thymidylate synthesis is depressed, reducing DNA synthesis. Reduction in hepatic S-adenosylmethionine (SAM) is thought to be associated with neurological damage resembling subacute combined degeneration.

Nitrous oxide causes a fall in methionine transferase activity, and serum methionine levels fall after 1 h, remaining low for 24 h after cessation of breathing nitrous oxide. At the same time, serum valine increases after 3 h of nitrous oxide inhalation.

Tissue methylcobalamin depletion occurs and availability of 5,10-methylenetetrahydrofolate is reduced. This latter substance is the essential carbon donor for the conversion of deoxyuridylate to thymidylate, again reducing DNA synthesis.

The dU-suppression test is abnormal (vitamin B_{12} deficiency pattern) in a high proportion of patients exposed to nitrous oxide, the abnormality being directly related to the duration of exposure. Also the more severely ill the patient, the sooner abnormalities appear. With clinical recovery the dU-suppression test abnormality becomes that found in folate deficiency. The concentration of nitrous oxide in the surgical theatre atmosphere around anaesthetists should not exceed 200 ppm.

References
Amos, R. J., Amess, J. A. L., Hinds, C. J. *et al.* (1982) *Lancet* **2**, 835
Chanarin I. (1980) *J. Clin. Pathol.* **33**, 909
England, J. M. and Linnell, J. C. (1980) *Lancet* **ii**, 1072
Hayden, P. J., Hartemink, R. J. and Nicholson, G. A. (1983) *Burns* **9**, 267
Layzer, R., Fishman, R. A. and Schafer, J. A. (1978) *Neurology* **28**, 504
Sharer, N. M., Nunn, J. F., Royston, J. P. *et al.* (1983) *Br. J. Anaesth.* **55**, 693

2. *Conditions with methylmalonic aciduria (MMA)*

• Vitamin B_{12} deficiency after a loading dose of L-valine

This is not a useful diagnostic test, but demonstrates the metabolic block between propionic acid and succinic acid when vitamin B_{12} is deficient.

• Some rare congenital metabolic disorders

Associated with failure to thrive, ketosis and mental handicap [R]:

1. Methylmalonyl-CoA mutase apoenzyme:
   (a) absent;
   (b) abnormal form.
2. Cob(I)alamin: ATP adenosyltransferase deficiency.
3. Intramitochondrial cob(III)alamin or cob(II)-alamin reductase deficiency.
4. Unidentified cobalamin metabolism.
5. Associated with a variety of homocystinuria. Clinically these conditions:
   (a) respond to vitamin B_{12} therapy;
   (b) do not respond to vitamin B_{12} therapy.

References
Matsui, S. M., Mahoney, M. J. and Rosenberg, L. E. (1983) *N. Engl. J. Med.* **308**, 857
Norman, E. J., Martelo, O. J. and Denton, M. D. (1982) *Blood* **56**, 1128

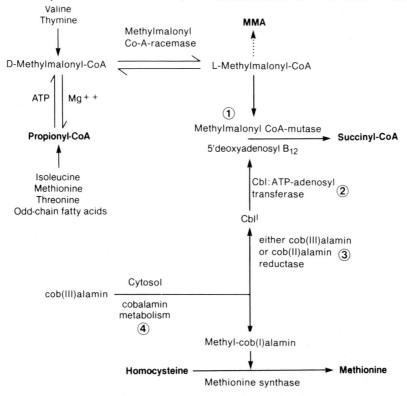

Inherited methylmalonic aciduria (MMA): ① methymalonyl CoA-mutase deficiency; ② cob(I)alamin: ATP adenosyl transferase deficiency; ③ intramitochondrial cob(III) alamin or cob(II)alamin reductase deficiency; ④ unidentified defects in cobalamin metabolism. CbI = cobalamin.

3. *Methionine synthase deficiency [R]*

Neonatal megaloblastic anaemia and homocystinuria with neurological dysfunction, but no methylmalonic aciduria, was found in an infant with methionine synthase deficiency. Cobalamin was able to enter the infant's cells, but intracellular methylcobalamin was abnormally reduced. Complete recovery, with subsequent normal neurological development, followed cyanocobalamin therapy.

Reference
Hallam, L. J., Sawyer, M., Clark, A. C. L., and van der Weyden, M. B. (1987) *Blood* **67**, 1128

Tests of faulty absorption of vitamin B_{12}

After an oral dose of vitamin B_{12} containing a radioactive isotope of cobalt the following can occur.

Serum levels

After an oral dose of vitamin B_{12}, serum levels rise after 2 h, to reach plateau results by 8 h.

Faecal excretion

After oral radioactive vitamin B_{12} the stools are collected for 7 days, and the radioactivity measured. Normally less than 50% of the test dose is recovered, whereas in pernicious anaemia more than 70% of the test dose is recovered, if all the stools have been collected.

Urine excretion

- Schilling test

A small dose of radioactive vitamin B_{12} is given by mouth, followed later by a large dose of non-radioactive vitamin – the so-called 'flushing dose'. Peak plasma levels are found at 8 h.

In normal subjects radioactive vitamin B_{12} is excreted in the urine during the next 24 h. In pernicious anaemia, little or no radioactive vitamin B_{12} is excreted in the urine. Low urine ouput of radioactive B_{12} with satisfactory plasma levels occur: (1) faulty urine collection; (2) renal damage.

Following gastrectomy, even though intrinsic factor may still be formed, intestinal hurry may cause incomplete absorption of the radioactive vitamin B_{12}.

- Dicopac test

In this test, free vitamin B_{12} tagged with ^{58}Co is given with an equal amount of vitamin B_{12}–IF complex, the vitamin B_{12} being tagged with ^{57}Co. After a 'flushing dose' of non-radioactive vitamin B_{12}, the ratio of $^{57}Co:^{58}Co$ is estimated in subsequent urine samples.

In normal subjects, since both forms of vitamin B_{12} are absorbed, the ratio is 1:2 (there being slightly higher absorption of ^{57}Co bound to IF). In pernicious anaemia, the ratio is usually greater than 2.0.

Unfortunately, overlap of results between normal and abnormal occurs, and results may become complicated, if there is renal impairment. In malabsorption, the ratio falls into the normal range, but the actual excretion of either form of vitamin B_{12} is low, as its absorption is low. A normal Dicopac ratio ($^{57}Co:^{58}Co$) is found when antibodies are present in both the serum and the gastric juice (e.g. atrophic gastritis without pernicious anaemia).

Reference
Knudsen, L. and Hippe, E. (1974) *Scand. J. Haematol.* **13**, 287

Some authorities prefer the single-dose Schilling test in the diagnosis of pernicious anaemia. Probably it is true that with more sophisticated blood-counting machines, with accurate MCV and MCH estimations (as with the Coulter 'S' counter), cases in the earlier stages of the disease are being detected, with moderately reduced rates of absorption of vitamin B_{12}.

Folic acid

Occurrence and daily requirement

Folic acid (pteroylglutamic acid), in the form of polyglutamates, is present in green vegetables (especially spinach and cabbage), nuts, cereals, crude yeast extracts, liver and kidney.

The daily requirement is about 100–200 μg, rising to 300–500 μg in pregnancy, and increasing in any condition where there is rapid cell division.

Absorption

Specific folate-binding protein occurs in the jejunal and, to a lesser extent, in the rest of the small intestinal mucosa. The folate polyglutamate chain is deconjugated, probably extracellularly, until a folate monoglutamate remains, and this is reduced and methylated to produce N^5-methyltetrahydrofolate, in which form it is absorbed and transported.

Specific folate-binding protein also occurs in saliva, bile and milk. Folate 60–90 μg is secreted in the bile and reabsorbed each day in the small intestine.

Transport in plasma

Much of 5-methyl-THF is bound to α_2-macroglobulin, albumin and transferrin, with some bound firmly to specific folate-binding protein. Folate is transported into bone marrow cells, reticulocytes, hepatocytes, renal tubular cells and the cerebrospinal fluid by an energy-dependent process via folate receptors in cell membranes, and more folate is taken up by reticulocytes than by mature erythrocytes. It can only cross the cell membrane as a monoglutamate, and is only retained inside the cell as a polyglutamate, predominantly pentaglutamate in humans. Inside the cell, 5-methyl-THF monoglutamate is converted to tetrahydrofolate, as only tetrahydrofolate can be converted to pentaglutamate. This enables intracellular folate levels to reach 30 times the plasma folate concentration, and explains the greater clinical value of red cell folate estimations in the detection of folate deficiency. The specific binding of folate in milk may have an antibacterial function by making folate unavailable to micro-organisms. The placenta also contains folate-binding receptors to facilitate transfer of folate from the mother's circulation to the fetus.

Functions

All folates are derived from a pteridine moiety linked by a methylene bridge to *p*-aminobenzoic acid which is joined by a peptide bond to glutamic acid. The number of glutamate residues varies from one to eight, and various one-carbon groups (methyl, formyl, formimino and methylene) may be attached. The various substances formed in this way are interconvertible, and are used in different reactions shown in the figure on p. 32.

Folates are directly involved in the transfer of one-carbon units from serine to glycine, the imidazole ring of histidine, and the utilization of formate. Folates are also essential for the de novo synthesis of purine nucleotide, providing carbon atoms 2 and 8 in the purine ring, and for pyrimidine nucelotide synthesis to produce dTMP from dUMP, i.e. DNA synthesis. With vitamin B_{12}, it controls the conversion of homocysteine to methionine. They are also responsible for the methylation of transfer RNA.

DNA synthesis is abnormal when the intracellular folate falls to $0.2–0.5$ ng/10^6 cells, and is markedly abnormal when it falls below 0.1 ng/10^6 cells. Megaloblastic changes develop when the intracellular folate falls below 0.06 ng/10^6 cells in tissue culture.

Reference
Steinberg, S. E., Fonda, S., Campbell C. L. *et al.* (1983) *Br. J. Haematol.* **54**, 605

Folate values

- Serum folate: normal $ = >2.2$ μg/l.
- Red cell folate: normal $ = >125$ μg/l.

Most of the red cell folate and some of the serum folate exists as polyglutamates. For accurate assay, whether by radio-immunoassay or by microbiological methods, folate in samples should be converted to the monoglutamate state before estimation.

There is poor correlation between red cell folate and serum folate, because serum folate fluctuates with the amount of folate in the diet and the time of its absorption in relation to sampling time.

- White blood cell folate: $263–1028$ μg/l packed cells. Lymphocytes contain three to four times the amount of folate present in polymorphs.
- Platelet folate: $40–170$ μg/l packed cells.
- Cerebrospinal fluid folate: $19–39$ μg/l. Selective concentration occurs in the CSF even during folate deficiency. Anticonvulsant therapy causes some reduction in CSF folate.

The normal red cell and serum folate levels are raised at birth, falling to low levels by 3 months, when the folate stores laid down during pregnancy are depleted.

References
Bain, B. J., Wickramasinghe, S. N., Broom, G. H. *et al.* (1984) *J. Clin. Pathol.* **37**, 888
Shane, B., Tamura, T. and Stokstad, E. L. R. (1980) *Clin. Chim. Acta* **100**, 13

Serum folate

Pathological

Increase

1. Pharmacological doses of folic acid.
2. Very rare inherited diseases:
   (a) glutamate formiminotransferase deficiency;
   (b) methenyl-tetrahydrofolate cyclohydrolase deficiency;
   (c) N^5-methyl-tetrahydrofolate transferase deficiency (the vitamin B_{12} reaction involved in the conversion of homocysteine to methionine);
   (d) methylene-tetrahydrofolate reductase deficiency.
3. Intestinal blind loop syndrome: many of the folic acid compounds formed by organisms in the gut, and absorbed, are not utilizable by the human body, but are estimated (as with many cobalamin forms).

References
Arakawa, T., Fujii, M., Ohara, K. *et al.* (1966a) *Tohoku J. Exp. Med.* **88**, 35
Arakawa, T., Fujii, M. and Ohara, K. (1966b) *Tohoku J. Exp. Med.* **88**, 195
Erbe, R. W. (1975) *N. Engl. J. Med.* **293**, 753, 807
Hoffbrand, A. V., Tabaqchali, S. and Mollin, D. L. (1966) *Lancet* **i**, 1939

Serum and red cell folate

Pathological

Decrease

1. INADEQUATE INTAKE

- Poor diet, e.g. poverty, alcoholism, mental illness, kwashiorkor.

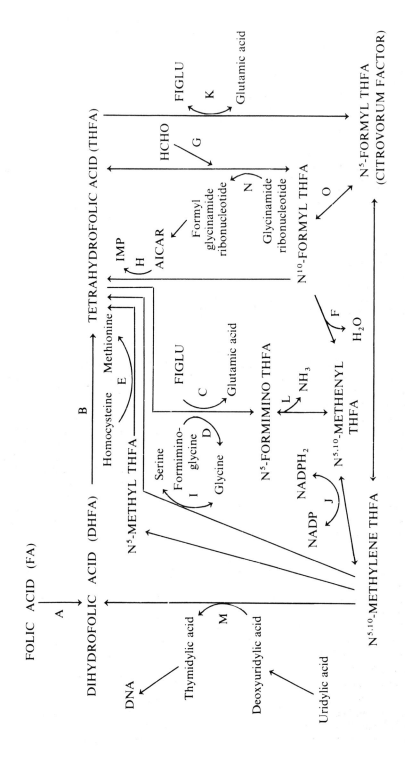

Reaction	Enzyme	Coenzyme or cofactor
A	Folate acid reductase	
B	Dihydrofolic acid reductase	
C	Glutamate formiminotransferase	
D	Glycine formiminotransferase	
E	N^5-Methyltetrahydrofolate transferase	Vitamin B_{12}
F	Methenyltetrahydrofolate cyclohydrolase	
G	Formyltetrahydrofolate synthase (formate-activating enzyme)	
H	Formyltetrahydrofolate deformylase	
I	Serine hydroxymethyl transferase	Vitamin B_6
J	$N^{5,10}$-Methylenetetrahydrofolate dehydrogenase	NADP
K	Formylglutamate formyl transferase	
L	Formiminotetrahydrofolate cyclodeaminase	
M	Thymidylate synthase	Vitamin B_{12}
N	Glycinamide ribonucleotide formylase	
O	N^4-formyltetrahydrofolate isomerase	ATP

DNA = deoxyribonucleic acid.
NADP = coenzyme II.
FIGLU = Formiminoglutamic acid.
AICAR = 5-amino-4-imidazole carboxamide ribotide.
IMP = inosine monophosphate.
Congenital deficiencies of enzymes C, E and F are associated with megaloblastic anaemia.
Antifolate antimetabolites (e.g. 6-mercaptopurine) inhibit enzymes A and B.

- Special diets without added folic acid – for example, early special amino acid controlled diets for phenylketonuric patients and patients with maple syrup disease, hopefully now only of historical interest.
- Infants fed on goats' milk for long periods before weaning. Goats' milk is deficient in both folic acid and vitamin B_{12}.

2. INCREASED UTILIZATION OF FOLATE, INCREASING FOLATE REQUIREMENTS (Deficiency accelerated by poor diet.)

- Pregnancy and lactation: increased folate required from the sixth month of pregnancy onwards. If there is a shortage of folate, the fetus takes metabolic priority, and the mother becomes deficient.
- Prematurity and infancy: rapid growth leads to greater folate requirements, becoming overt if the mother is folate deficient.
- Haemolysis: rapid replacement of red cells with shortened lives.
- Myelosclerosis, malignancy, sideroblastic anaemia and inflammatory disease: rapid cell turnover increases folate requirement.

3. DEFECTIVE ABSORPTION
- Idiopathic steatorrhoea.
- Tropical sprue.
- Coeliac disease – megaloblastic anaemia rare.
- Blind or stagnant intestinal loop.
- Tuberculous enteritis.

- Crohn's regional ileitis.
- Lymphoma and lymphosarcoma affecting the small intestine [R].
- Intestinal resection, especially of jejunum.
- Systemic bacterial infection.
- Anticonvulsants: phenytoin, primidone, phenobarbitone and other anticonvulsants interfere with the absorption of folate by the intestinal mucosa. At the same time, pharmacological doses of folic acid similarly interfere with the absorption of oral anticonvulsants, leading to more fits. Regular yeast tablets give a cheap and safe prophylaxis against folate deficiency in epileptics on long-term anticonvulsant therapy.

Reference
Eastham, R. D., Jancar, J. and Cameron, J. D. (1975) *Br. J. Psychiatr.* **126**, 263

4. INCREASED LOSS OF FOLATE

- Congestive cardiac failure.
- Liver necrosis.
- Haemodialysis, in the dialysate.
- Peritoneal dialysis, in the dialysate.

5. INTERFERENCE WITH FOLATE METABOLISM

1. Folate antagonists:
   (a) 4-aminopteroylglutamic acid;
   (b) methotrexate;
   (c) 6-mercaptopurine;

(d) ethanol – serum N^5-methyl-THF falls and liver folate is depleted. Following ethanol infusions, serum folate falls and does not return to normal until the infusion is stopped. Megaloblastic anaemia rapidly develops in chronic alcoholics eating a poor diet;

(e) pyrimethamine – malarial prophylactic;

(f) rarely caused by oral contraceptives, when they interfere with pteroylpolyglutamate hydrolase in the intestinal brush border;

(g) homocystinuria due to cystathionine synthase deficiency;

(h) following oral methionine 8 g daily for 4 days – paracetamol poisoning treatment;

(i) liver folate dihydrofolate reductase deficiency [R].

Reference
Tauro, G. P., Danks, D. M., Rowe, P. B. *et al.* (1976) *N. Engl. J. Med.* **294**, 466

Urine excretion of folic acid

- Normal – up to 20 μg/day.
- Increased – liver disease and liver damage secondary to congestive cardiac failure.
- Reduced – pernicious anaemia.

This estimation is of no clinical value.

Urine excretion of formiminoglutamic acid (FIGLU)

Following an oral histidine load, the intermediate metabolite in its catabolism, FIGLU, is excreted in excess in the urine if folate is deficient. This test is no longer used in clinical practice, because estimations of serum and red cell folate are rapid and relatively simple.

Oral folate absorption test

This test is obsolete. Pharmacological doses of THF-monoglutamate do not test intestinal absorption.

Folate clearance test

Estimation of serum folate 15 min after an intravenous injection of folic acid is no longer thought to be clinically useful.

Deoxyuridine suppression test

Deoxyuridine (dU) is added to normoblastic, short-term, human bone marrow cultures. dU enters deoxyuridine monophosphate (dUMP), which in the presence of: (1) N^5,N^{10}-methylene-THF, (2) methyl-cobalamin and (3) thymidylate synthase is converted to thymidine monophosphate (dTMP), and then to thymidine triphosphate (dTTP), to be converted in turn to thymine and incorporated in DNA. Later, tritiated thymidine ([^{3}H]thymidine) is added to the marrow. In normoblastic normal bone marrow, only a little of the [^{3}H]thymidine ($<10\%$) is then incorporated as radioactive thymine in DNA.

In vitamin B_{12} or folate deficiency less deoxyuridine is utilized, and more [^{3}H]thymidine is incorporated as radioactive thymine in DNA.

If the marrow is folate deficient, then folic acid, folinic acid (5-formyl-THF) and 5-methyl-THF will correct the dU suppression. Folinic acid also corrects marrows which are deficient in vitamin B_{12}, or deficient in both vitamin B_{12} and folate. Vitamin B_{12} only corrects dU suppression in vitamin B_{12} deficiency, but not in folate deficiency.

In patients treated with anticonvulsants a high dU suppression rate represents folate deficiency, and not interference with methylation of deoxyuridylate.

Following prolonged nitrous oxide anaesthesia (more than 5–6 h), the dU suppression test becomes abnormal, as nitrous oxide oxidizes active methylcob(I)alamin which acts normally as a cofactor with methionine synthase, to inactive methylcob(II)alamin and methylcob(III)alamin forms. In seriously ill patients, this effect occurs within 2 h exposure to nitrous oxide. This change to megaloblastic haemopoiesis can be prevented by giving 30 mg folinic acid intravenously every 5 h of nitrous oxide exposure.

Fifty per cent of kwashiorkor (protein–energy malnutrition) cases have abnormal dU suppression tests.

The suspected deficiency can be tested for by adding:

1. 1 μg 5-formyltetrahydrofolate ⎫
2. 50 μg hydroxycobalamin   ⎬ per ml of marrow culture
3. 100 μg thiamine hydrochloride ⎭

The deoxyuridine suppression test is not useful in simple folate or vitamin B_{12} deficiency, but is used in the investigation of rare enzyme deficiencies causing megaloblastic anaemia, and/or interference in folate or vitamin B_{12} metabolism.

References
Ganeshaguru, K. and Hoffbrand, A. V. (1978) *Br. J. Haematol.* **40**, 29
O'Sullivan, H., Jennings, F., Ward, K. *et al.* (1981) *Anaesthesiology* **55**, 645
Skacol, P. O., Chanarin, I., Hewlett, A. *et al.* (1982) *Anaesthesiology* **57**, 557
Wickramasinghe, S. N. (1981) *Clin. Lab. Haematol.* **3**, 1
Wickramasinghe, S. N., Akinyanju, O. O., Grange, A. *et al.* (1983) *Br. J. Haematol.* **53**, 135

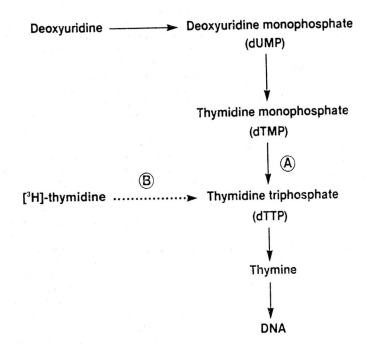

Deoxyuridine suppression test: in the presence of adequate vitamin B_{12}/folate. [^{3}H]thymidine does not form labelled thymine in DNA in short-term normoblast cultures. In vitamin B_{12}/folate deficiency [^{3}H]thymidine enters to form labelled thymine in DNA in short-term normoblast cultures.

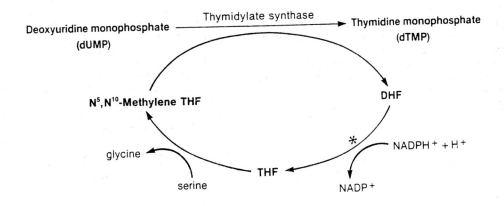

Folate metabolism and synthesis of thymidine (and hence DNA). * = site of inhibition by methotrexate.

The effects of vitamin B_{12} deficiency and/or folate deficiency

Each cell division requires a two-fold increase in nuclear DNA, as the chromosomes are duplicated. Following cell division, RNA synthesis also occurs to duplicate the amount of RNA present in the original cell, and now in two cells. Both vitamin B_{12} and folate are essential for DNA synthesis and RNA synthesis. Whilst folate deficiency results directly in a reduction in intracellular folate, especially in the active pentaglutamate forms, vitamin B_{12} also causes intracellular folate deficiency as a result of the 'folate trap'.

The 'folate trap'

Vitamin B_{12} is necessary for the conversion of folate monoglutamate, the form in which it is able to enter the cells, to pentaglutamate, the form in which the various folate forms are active in the cell. Lack of conversion of N^5-methyl-THF-monoglutamate to THF-pentaglutamate results in a deficiency of N^5,N^{10}-methylene-THF, which is essential for thymidine formation, impeding DNA synthesis. Conversion of THF to formyl-THF requires a 1-carbon unit from methionine, which is not being produced from homocysteine if vitamin B_{12} is deficient. Intracellular N^5,N^{10}-methylene-THF, N^5,N^{10}-methenyl—THF, N^{10}-formyl-THF and THF are all reduced in vitamin B_{12} deficiency, as well as in folate deficiency.

Megaloblastic changes in the bone marrow and peripheral blood

Protein synthesis is affected, with both plasma albumin and globulins falling, reflecting impaired RNA synthesis. Similarly, histone synthesis is impaired, and the very basic histones are responsible for the normal tight binding of the strongly acidic DNA strands. This probably explains the clumped and finely dispersed chromatin seen in the affected cell nuclei. The deficiency in DNA results in a long resting phase between each mitosis, and each mitosis takes longer than normal. The result is that many mitoses in various stages are visible in stained marrow films, suggesting an active marrow, but which is a picture of a queue of cells waiting for DNA. Large filamentous strands of DNA, delicately fenestrated chromatin and filamentous chromosomes are formed, giving the characteristic appearance of the megaloblastic nuclei.

Normal erythroblasts develop through stages recognized as:

$$E_1 \rightarrow E_2 \rightarrow E_3 \rightarrow E_4 \text{ (early polychromatic)}$$

doubling in number at each stage.

In pernicious anaemia there is failure to double from $E_1 \rightarrow E_3$, with intramedullary cell death. There is arrest of cell proliferation at all stages of interphase, with the polychromatic megaloblast being the largest site of ineffective erythropoiesis. The abnormality persists after treatment has started, and the reticulocytosis represents maturation of a new generation of erythroblasts or of the most immature basophilic erythroblasts.

Giant metamyeloctyes also die in the marrow (ineffective myelopoiesis).

The red cells formed in megaloblastic anaemia are abnormal and survive approximately 40 days (i.e. combination of haemolysis and decreased resistance to destruction). In severe megaloblastic anaemia the red cell membrane protein is abnormal, lacking bands 1, 2 and 3 on gel electrophoresis. The pattern is normal in mild megaloblastic or severe iron-deficiency anaemia. This destruction is reflected by extremely high serum lactate dehydrogenase levels without other evidence suggesting liver damage, the lactate dehydrogenase probably being derived from erythrocytes. Erythropoiesis is increased to about three times the normal rate, with increased excretion of coproporphyrin I in the urine.

The bone marrow appearances in vitamin B_{12} deficiency, folic acid deficiency or vitamin B_{12} plus folic acid deficiency are indistinguishable. In the peripheral blood, in folic acid deficiency, the macrocytosis is not so marked and both leucopenia and thrombocytopenia are inconstant, when compared with the findings in vitamin B_{12} deficiency. Thus in megaloblastic anaemia of pregnancy, the total white cell count may be normal or raised, the MCV may be normal with a normal MCH and a progressively falling haemoglobin level. In such cases it is a very useful and simple test to examine 'buffy layer' preparations of the peripheral blood, when nucleated red cells and some megaloblasts are found.

The more active the patient, the more likely are nucleated red cells and megaloblasts to be found in 'buffy layer' preparations of the peripheral blood of patients with megaloblastic anaemia.

Rapid estimation of red cell folate and serum vitamin B_{12}, earlier detection of deficiencies in vitamin B_{12} or folate are making the appearance of advanced megaloblastic anaemia uncommon. It is important to appreciate that pernicious anaemia manifests in Latin Americans and Blacks a decade earlier than in White US citizens. Vitamin B_{12} or folate deficiency cannot be predicted from the MCV.

References
Broin, S. D. O., Kelleher, B. P. McCann, S. R. *et al.* (1990) *Clin. Lab. Haematol.* **12**, 247
Carmel, R., Johnson, C. S. and Weiner, J. M. (1987) *Arch. Intern. Med.* **147**, 1995

Plasma enzymes

Isolated increase in lactate dehydrogenase suggests megaloblastic change in undiagnosed macrocytic anaemia. Serum alkaline phosphatese is reduced in cobalamin deficiency.

Reference
Carmel, R., Lau, K-H. W., Baylink, D. J. *et al.* (1988) *New Engl. J. Med.* **319**, 70

Nervous system damage

Whilst folate deficiency may be associated with increasing forgetfulness, irritability and slowing of mental processes, neuropathy is uncommon. Folate deficiency in patients treated with long-term anticonvulsants can be repaired simply and safely with daily oral yeast tablets.

In prolonged vitamin B_{12} deficiency, nervous system damage may be more severe, especially if folate is given. In addition to reversible peripheral neuropathy, irreversible subacute combined degeneration of the spinal cord may develop. The mechanisms for these changes are still a matter for debate, but the metabolic block at propionic acid in the metabolism of fatty acids with odd numbers of carbon atoms, and of valine and isoleucine, is suspected. The depleted synthesis of methionine from homocysteine may also be important, since a methylgroup from methionine is normally incorporated in the formation of choline, on which the synthesis of phospholipids and sphingomyelin depend. Phospholipids and sphingomyelin are essential components in the nerve sheath.

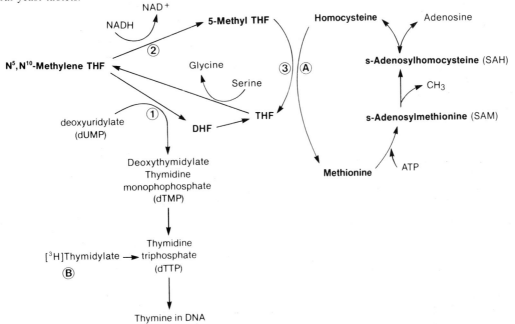

Interrelationships between vitamin B_{12} and folate metabolism, linking the active methyl cycle and thymine synthesis: ① thymidylate synthase; ② methylene-THF reductase; ③ methyl-THF: homocysteine methyltransferase; Ⓐ methylcobalamin; Ⓑ [³H]thymidine for dU suppression test.

Causes of megaloblastic anaemia

- Vitamin B_{12} deficiency
- Folate deficiency
- Vitamin B_{12} and folate defriciency

Causes other than vitamin B_{12} and/or folate deficiency

Inherited

- Sideroblastic anaemia (megaloblasts may be seen in the marrow).

- Orotic aciduria [R].
- Lesch–Nyhan disease [R].
- Thiamine-responsive megaloblastic anaemia [R].
- Congenital dyserythropoietic anaemia, type I.

Reference
Porter, F. S., Rogers, L. E. and Sidbury, J. B. (1969) *J. Pediatr.* **74**, 494

Acquired

1. Sideroblastic anaemia (megaloblasts may be seen

2. Erythroleukaemia
3. Drug action:
   (a) Pyrimidine inhibition: fluorodeoxyuridine – inhibits thymidylate synthetase; 6-azauridine – inhibits orotic carboxylase;
   (b) Purine inhibition: 6-mercaptopurine; thioguanine; azathioprine.
   (c) Ribonucleotide reductase inhibition: cytosine arabinoside; hydroxyurea; azarabine causes mild megaloblastic anaemia during treatment of psoriasis. Uridine corrects the anaemia but exacerbates the psoriasis.

Reference
Cornall, R. C. et al. (1976) Arch. Dermatol. **112**, 1717

4. Arsenic intoxication, with normal serum folate and vitamin B$_{12}$ levels.

Reference
Westhoff, D. D., Samaha, R. J. and Barnes, A. Jr. (1975) Blood **45**, 241

5. Megaloblastic anaemia with hepatocellular carcinoma, markedly increased TC-I and virtually absent TC-II.

Reference
Nexo, E., Olesen, H., Norredam, K. et al. (1975) Scand. J. Haematol. **14**, 320

6. 'Achrestic anaemia' found in the older literature is no longer a satisfactory diagnosis.

(Macrocytosis due to pernicious anaemia may be masked by the presence of α-thalassaemia in the same patient.)

Reference
Green, P., Kuhl, W., Jacobson, R. et al. (1982) N. Engl. J. Med. **307**, 1322

Megaloblastic anaemia in infants and children

Due to vitamin B$_{12}$ deficiency

First few months
• Congenital deficiency of plasma TC-II. Responds to pharmacological doses of vitamin B$_{12}$ which have to be given for life.
• Vitamin B$_{12}$ deficiency associated with maternal deficiency of vitamin B$_{12}$, although there is preferential transfer of vitamin B$_{12}$ from the mother to the fetus during pregnancy.

After 6 months
• Congenital deficiency of intrinsic factor.
• Congenital abnormality of intrinsic factor.
• Juvenile pernicious anaemia. 'Autoimmune' with antibodies present, but free gastric acid.

Reference
Maurer, H. S., Choi, H. S., Forman, E. N. et al. (1973) J. Pediatr. **83**, 832

• Selective malabsorption of vitamin B$_{12}$, and proteinuria (Imerslund–Gräsbeck syndrome). The defect is after IF–B$_{12}$ complex binds to ileal mucosal cells and before vitamin B$_{12}$ binds to TC-II.

Reference
Mackenzie, I. L., Donaldson, R. M. Jr., Trier, J. S. et al. (1972) N. Engl. J. Med. **286**, 1021

• Associated with ketosis: (1) methylmalonic aciduria, vitamin B$_{12}$ responsive; (2) methylmalonic aciduria associated with homocystinuria; (3) pernicious anaemia with polyendocrinopathy.

Due to folate deficiency

Premature infants

Congenital enzyme deficiencies
• Glutamate formiminotransferase deficiency.
• Methenyl-tetrahydrofolate cyclohydrolase deficiency.
• N^5-methyl-tetrahydrofolate transferase deficiency.

After 6 months

Malnutrition:
• Associated with kwashiorkor.
• Associated with scurvy.
• Goats' milk anaemia.
• Associated with special diets deficient in folic acid.
• Specific folate malabsorption.
• As in adults: anticonvulsant therapy; coeliac disease etc; chronic haemolytic states.

Reference
Chanarin, I. (1983) Br. J. Haematol. **53**, 1

Not due to vitamin B$_{12}$ or folate deficiency alone
• Orotic aciduria [R] – treat with uridine.
• Responding to thiamine.

Reference
Mandel, H., Berant, M., Hazani, A. et al. (1984) N. Engl. J. Med. **311**, 836

• Responding only to massive doses of both vitamin B$_{12}$ and folic acid.
• Lesch–Nyhan syndrome.

Vitamin B$_{12}$ deficiency in teenagers
• Congenital intrinsic factor deficiency [R].
• Abnormal intrinsic factor [R].
• Imerslund–Gräsbeck syndrome [R].
• Early expression of adult form of pernicious anaemia [R].

Low serum vitamin B_{12} levels in the absence of vitamin B_{12} deficiency

With clinical signs of deficiency

Folic acid deficiency.

Without clinical signs of deficiency

- Normal pregnancy (low levels in 14–28%).
- Patients taking the contraceptive pill.
- Transcobalamin I deficiency [R].
- 75% of strict vegetarians.
- No apparent cause (?unsuspected transcobalamin I deficiency).
- Technical problems.

Interfering agents in serum:

- Gallium–67 (^{67}Ga) in serum interfering with isotope assay.
- Antibiotics in serum interfering with microbiological assay.

Reference
Lindenbaum, J. (1983) *Blood* **61**, 624

Tissue vitamin B_{12} depletion in the absence of low serum vitamin B_{12} levels

- 10–20% of cobalamin deficiency.
- Nitrous oxide exposure.
- Transcobalamin II deficiency [R].
- Inborn errors of cobalamin metabolism. Check for methylmalonic aciduria [R].
- Cobalamin deficiency in chronic myeloid leukaemia.

Erythropoietin

Erythropoietin is a glycoprotein which is produced mainly in the kidney, but to a lesser extent in the liver, and by the macrophages. It is produced in response to anoxia and/or falling haemoglobin concentration, and its actions are thought to include:

- Stimulation of erythropoietin-sensitive marrow stem cells (CFU-E) to produce increased numbers of pronormoblasts.
- Increases the maturation rate, haemoglobin synthesis and release of red cells into the circulation.
- Commits the stem cell in the marrow to the erythroid line.

Reference
Rich, I. N., Heit, W. and Kubanek, B. (1982) *Blood* **60**, 1007

- In the steady state proerythroblasts derived from progenitors are only responsible for a small fraction of reticulocytes. After blood loss, progenitors, stimulated by erythropoietin burst-promoting activity, replicate rapidly and produce large numbers of proerythroblasts, resulting in a reticulocytosis.

Reference
Nathan, D. G. and Sytkowski, A. (1983) *N. Engl. J. Med.* **308**, 520

Serum erythropoietin assay is difficult, and discrepancies have been found between biological methods of assay which directly measure erythropoietin activity, and immunoreactive systems.

Reference
de Klerk, G., Vet, R. J. W. M., Rosengarten, P. C. J. *et al.* (1980) *Blood* **55**, 955

Physiological increase

- Normal pregnancy.
- High altitude acclimatization. The haemoglobin increases by +1 g/dl per 3–4% decrease in arterial oxygen concentration.

Pathological increase

Compensatory

1. Acute blood loss. Immunoreactive erythropoietin increases when 75 ml of blood are lost rapidly.

Reference
Miller, M. E., Cronkite, E. P. and Garcia, J. F. (1982) *Br. J. Haematol.* **522**, 545

2. Anaemia:
   (a) haemolysis;
   (b) iron-deficiency anaemia;
   (c) megaloblastic anaemia;
   (d) some cases of aplastic anaemia.
3. Cardiovascular shunt, e.g. congenital cardiac anomaly.
4. Chronic pulmonary disease.
5. Low red cell 2,3-DPG with increased affinity of haemoglobin for oxygen:
   (a) hexokinase deficiency [R];
   (b) diphosphoglycerate mutase deficiency [R].
6. High oxygen-affinity haemoglobinopathies.
7. Drugs:
   (a) androgens;
   (b) cobalt.

Inappropriate

1. Tumours (producing erythropoietin or erythropoietin-like substances);
   (a) renal carcinoma;
   (b) cerebellar haemangioblastoma;
   (c) hepatoma;
   (d) ovarian carcinoma;
   (e) adrenocortical adenoma;
   (f) uterine fibroma (uncommon).
2. Renal disease:
   (a) hydronephrosis;
   (b) renal cyst;
   (c) renal transplant.

3. Familial inappropriate secretion of erythropoietin [R] [AD].

Reference
Distelhorst, C. W., Wagner, D. S., Goldwasser, E. *et al.* (1981) *Blood* **58**, 1155

Normal or low serum erythropoietin

- Polycythaemia vera. There is evidence that some erythroid progenitors are excessively sensitive to erythropoietin in the presence of serum.

Reference
Casadevall, N., Vainchenke W., Lacombe, C. *et al.* (1982) *Blood* **59**, 447

- Progressive renal damage. Anaemia in uraemia.
- Refractory anaemia of chronic disease.
- Starvation anaemia.
- Haemoconcentration.

Erythropoiesis inhibiting factor

An erythropoiesis inhibiting factor appears in the plasma after over-transfusion, and also in renal failure. It is probably synthesized in the kidney.

Reference
Moriyama, Y. and Shimotori, T. (1970) *Acta. Haematol.* **44**, 321

Refractory normoblastic anaemia

1. Aplastic or hypoplastic anaemia.
2. Megaloblastic anaemia, other than true pernicious anaemia. Megaloblastic anaemia of pregnancy may present with a peripheral blood picture of normoblastic anaemia.
3. Thalassaemia.
4. In relation to leukaemia:
   (a) aleukaemic phase of leukaemia;
   (b) leukaemia superimposed on pre-existing anaemia;
   (c) 'preleukaemic phase' of leukaemia;
   (d) di Guglielmo's disease (erythraemic myelosis).
5. Pyridoxine deficiency [R].
6. Anaemia of infection.
7. Anaemia following burns.
8. Rheumatoid arthritis and other collagen disorders.
9. Refractory anaemia with dysproteinaemia in elderly.
10. Anaemia in uraemia:
    (a) dilutional anaemia;
    (b) red cell life reduced;
    (c) red cell iron utilization reduced;

(d) decreased response to erythropoietin;
(e) loss from bleeding;
(f) disordered red cell production.

References
Douglas, S. W. and Adamson, J. W. (1975) *Blood* **45**, 55
Hume, R., Dagg, J. H. and Goldberg, A. (1973) *Blood* **41**, 27
Lee, G. R. (1983) *Semin. Haematol.* **20**, 61
Samson, D. (1983) *Postgrad. Med. J.* **59**, 543 (review)
Samson, D., Halliday, D. and Gumpel, J. M. (1977) *Ann. Rheum. Dis.* **36**, 181

Sideroblastic anaemia

This is a refractory dyserythropoietic anaemia with an excesss of iron and with abnormal 'ring' sideroblasts present in the bone marrow. These abnormal sideroblasts have iron deposited in a perinuclear ring, aggregating in the mitochondria.

Primary

1. Hereditary sex-linked sideroblastic anaemia

This X-linked, partly recessive condition is found mainly in males, with its onset in childhood or adolescence. Females are usually only mildly affected. The peripheral blood count reveals a hypochromic microcytic picture (low MCV and MCH) with a few circulating siderocytes and nucleated red cells. Serum iron is increased with normal TIBC levels. Iron clearance and utilization are reduced. The bone marrow shows erythroid hyperactivity. Some cases respond to long-term pyridoxine therapy, while others are refractory.

2. Primary acquired sideroblastic anaemia

This condition presents in middle-aged and elderly males and females. The peripheral blood count reveals macrocytosis with increased MCV and MCH, with a dimorphic appearance in the blood films (a few hypochromic microcytic cells are present). Megaloblastic changes are found in up to 20% associated with folate deficiency. The condition is heterogeneous, with some cases responding to pyridoxine and others refractory. Ferrochetolase activity has been found to be reduced in some cases and δ-aminolaevulinic acid synthase activity reduced in others. Some other cases have coproporphyrinogen oxidase deficiency, whilst no deficiency has been defined in many other cases.

References
Bottomly, S. S. (1982) *Clin Haematol.* **11**, 389–409
Buchanan, G. R., Bottomley, S. S. and Nitschke, R. (1980) *Blood* **55**, 109

Secondary

1. Antituberculous treatment may cause sideroblastic anaemia:

(a) isoniazid (interfering with pyridoxine metabolism);

(b) pyrazinamide;

(c) cycloserine (now out of date as therapy for tuberculosis);

(d) Ethionamide.

2. Chloramphenicol.

3. Lead poisoning: lead causes spatial alteration in the red cell membrane proteins, leading to crenation and marked selective loss of potassium. Red cell pyrimidine-5'-nucleotidase activity is reduced, and this probably has the effect of leading to punctate basophilia. Red cell survival is decreased. Haem synthesis is interfered with, and it is at this point probably that 'ring' sideroblasts result. In addition, globin synthesis is depressed.

4. Alcohol: red cell and serum pyridoxine levels are reduced. Response to pyridoxal phosphate is more than to pyridoxine.

5. Sideroblastic anaemia rarely occurs during chemotherapy of myeloma, and Hodgkin's disease.

Pyridoxine metabolism

Pyridoxine (present in fruit, vegetables and cereals), and pyridoxamine and pyridoxal (present in meats) are essential substances. Pyridoxine is converted by pyridoxine kinase to pyridoxine phosphate, in turn converted by an oxidase to pyridoxal phosphate. Pyridoxal phosphatase converts pyridoxal phosphate to active pyridoxal.

Pyridoxal is involved in decarboxylation, deamination, transamination, transulphuration and desulphuration, acting as an essential cofactor to various enzymes. The daily requirement is normally 0.5–2.0 mg of pyridoxine. Pharmacological doses are required in pyridoxine dependency (i.e. large amounts of the vitamin enable abnormally structured enzymes to function, as in some forms of sideroblastic anaemia). It is important to remember that large doses of pyridoxine may be toxic.

There may be an increased number of siderocytic granules in the nucleated red cells in the marrow, with an increase in the size of the granules. The number of granules is usually less than 6 per cell, and the granules show no particular relationship with the nucleus. There appears to be a direct relationship between the number and size of the iron-staining granules and the degree of saturation of the serum iron-binding capacity:

- Haemolytic anaemia.
- Megaloblastic anaemia.
- Thalassaemia.

- Myeloproliferative disorders, including leukaemia.
- Aplastic anaemia.
- Haemochromatosis.

See Sideroblasts, p. 12.

Dyserythropoietic anaemia (ineffective erythropoiesis)

Anaemia with low reticulocyte counts associated with a cellular bone marrow (increased erythroid cells), increased excretion of pre-haemoglobin, stercobilinogen-like substances and resistance to treatment in some conditions.

- Iron-deficiency anaemia: if a small dose of iron is given, urine iron excretion following desferrioxamine is markedly reduced. Full iron therapy is effective.
- Megaloblastic anaemia: there is full response to treatment with the appropriate substance in vitamin B_{12} deficiency or folate deficiency.
- Thalassaemia.
- Sideroblastic anaemia: some cases respond to treatment with pyridoxine.
- Refractory normoblastic anaemia.
- Congenital erythropoietic porphyria.
- Congenital erythropoietic protoporphyria.
- Congenital dyserythropoietic anaemia.

Congenital dyserythropoietic anaemia

1. Type I [AR] [R]

Whilst hererozygotes are not detectable, homozygotes may be diagnosed by chance from a routine blood count, or because of symptoms of anaemia or iron overload. They suffer from jaundice, hepatomegaly and splenomegaly. There is a defect in DNA synthesis affecting development of basophilic erythroblasts into polychromatic erythroblasts. The erythroblasts appear megaloblastoid with internuclear bridging with bundles of microtubules. Apart from the persistence of microtubules in the cytoplasm, cytoplasmic maturation appears to be normal. Cytoplasmic organelles are found in the nuclear area on electron microscopy.

2. Type II [AR] [R]

These patients also suffer from jundice, hepatomegaly, splenomegaly and iron overload with cirrhosis and diabetes. Hereditary erythroblastic multinuclearity associated with a positive acidified serum test (HEMPAS) is the most frequently found variety, and occurs more often in north-west Europe, Italy and north Africa. The red cells are deficient in sialic acid, an essential component of the red cell membrane. Multinucleate erythroblasts are found in the marrow, with a defect in maturation of polychromatic erythroblasts into orthochromic erythroblasts. The red cells are lysed by normal acidified sera which contain IgM anti-HEMPAS antibody (30% of normal people). The patient's acidified serum does not lyse the red cells, and the cane sugar-lysis test is negative (compare paroxysmal nocturnal haemoglobinuria).

3. Type III [AD] [R]

This rarest variety presents with a macrocytic anaemia, increased urine urobilinogen, raised serum bilirubin and multinucleate erythroblasts with some gigantoblasts in the marrow. In all vertebrate cells, except during periods of DNA synthesis or in malignant tissue, DNA content per diploid set is constant. In this condition, there is great deviation in the DNA content of erythroblast nuclei. The red cells are haemolysed by anti-I and anti-i sera, but not by acidified sera.

4. A variant resembling type III

This has been described with a membrane transfer defect of 5-methyl-THF.

References
Bethlenfalavy, N. C., Hadnagy, G. and Heimpel, H. (1985) Br. J. Haematol. 60,541
Howe, R. B., Branda, R. F., Douglas, S. D. et al. (1979) Blood 54, 1080
Valentine, W. N., Crookston, J. H., Paglia, D. E. et al. (1972) Br. J. Haematol. 23,107
Verwillghen, R. L., Lewis, S. M., Dacie, J. V. et al. (1973) Q. J. Med. 42, 257

Anaemia in infancy

Normally erythropoiesis continues in the newborn infant for the first 3 days after birth. Then erythropoiesis ceases until the haemoglobin level has fallen to 11–12 g/dl, i.e. falling about 1% per day for 6–8 weeks. Red cell regeneration restarts to maintain the infant haemoglobin level at 11–12 g/dl for 18 months.

At the moment of birth the average infant contains about 370 ml of blood, and the placenta and cord contain a further 100 ml. During the first year of life, when the body weight increases by about 7 kg, 245 mg of iron are required for this growth.

Anaemia of prematurity

Excessive postnatal fall

The haemoglobin level may fall to 8 g/dl before erythropoiesis is restarted.

Iron deficiency

Marrow-stainable iron disappears in infants of less than 1400 g within 6–8 weeks of birth, whereas marrow-stainable iron disappears in infants of more than 1400 g within 8–12 weeks of birth. The iron

required per kg of growth, when the haemoglobin level is 11 g/dl, is 35 mg. Thus an underweight pre-term infant requires iron more rapidly than does a normal infant.

Reference
Gaisford, W. and Jennison, R. F. (1955) Br. Med. J. 2, 700

In the presence of iron stores, the rate of release of iron from these stores in low-birth-weight infants may not be rapid enough to maintain optimal erythropoiesis. Both free red cell protoporphyrin and serum ferritin are raised at the same time.

Reference
Faldella, G., Alessandroni, R., Salvioli, G. P. et al. (1983) Arch. Dis. Child. 58, 216

Blood counts in extremely low-birth-weight infants

Reference
McIntosh, N., Kempson, C. and Tyler, R. M. (1988) Arch. Dis. Child. 63, 74

Haemolytic anaemia

Haemolytic disease due to maternal immunization

Ninty per cent due to anti-D; also due to: anti-C, anti-E, anti-Kell, anti-Duffy.
Severe ABO-haemolytic disease is uncommon.

Reference
Desjardins, L., Blajchman, M. A., Chintu, C. et al. (1979) J. Pediatr. 95, 447

Hereditary spherocytosis

Only rarely presenting in the first few days of life, it mimics haemolytic disease due to ABO incompatibility immunization. Spherocytes and increased red cell osmotic fragility occur in both.

Toxic agents

- Naphthalene (from napkins stored in mothballs).
- Resorcin (in ointments and lotions).
- Excess vitamin K analogues (e.g. Synkavit).

Fetal blood loss

Bleeding into the maternal circulation

This can be detected when the maternal blood contains more than 2% fetal haemoglobin.

Bleeding from one twin to another

This can occur but is very rare.

Placental bleeding or bleeding from umbilical vessels

- Premature separation of the placenta.
- Abnormal siting of the placenta, e.g. placenta praevia.
- Abnormal arrangement of umbilical vessels, e.g. velamentous insertion, especially if associated with placenta praevia.

- Damage to the placenta during surgical induction of labour.
- Damage to the placenta at caesarean section (the placenta may be cut during the uterine incisions).

Note: It is important to test blood samples from antepartum haemorrhage for the presence of fetal haemoglobin.

Reference
Mitchell, A. P. B., Anderson, G. S. and Russell, J. K. (1957) *Br. Med. J.* **1**, 611 (rapid method for detecting fetal haemoglobin)

Congenital hypoplastic anaemia

Anaemia develops in early infancy. There appears to be a maturation arrest at the late normoblast stage, and it has been suggested that the condition is due to an inborn error of metabolism. Steroid therapy has been effective in some cases.

Reference
Reinhold, J. D. L., Neumark, E., Lightwood, R. *et al.* (1952) *Blood* **7**, 915

Copper deficiency

- Cows' milk contains little copper. A pure milk diet may lead to copper deficiency. Both copper and iron should be given for successful treatment.

Reference
Williams, D. M. (1983) *Semin. Haematol.* **20**, 118

- Nephrosis: copper is lost with protein in the urine.
- Sprue syndrome: copper is not absorbed properly from the diet.

Megaloblastic anaemia

Milk contains very little folic acid and, therefore, on a strictly milk diet folic acid deficiency may develop. Goats' milk contains little folic acid and very little vitamin B_{12}. Megaloblastic anaemia due to these causes must be rare, because a variety of different foodstuffs is added to the normal infant's diet at an early age.

When megaloblastic anaemia does occur, it appears at the seventh to eighth month, and is associated with increased urine excretion of formiminoglutamic acid. On recovery, following treatment with folic acid, the formiminoglutamic acid disappears from the urine.

Haemolytic anaemia

The maintenance of normal erythrocyte integrity depends on:

- Normal red cell membrane structure.
- Cell membrane sodium pump activity which keeps the intracellular sodium concentration low and the potassium concentration high relative to the surrounding plasma, with its high sodium and low potassium concentrations.

- Normal intracellular glycolysis leading to adequate synthesis of NADH, NADPH and ATP.
- Maintenance of adequate reduced glutathione at the cell surface to combat the action of anti-oxidants. This involves both the synthesis of glutathione and maintenance of reduced glutathione.
- Absence of unstable haemoglobins.
- Synthesis of normal fetal and, later, adult haemoglobins.

Red cell defects

1. MEMBRANE DEFECTS

- Paroxysmal nocturnal haemoglobinuria (PNH)

An acquired stem cell disorder results in production of red cells without the necessary molecular anchors to attack molecules which regulate activation of complement, important molecules involved in resistance to infection, and enzymes erythrocyte cholinesterase, 5'-ecto nucleotidase and leucocyte alkaline phosphatase. The PNH red cells are abnormally sensitive to haemolysis in the presence of complement at reduced pH (i.e. during sleep). Platelets and granulocytes also have similar membrane abnormalities.

The majority of patients are adult. Sudden exacerbations of haemolysis may occur, with bone marrow failure in some patients, especially in children and adolescents, an increased liability to bacterial infections and an increased tendency to develop venous thrombosis.

References
Rosse, W. F. and Parker, C. J. (1985) In: Schrier, S. L. Ed. *Clinics in Haematology,* Vol. 14, p. 105. London. W. B. Saunders
Rotoli B. and Luzzatto L. (1989) In: Gordon-Smith, E. G., Ed. *Ballière's Clinical Haematology,* Vol. 2, No. 1, p. 113. London. Baillière Tindall
Ware, R. E., Hall, Sharon and Rosse, W. F. (1991) *New Engl. J. Med.* **325**, 991

Abnormal accumulation of phosphatidyl choline in the red cell membrane [R]

Haemolytic anaemia occurs in this very rare condition, as a result of abnormal accumulation of phosphatidyl choline in the red cell envelope, due to defective catabolism of phosphatidyl choline, with excess cation permeability and excess diversion of glycolytic energy to sodium pump.

References
Shohet, S. B., Livermore, B. M., Nathan, D. G. *et al.* (1971) *Blood* **38**, 445
Shohet, S. B., Nathan, D. G., Livermore, B. M. *et al.* (1973) *Blood* **42**, 1

- Vitamin E deficiency anaemia [R]

Rarely normal newborn infants, and especially preterm male infants, have developed haemolytic anaemia

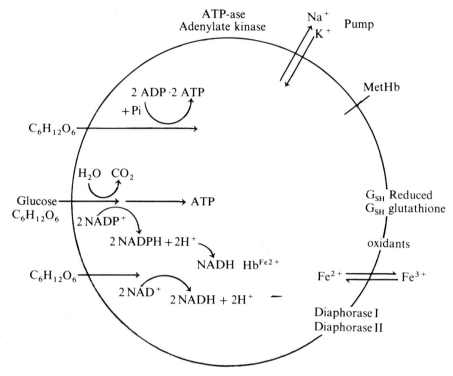

a. Hb in solution in cell. Fe^{2+} easily oxidized. System for continuous reduction.
b. Osmotic control.—Sodium pump. ATP-ase, etc. (N.B. Complement holes.)
c. Intact lipoprotein membrane—reduced glutathione.

following feeding with an artificial milk formula deficient in vitamin E. The red cell membrane is damaged by faulty repair with saturated fatty acids in place of unsaturated fatty acids and in phospholipid, with increased haemolysis and reticulocytosis. There is rapid recovery to normal following treatment with vitamin E.

● 'Spur cell' anaemia

Acquired haemolytic anaemia occurs in severe liver disease (usually alcoholic) due to changes in red cell membrane cholesterol/phospholipid ratio.

References
Cooper R. A. (1969) *J. Clin. Invest.* **48**, 1820
Cooper, R. A., Arner, E. C., Wiley, J. S. *et al.* (1975) *J. Clin. Invest.* **55**, 115

● Red cell sialic acid deficiency and reduced red cell life [R]

Case described with abnormally reduced red cell life, with polyagglutinability of red cells, leucocytes and platelets due to red cell membrane sialic acid deficiency.

Sialic acid present in red cell surface is essential to the survival of red cells in the circulation. With increasing age sialic acid is lost (mechanism unknown) and the red cells can then be coated with immunoglobulin IgG and then phagocytosed.

References
Durocher, J. R., Payne, R. C. and Conrad, M. E. (1975) *Blood* **45**, 11
Lalezari, P. and Al-Mondhiry, H. (1973) *Br. J. Haematol.* **25**, 399

2. DEFECT IN CELL MEMBRANE SODIUM PUMP

Haemolytic anaemia due to leaking red cells in a heterogeneous group.

References
Lande, W. M. and Mentzer, W. C. (1985) In: Schrier, S. L. Ed. *Clinics in Haematology*, Vol. 14, p. 89. London: W. B. Saunders
Oski, F., Naiman, J. L., Blum, S. F. *et al.* (1969) *N. Engl. J. Med.* **280**, 909

Associated with abnormal red cell shape

- Spherocytosis – see p. 11.
- Elliptocytosis [R] – see p. 11.
- Pyropoikilocytosis, congenital haemolytic anaemia with marked poikilocytosis and microspherocytosis [R] – see p. 10.
- Stomatocytosis [R] [AD] – see p. 12.

Associated with normal red cell shape

- Hereditary erythrocyte adenylate kinase deficiency [R]

A rare congenital non-spherocytic haemolytic anaemia results from this deficiency.

$$2ADP \rightleftharpoons AMP + ATP$$

References
Boivin, P., Galand, C., Hakim, J. *et al.* (1971) *Presse méd.* **79**, 215
Szeinberg, A., Kahana, D., Gavendo, S. *et al.* (1963) *Acta Haematol.* **42**, 111

- Adenosine triphosphatase deficiency [R]

$$ATP \rightarrow ADP + P_i$$

One form of adenosine triphosphatase present in red cells requires the presence of magnesium ions. A second form of adenosine triphosphatase present in red cells requires the presence of magnesium, sodium and potassium ions, and deficiency of this enzyme is associated with haemolytic anaemia.

References
Hanel, K. H. and Cohn, J. (1972) *Scand. J. Haematol.* **9**, 28
Harvald, B., Hanel, K. H., Squires, R. *et al.* (1964) *Lancet* **ii**, 18

- Red cell adenosine triphosphate deficiency with normal adenylate kinase and normal adenosine triphosphatase [R]

A non-spherocytic haemolytic anaemia associated with abnormally low red cell ATP concentration, apparently due to increased ATP catabolism with normal red cell adenosine triphosphatase and adenylate kinase activities has been described.

Reference
Mills, G. C., Levin, W. C. and Alperin, J. B. (1968) *Blood* **32**, 15

- Non-spherocytic haemolytic anaemia due to ribose phosphate pyrophosphokinase deficiency [R]

$$Ribose-5-phosphate + ATP \rightarrow AMP$$
$$+ 5\text{-Phosphoribosyl-l-pyrophosphate}$$

Anaemia is associated with erythrocyte stippling, increased reduced glutathione, and increased total ADP plus ATP in the red cells.

Reference
Valentine, W. N., Bennett, J. M., Krivit, W. *et al.* (1973) *Br. J. Haematol.* **24**, 157

3. DEFECTS IN GLYCOLYSIS IN ERYTHROCYTES DUE TO SPECIFIC ENZYME DEFICIENCIES, ASSOCIATED WITH HAEMOLYTIC ANAEMIA

Beutler reviews the red cell enzyme deficiencies and concludes that:

- Glucose-6-phosphate dehydrogenase deficiency is the most common of these conditions (affecting millions of people).
- Pyruvate kinase deficiency is the next most common deficiency, but unless great care is taken in the laboratory, cases can be missed.
- The next most frequently found (but uncommon) deficiencies are those of glucose isomerase and of 5′-nucleotidase deficiencies.
- A number of patients suffered from chronic haemolytic anaemia for which no cause was yet discovered.

Reference
Beutler, E. (1979) *Blood* **54**, 1

- Glucose-6-phosphate dehydrogenase (G6PDH) deficiency

It is thought that approximately 100 000 000 people have some form of G6PDH deficiency. On electrophoresis it has been found that the enzyme exists in a fast-moving form, Gd^A, and a slower-moving form, Gd^B. In Caucasians the enzyme is present only in the Gd^B form, and inheritance of the enzyme is sex linked to the X chromosome.

AFRICAN NEGROES

From 7% to 15% of the population have a third defective form of the enzyme, Gd^{A-}. In malarial areas it appears that low parasite counts are found in Negro males of the type Gd^A, whereas low parasite counts are found in Negro females of the type Gd^B/Gd^{A-}. If low parasite counts represent protection from the effects of malarial infection, then in the absence of elimination of malaria a polymorphic population containing Gd^A, Gd^B and Gd^{A-} would be maintained.

Affected Negro males (Gd^{A-}) remain symptom free until exposed to severe infections, diabetic ketosis or oxidant drugs capable of catalysing degradative oxidation of haemoglobin and oxidation of reduced glutathione in the red cell membrane (e.g. primaquine, sulphonamides, sulphones, nitrofurantoin etc.).

MEDITERRANEAN PEOPLES

Sardinians, Greeks and Sephardic Jews develop haemolytic anaemia when exposed to oxidant drugs, and chloramphenicol, and to fava beans (favism). This form of enzyme deficiency can be associated with neonatal haemolytic anaemia in an affected infant. Broad beans contain divicine and isoramil and these, in their oxidized forms, readily deplete reduced glutathione in the red cells of G6PDH-deficient individuals. During fava bean haemolysis, the red cell calcium increases ten-fold.

Untreated G6PDH-deficient red cells and normal red cells support in vitro growth of *Plasmodium falciparum*. Pre-treatment of G6PDH-deficient red cells with isouracil (a fava bean extract) results in their inability to support *P. falciparum* growth. This does not happen with normal red cells when they are pre-treated with the extract.

References
Clark, I. A., Cowden, W. B., Hunt, N. H. *et al.* (1984) *Br. J. Haematol.* **57**, 479
Golenser, J., Miller, J., Spira, D. T. *et al.* (1983) *Blood* **61**, 507
Roth, E. F. Jr, Schulman, S., Vandenberg, J., Olson, J. and Golenser *et al.* (1986) *Blood*, **67**, 827
Turrini, F., Naitana, A., Mannuzzi, L. *et al.* (1985) *Blood* **68**, 302

MILDER VARIETY

A milder variety is found in some Italians and Greeks, with a few cases occurring in Austria. Enzyme activity in male hemizygote found to be 25–75% of normal.

CANTON VARIETY

This form has a clinical severity midway between the Mediterranean and Negro varieties, with favism and occurrence of haemolytic attacks in the newborn.

NORTH EUROPEANS

Very low red cell G6PDH activity in red cells is associated with severe non-spherocytic haemolytic anaemia in this uncommon form.

JAPANESE VARIETY

References
Nakai, T. and Yoshida, A. (1974) *Clin. Chim. Acta.* **51**, 199
Yoshida, A., Bautler, E. and Motulsky, A. G. (1971) *Bull. WHO* **45**, 243

NORMAL NEWBORN INFANT

Especially if early for dates the normal newborn has a low red cell G6PDH activity, and following exposure to oxidant drugs, such as vitamin K analogues, or chemicals, such as naphthalene, can develop non-immune haemolytic anaemia.

• Pyruvate kinase deficiency

The majority of cases of 'type II' non-spherocytic haemolytic anaemia were probably caused by this deficiency. The defective enzyme is inherited by means of a recessive character, and the homozygote is severely anaemic. Variants of the abnormal enzyme have been found by electrophoresis, with different activities, which probably explains the absence of correlation between *in vitro* enzyme activity and the clinical severity. Red cell 3-phosphoglycerate is markedly increased in pyruvate kinase deficiency, and this is much easier to estimate than pyruvate kinase activity, since pyruvate kinase estimation can be interfered with by a reticulocytosis. In this condition,

some red cells may be irregularly contracted, resembling acanthocytes. The red cells have an abnormally low ATP concentration, and a raised concentration of 2,3-diphosphoglycerate, and the consequent 'shift to the right' of the haemoglobin oxygen-dissociation curve results in as much oxygen being available to the tissues from 9 g of haemoglobin/100 ml of blood as is available from normal non-anaemic blood. Therefore blood transfusion is not indicated unless very severe anaemia develops. There is clinical improvement following splenectomy, with increased reticulocytosis up to 50%, with siderocytes and Peppenheimer bodies.

References
Lestas, A. N., Kay, L. A. and Bellingham, A. J. (1987) *Br. J. Haematol.* **67**, 485
Miwa, S., Nakashima, K., Ariyoshi, K. *et al.* (1975) *Br. J. Haematol.* **29**, 157
Staal, G. E. J., Rijksen, G., Vlug, A. M. *et al.* (1982) *Clin. Chim. Acta* **118**, 241

• Hexokinase deficiency [R]

Cases suffer from moderate anaemia, with reticulocytosis, low cell 2,3-diphosphoglycerate concentrations with consequent 'shift to the left' of the haemoglobin oxygen-dissociation curve. There is clinical improvement following splenectomy. It has been found by electrophoresis of red cell hexokinase in agarose that there are two major (1 and 2) bands, and two minor (3 and 4) bands, and absence of bands 2, 3 and 4 results in haemolysis with low enzyme activity and reduced red cell glycolysis.

Reference
Altay, C., Alper, C. A. and Nathan, D. G. (1970) *Blood* **36**, 219

• Phosphohexose isomerase deficiency [R]

In addition to haemolytic anaemia, progressive neurological degeneration may occur. Following splenectomy, haemoglobin levels increase.

• Phosphofructokinase deficiency [R]

Electrophoresis of the enzyme suggests that there are two distinct isoenzymes in the red cell. Deficiency of one isoenzyme is associated with muscle disease (i.e. the same enzyme is deficient in muscle in glycogen storage disease type VII), whilst deficiency of the other isoenzyme in red cells is associated with haemolytic anaemia alone. The haemolytic anaemia results in splenomegaly with attacks of jaundice.

Clinical varieties include:

• Profound muscle enzyme deficiency with mild red cell enzyme deficiency.
• No muscle enzyme deficiency: moderate red cell enzyme deficiency.
• No muscle enzyme deficiency: severe red cell enzyme deficiency.

Reference
Miwa, S., Sato, T., Murao H. *et al.* (1972) *Acta Haematol. Jap.* **35**, 113

● Triose-phosphate isomerase deficiency [R]

This rare condition occurs as a compensated haemolytic anaemia associated with severe neurological disease in children. The enzyme deficiency occurs in many tissues, including red cells, white blood cells, cerebrospinal fluid and muscle. Red cells show anisocytosis and poikilocytosis with occasional irregular contracted red cells resembling acanthocytes.

● Glyceraldehyde-3-phosphate dehydrogenase deficiency [R]

This rare condition occurs as a well-compensated haemolytic anaemia.

● 2,3-Diphosphoglycerate mutase deficiency [R]

In this rare autosomal recessive condition the urine is found to contain mesobilifuchsin.

● Phosphoglycerate kinase deficiency [R]

No cation transport studies across the red cell membrane have been reported yet, even though the enzyme is sited in the red cell membrane; when the enzyme is sited in the red cell membrane and when the enzyme is defective, there is gross impairment of ATP generation.

● 2,3-Diphosphoglycerate phosphatase deficiency [R]

A rare non-spherocytic haemolytic anaemia.

● Enolase deficiency [R]

Chronic haemolytic anaemia exacerbated by ingestion of nitrofurantoin, associated with red cell deficiency, has been reported.

Reference
Stefanini, M. (1972) *Am. J. Clin. Pathol.* **58**, 408

● 6-Phosphogluconate dehydrogenase deficiency [R]

Patients suffering from this deficiency may suffer exacerbations of haemolysis if exposed to primaquine.

● Aldolase deficiency [R]

One case has been described [AR] in a moderately mentally handicapped patient with increased liver glycogen and mild chronic non-spherocytic haemolytic anaemia.

Reference
Beutler, E., Scott, S., Bishop, A. *et al.* (1974) *Trans. Assoc. Am. Physicians* **86**, 154

● Acquired defect in glycolysis associated with haemolysis

Gross hypophosphataemia with hypomagnesaemia, interfering with red cell glycolysis, has been described, associated with haemolysis.

Reference
Jacob, H. S. and Amsden, T. (1971) *N. Engl. J. Med.* **285**, 1446

4. HAEMOLYTIC ANAEMIA ASSOCIATED WITH DEFECTS IN THE MAINTENANCE OF REDUCED GLUTATHIONE IN THE RED CELL MEMBRANE

● γ-Glutamyl-cysteine synthase deficiency [R]

$$\text{Glutamic acid} + \text{Cysteine} \xrightarrow{+\text{ATP}}$$
$$\text{Glutamyl-cysteine (GC)}$$

Well-compensated, life-long haemolytic anaemia due to this deficiency in homozygotes has been described, with detection of clinically unaffected heterozygotes.

Reference
Konrad, P. N., Richards, F. II., Valentine, W. N. *et al.* (1972) *N. Engl. J. Med.* **286**, 557

● Glutathione synthase deficiency [R]

$$\gamma\text{-Glutamyl-cysteine} + \text{Glycine} \xrightarrow{+\text{ATP}} \text{Glutathione}$$

In this autosomal recessive condition, red cell glutathione concentration is reduced in the presence of a well-compensated haemolytic anaemia, aggravated by primaquine (and possibly fava bean).

Reference
Boivin, P., Galand, C., André R. *et al.* (1966) *Nouv. Rev. Fr. Hematol.* **6**, 859

● Glutathione reductase deficiency [R]

$$\text{Glutathione (GS-SG)} + \text{NADPH} \rightarrow$$
$$\text{Reduced glutathione (GSH)} + \text{NADP.}$$

Deficiency of this riboflavin-dependent enzyme with haemolytic anaemia is inherited by a dominant autosomal character. When enzyme activity is below 40–50% of normal, the red cells are susceptible to haemolysis following exposure to oxidant drugs. Thrombocytopenia has also been described in some cases, and the enzyme deficiency has been found in red cells, white blood cells and platelets. In addition, it appears that the nervous system may be affected, since some cases suffer from spasticity, and an oligo-phrenic family has been described.

Reference
Waller, H. D., Lohr, G. W., Zysno, E. *et al.* (1965) *Klin. Wochenschr.* **43**, 413

● Glutathione peroxidase deficiency [R]

Acute haemolytic attacks may develop in homozygotes in this autosomal recessive condition, following exposure to oxidant drugs, such as sulphonamides and nitrofurantoin.

Reference
Necheles, T. F., Steinberg, M. H. and Cameron, D. (1970) *Br. J. Haematol.* **19**, 605

- Glutathione deficiency [R]

In this autosomal recessive condition, increased haemolysis follows exposure to fava beans and to primaquine. Red cell glyoxalase activity is markedly reduced, and reduced glutathione is an essential cofactor for this enzyme.

Reference
Prins, H. K., Oort, M., Loos, J. A. *et al.* (1966) *Blood* **27**, 145

- Erythrocyte pyrimidine-5-nucleotidase deficiency [R]

This chronic, non-spherocytic, haemolytic anaemia with moderate splenomegaly is characterized by marked basophilic stippling of the red cells, due to accumulation of abnormal forms of RNA. In the normal reticulocyte the ribosome is degraded and RNA is converted to 5-pyrimidine nucleotide, which is broken down further by pyrimidine-5-nucleotidase. Normal enzyme activity in reticulocytes = 1755 mU/g Hb, and in adult red cells = 50 mU/g Hb. In this deficiency state the red cells contain only 6 mU/g Hb. There is decreased pentose shunt activity, and therefore increased susceptibility to Heinz body formation and the Heinz body provocation test is positive.

References
Tomoda, A., Noble, N. A., Lachant, N. A. *et al.* (1982) *Blood* **60**, 1212
Torrance, J. D., Whittaker, D. and Jenkins, T. (1980) *Br. J. Haematol.* **45**, 585
Valentine, W. N., Fink, K., Paglia, D. E. *et al.* (1974) *J. Clin. Invest.* **54**, 866

Identification of the enzyme deficiency causing haemolytic anaemia

Although these conditions are rare (apart from glucose-6-phosphate dehydrogenase deficiency, pyruvate kinase deficiency and acholuric jaundice), it is possible by means of simple tests to cut down the number of different enzyme estimations.

'SUGAR WATER' LYSIS TEST

This is almost diagnostic for paroxysmal nocturnal haemoglobinuria.

ABNORMAL CELLS VISIBLE IN THE PERIPHERAL BLOOD

- Congenital spherocytic haemolytic anaemia – spherocytes.
- Elliptocytosis – elliptocytes.
- Stomatocytosis – stomatocytes (follow by estimation of red cell sodium and potassium). Glyceraldehyde-3-phosphate dehydrogenase – 'burr' cells, target cells and pear-drop cells.
- Triose phosphate isomerase – anisocytosis, poikilocytosis and some contracted cells.

STANDARD ENZYME ESTIMATIONS, OR SCREENING TESTS AVAILABLE

Glucose-6-phosphate dehydrogenase deficiency; pyruvate kinase deficiency. (The two most common deficiencies.)

SALINE OSMOTIC FRAGILITY TEST USING PATIENT'S FRESH RED CELLS

Abnormal lysis is found in:

- Congenital spherocytic haemolytic anaemia.*
- Elliptocytosis (homozygote).*
- Stomatocytosis.*
- Hexokinase deficiency (slight increase).

AUTOHAEMOLYSIS OF DEFIBRINATED BLOOD INCUBATED AT 37°C

1. Lysis corrected by added glucose, ATP:
   (a) congenital spherocytic haemolytic anaemia;*
   (b) elliptocytosis;*
   (c) stomatocytosis;*
   (d) triose phosphate isomerase deficiency;
   (e) 2,3-diphosphoglycerate mutase deficiency.
2. Lysis corrected by added ATP, but not by added glucose: glucose-6-phosphate dehydrogenase deficiency.*
3. Lysis corrected by added ATP, but not by added glucose:
   (a) pyruvate kinase deficiency;*
   (b) hexokinase deficiency;
   (c) adenosine triphosphatase deficiency.
4. Effect of glucose or ATP ±:
   (a) glucose-6-phosphate isomerase deficiency;
   (b) phosphoglycerate kinase deficiency;
   (c) reduced glutathione deficiency;
   (d) hereditary adenylate kinase deficiency.

HEINZ BODY PROVOCATION TEST POSITIVE

- Glucose-6-phosphate dehydrogenase deficiency.
- Glutathione reductase deficiency.
- Adenosine triphosphatase deficiency.
- Reduced glutathione deficiency.
- γ-Glutamyl-cysteine synthase deficiency.
- 6-Phosphogluconate dehydrogenase deficiency.
- Glutathione synthase deficiency.

5. SYNTHESIS OF ABNORMAL HAEMOGLOBIN

Associated with Heinz body haemolytic anaemia

- α-thalassaemia (major)

Excess of haemoglobin H (tetramers of β-chains), present in the red cells producing a fine dispersed precipitate, and also Heinz bodies.

*Presumptive diagnosis made in earlier test.

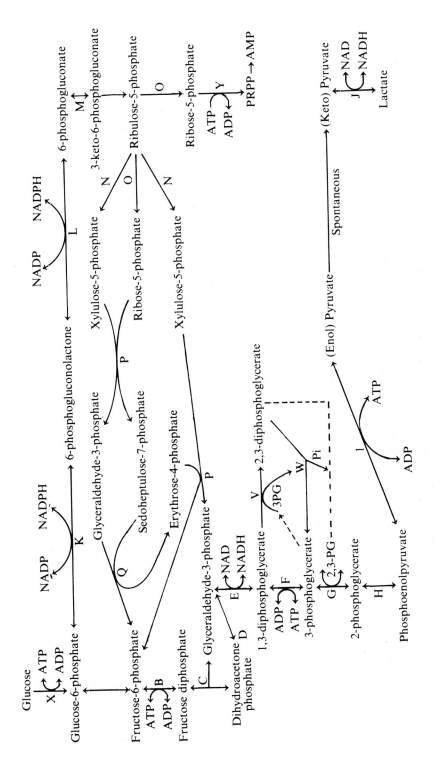

Catabolism of glucose in erythrocytes.

Adenylate kinase

$$2\,ADP \underset{}{\overset{b}{\rightleftharpoons}} ATP + AMP$$

Adenosine triphosphatase

$$2\,ATP \xrightarrow{\quad c \quad} ADP + Pi$$

$$C_6H_{12}O_6 \xrightarrow[\substack{2\,NAD^+\ 2\,NADH \\ +\ 2H^+}]{\substack{2\,ADP\ 2\,ATP \\ +\,Pi}} CO_2 + H_2O$$

$$C_6H_{12}O_6 \xrightarrow[\substack{2\,NADP^+\ 2\,NADPH \\ +\ 2H^+}]{\substack{H_2O\ \ CO_2}} Xylulose\text{-}5\text{-}P$$

Catabolism of glucose in erythrocytes.

Enzymes

A = phosphohexose isomerase*
B = phosphofructokinase
C = aldolase
D = triose phosphate isomerase*
E = glyceraldehyde-3-phosphate dehydrogenase*
F = phosphoglycerate kinase*
G = phosphoglyceromutase
H = enolase
 I = pyruvate kinase*
K = glucose-6-phosphate dehydrogenase*
L = gluconolactone hydrolase
J = lactate dehydrogenase
M = 6-phosphogluconate dehydrogenase
N = ribulose-5-phosphate epimerase
O = ribose-5-phosphate ketoisomerase
P = transketolase
Q = transaldolase
R = glutathione reductase*
S = glutathione peroxidase*

*Deficiency associated with haemolytic anaemia.

• Haemoglobin zurich [R]

Symptom-free heterozygotes with a compensated haemolytic anaemia, develop severe haemolysis with Heinz bodies in circulating red cells, when exposed to sulphonamides.

• Haemoglobin Köln [R]

Moderately severe haemolytic anaemia with splenomegaly. Following splenectomy 80% of the red cells contain Heinz bodies. During attacks of haemolysis, the urine contains dipyrroles and is darkly pigmented.

• Other unstable haemoglobins including [R]

Ube 1   Hammersmith
Seattle   St. Mary's
Geneva   Torino
Sidney   Puerto Rico, and others.
Bibba

Heinz bodies are present either in fresh blood, or in incubated blood. There is moderate, non-spherocytic, haemolytic anaemia with dark urine. Amino acid residue substitutions occur in the region of the haem pocket.

• Haemolytic anaemia due to unstable haemoglobins

Affected patients are heterozygotes, and homozygotes are not found. The clinical severity varies with the abnormality. Drug-induced haemolytic episodes are rare. Splenectomy sometimes results in clinical improvement. Many haemoglobins appear as precipitates of denatured haemoglobin in Heinz body preparations, and the abnormal haemoglobins precipitate at 50–60°C. Often the HbA$_2$ level is increased.

• Associated with unstable haemoglobins, without Heinz bodies

• *Haemoglobin S.*
• *Haemoglobin C.*
• *Haemoglobin D.*
• *Haemoglobin E.*
• *Haemoglobin M, etc.* [R]

Absence of normal switch from fetal haemopoiesis to adult haemopoiesis

• *β-Thalassaemia.*
• *α-Thalassaemia.*

Extracorpuscular factors

6. HAEMOLYSINS

Abnormal isoantibodies

• Incompatible blood transfusions

Anaesthesia may abolish early signs that incompatible blood is being transfused.

• Erythroblastosis fetalis (haemolytic disease of the newborn)

Haemolytic disease of newborn: 90% due to anti-D;

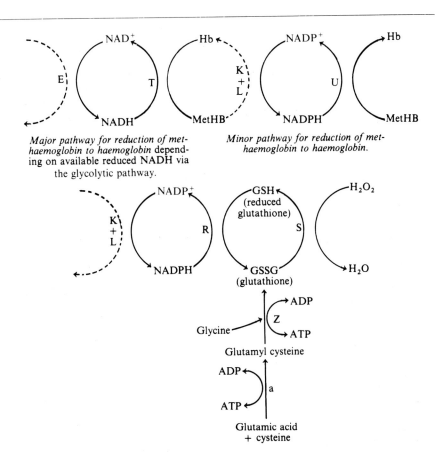

Major pathway for reduction of met-haemoglobin to haemoglobin depending on available reduced NADH via the glycolytic pathway.

Minor pathway for reduction of met-haemoglobin to haemoglobin.

Maintenance of erythrocyte stability by continuous supply of reduced glutathione.

T = diaphorase I†
U = diaphorase II†
V = 2,3-diphosphoglyceryl mutase*
W = 2,3-diphosphoglycerate phosphatase
X = hexokinase*
Y = ribose-5-phosphate pyrophosphokinase*
Z = glutathione sythase*
a = glutamyl cysteine*
b = adenylate kinase*
c = adenosine triphosphatase*

NAD^+ = nicotinamide adenine dinucleotide (coenzyme I, DPN); $NADP^+$ = dihydronicotinamide adenine dinucleotide phosphate (coenzyme II, TPN); ATP = adenosine triphosphate; ADP = adenosine diphosphate.

*Deficiency associated with haemolytic anaemia.
†Deficiency associated with methaemoglobinaemia.

also anti-C, anti-E, anti-Kell, anti-Duffy. Uncommonly ABO incompatibility.

7. ABNORMAL AUTOANTIBODIES

● 'Warm' autoantibodies

The indirect Coombs' test, related to antibodies to blood group antigens c, C, E, e, D, K, JK, F^y, is frequently positive. The antibody is usually immunoglobulin IgG (but may be IgM or rarely IgA). It is usually Rh specific, and does not fix complement, if the antibody is IgG (with λ or κ light chains). The damaged red cells are destroyed in the spleen.

The thermal range of the antibody is from 0 to 37°C

with the majority occurring at the warmer end of the range.

IDIOPATHIC

These cases are eight times as frequent as idiopathic cases with 'cold' autoantibodies. Persistent low platelet counts indicate a poor prognosis, i.e. Evan's syndrome–warm autoantibody plus antiplatelet antibody.

SECONDARY

These cases are eight times as frequent as idiopathic cases with 'cold' autoantibodies developing secondary to a disease process:

- Virus pneumonia and other virus infections.
- Chronic lymphatic leukaemia.
- Hodgkin's disease.
- Lymphosarcoma.
- Glandular fever.
- Lymphoma.
- Lupus erythematosus.

Warm autoimmune haemolytic anaemia responds to steroid therapy. Those cases which either fail to respond to steroids, or require excessively large doses, may respond to splenectomy.

Recently, such cases have been treated with vinca-alkaloid-loaded platelets. These are removed from the circulation by the mononuclear phagocytic system, and this results in suppression of uptake and destruction of antibody-coated red cells.

Reference
Ahn, Y. S., Harrington, W. J., Byrnes, J. J. *et al.* (1983) *JAMA* **249**, 2189

- 'Cold' autoantibodies

The 'cold' antibody may be active against the blood group antigens P, I, i or other group substances. The antibody is always an IgM immunoglobulin, with κ light chains only. Complement is fixed and intravascular haemolysis occurs, with red cell destruction in the liver (i.e. splenectomy ineffective). The thermal amplitude of the antibody is 0–28°C, with the majority occurring at the cooler end of the range.

IDIOPATHIC

In 'cold', antiimmune, haemolytic anaemia temporary improvement has followed plasmapheresis.

SECONDARY

- Acute virus pneumonia.
- Influenza A.
- Coxsackie virus A.
- Measles.
- Varicella.
- Encephalitis.
- Herpes simplex.

- Pleuropneumonia-like organism infection.
- *Listeria monocytogenes.*
- Infectious mononucleosis.
- Paroxysmal cold haemoglobinuria (i.e. Donath–Landsteiner test positive): (anti-P antibodies): congenital syphilis (affecting infants and young children); non-syphilitic (measles, mumps, virus pneumonia, myeloma, trypanosomiasis, spirillosis, cirrhosis, idiopathic).

8. PHYSICAL AGENTS

- Drugs

RELATED TO THE SIZE OF THE DOSE

1. Phenylhydrazine ⎫ i.e. direct damage to the red cells.
2. Naphthalene ⎭
3. Oxidants are particularly liable to cause haemolysis in:
   (a) glucose-6-phosphate dehydrogenase deficiency;
   (b) glutathione reductase deficiency;
   (c) haemoglobin Zurich;
   (d) haemoglobin H.

DRUG-INDUCED IMMUNE HAEMOLYSIS [R]

A rare but clinically serious condition. Various mechanisms have been described, including:

- A drug forms stable compounds with a plasma macromolecule. The resulting antigen reacts with its antibody to form immune complexes. These can form non-specific attachments to platelets leading to thrombocytopenia, or to red cells leading to haemolysis – the immune complex mechanism.
- A drug binds to the red cell membrane and to plasma proteins. Haemolysis results from reaction of antigen–antibody with the cell-bound drug – the drug adsorption mechanism.
- Development of red cell autoantibodies; mechanism unknown.
- Complement activation by drug–antibody complexes.

Any one or more of these mechanisms can develop in a patient for reasons yet unknown.

Reference
Patz, L. D. (1985) *N. Engl. J. Med.* **313**, 510

Vegetable poisons ⎫ Allergic
- Saponin. ⎪ response
- Castor oil (due to ricin). ⎬ red cell
- Fava bean ⎪ glutathione
- Pollen (Baghdad Spring fever) ⎭ metabolism
                                    abnormal.
- Animal poisons

Snake venom (in colubrine snakes, e.g. cobra, due to action of a lysolecithin on the red blood cells).

- Water

- Intravenous water in large volumes.
- Drowning in fresh water: water is absorbed rapidly from the lungs.

- Heat

In burns cases:

- Some red cells destroyed immediately, at the burns site, by direct heat action
- Other red cells are lysed during the next 24-h after the burns. These cells become spherocytic, with an increased osmotic fragility before lysis.

- Infections

BACTERIAL

Septicaemia due to:

- Haemolytic streptococci.
- *Staphylococcus pyogenes.*
- Clostridia, including *Clostridium perfringens.*
- Oroya fever: due to *Bartonella bacilliformis,* a flagellate bacillus.

- Protozoal
- *P. falciparum*–malignant tertian malaria.
- *P. vivax*–benign tertian malaria.
- *P. malariae*–quartan malaria.

- Virus

- Virus pneumonia ⎫
- Infectious mononucleosis ⎬ Rare

Mechanical

- Red cells damaged during passage through artificial heart valve.
- Red cells damaged in extracorporeal 'heart–lung' machines etc.
- March haemoglobinuria.

Microangiopathic haemolytic anaemia

Characterized by haemolytic anaemia with circulating fragmented red cells and 'burr' cells:

- Haemolytic–uraemic syndrome.
- Acute progressive malignant hypertension.
- Eclampsia, intrauterine death, amniotic fluid embolism.
- Thrombotic thrombocytopenic purpura.
- Carcinomatosis.
- Symptomatic

Some cases of:

- Cirrhosis of the liver.

- Renal disease and azotaemia.
- Lupus erythematosus.
- Collagen diseases.
- Metastatic carcinoma.
- Lymphoma.
- Leukaemias.
- Thrombotic thrombocytopenic purpura.

Fragmented red blood cells are present in the peripheral blood.

Haemolytic anaemia has been caused by the following substances (not listed in either severity or frequency of incidence):

Haemolysis occurs in some persons (not arranged in order of frequency)

- *p*-Aminosalicylates.
- Antimony, organic compounds.
- Benzedrine (amphetamine).
- Diphenylhydramine.
- Lead and tetraethyl lead (anti-knock).
- Mesantoin.
- Myanesin.
- Neoarsphenamine.
- Pamaquin.
- Pennyroyal.
- Phenacetin.
- Phenothiazine.
- Phenylsemicarbazide.
- Potassium chlorate.
- Primaquine.
- Pyribenzamine.
- Quinine.
- Sulphonamides.

Haemolysis due to direct destruction of red cells

- Acetanilide.
- Allyl-propyl-disulphide.
- Aniline.
- Arsine.
- Benzene (probably haemolytic, as well as causing marrow damage).
- Lead.
- Lecithin.
- Methyl chloride.
- Naphthalene.
- *β*-Naphthol.
- Nitrobenzenes (mono- and dinitrobenzenes).
- Phenacetin.
- Phenylhydrazine and its acetyl derivatives.
- Phosphorus.
- Ricin (from castor oil).
- Saponin.
- Silver, colloidal.

- Sulphones (promine, diaminodiphenylsulphone).
- Trinitrotoluene.
- Toluylenediamine.
- Xylene.

Laboratory findings in haemolytic anaemia

The clearing of haemoglobin from the plasma

Normally up to 0.7 g haemoglobin is released into the plasma each day. During extravascular haemolysis, free haemoglobin leaks back into the plasma, but during intravascular haemolysis free haemoglobin is released directly into the plasma.

A series of substances combine with, and help to remove, this circulating free haemoglobin. Plasma haptoglobins can normally bind 100–140 mg free haemoglobin per 100 ml plasma, the complex being removed by the reticuloendothelial system, with a clearance rate of approximately 15 mg Hb/100 ml plasma per hour. Haemopexin in the plasma binds free haemoglobin, the complex then being removed by the liver.

When the haptoglobin–haemopexin system is saturated, free haemoglobin is oxidized to meth-aemoglobin and binds to albumin, each albumin molecule binding up to two methaemoglobin molecules to form methaemalbumin. When the albumin pool is also saturated, haemoglobin escapes into the urine, being reabsorbed by the renal tubules and catabolized. The porphyrin and globin are rapidly metabolized, some of the iron returns to the capillary blood and the rest appears as haemosiderin in desquamated cells in the urine. Such iron-staining cells are evidence of chronic intravascular haemolysis. When the plasma haemoglobin level exceeds 30 mg/100 ml, free haemoglobin escapes in the urine; as free haemoglobin tetramers dissociate into α-β dimers, haemoglobin reaches the urine more easily.

Plasma haemoglobin (SI units = mg/l).

Normal range

- Less than 10 mg/l of plasma.
- When free haemoglobin released into plasma exceeds the haptoglobin binding capacity.

Pathological

Slight increase (50–100 mg/l):
- Sickle-cell thalassaemia.
- Haemoglobin C disease.

Moderate increase (100–250 mg/l)
- Acquired haemolytic anaemia (autoimmune).

- Sickle-cell anaemia.
- Thalassaemia major.
- Sickle-cell haemoglobin C disease.
- Prosthetic heart valve replacement. Haem is released, with lactate dehydrogenase (LDH), from cells which are lysed, and from red cells which are damaged but not lysed.
- March haemoglobinuria.
- After prolonged jogging.

Reference
Dale, J. and Myhre, E. (1972) *Acta. Med. Scand.* **191**, 133

Marked increase

- Incompatible blood transfusion; rarely Lewis antibodies with compatible ABO and Rh grouping.
- Transfusion of lysed blood (previously heated, frozen or grossly infected).

Reference
Sandler, S. G., Berry, E. and Zlotnick, A. (1976) *JAMA* **235**, 2850

- Paroxysmal nocturnal haemoglobinuria.
- Paroxysmal cold haemoglobinuria.
- Blackwater fever (falciparum malaria).

Plasma haemoglobin must exceed 250 mg/l before it gives the plasma a faint pink hue.

No increase in plasma haemoglobin occurs in hereditary spherocytosis, since red-cell breakdown occurs extravascularly in the spleen.

Note: It is important to avoid haemolysis either during or after the collection of the blood sample, otherwise the result is invalid.

Reference
Swolin, B., Roberts, D. and Waldenström, J. (1982) *Clin. Chim. Acta.* **121**, 389 (Method)

Plasma haptoglobins

Normal range

This is 0.3–1.9 g/l (30–190 mg/100 ml) of plasma, with slightly higher levels in normal men than in women.

Although the normal range is wide, the level appears to be constant in any one person, being determined genetically. The three haptoglobin groups are homozygotes (1-1) and (2-2), and heterozygote (2-1), with concentrations in group (1-1) > (2-1) > (2-2). Haptoglobins are not detectable in normal cord blood, and levels are low in children. They are absent from the plasma of some otherwise normal individuals. In normal women, haptoglobin levels fall at ovulation and rise at menstruation, varying by 20–40 mg/100 ml about the mean. There is no change during pregnancy, but there is an increase after parturition.

Haptoglobins are α-globulins, mucoproteins, synthesized by the liver, and 50% are replaced daily. Their rate of synthesis is limited and is modulated by glucocorticoids. Haptoglobins combine with free hae-moglobin, $\alpha\beta$-dimers preferentially to tetramers in the plasma, and the complexes are eliminated by the reticuloendothelial system. They can bind 100–140 mg Hb/+ 100 ml plasma, and the complexes can be eliminated at about 15 mg/100 ml plasma per hour. It is thought that, normally, 0.7 g haemoglobin escapes into the plasma each day, consuming 1 g haptoglobin. When the red cell life falls below 17 days, no hapto-globin is detectable in the plasma.

References
Eaton, J. W. Brandt, P., Mohoney, J. R. and Lee, J. T. Jr. (1982) *Science* **215**, 691
Hansson, L.-O., Kjellman, N. I. M., Ludvigsson, J. *et al.* (1983)*Scand. J. Clin. Lab. Invest.* **43**, 367
Kuriyama, M., Sonoda, K. and Igata, A. (1985) *Am. J. Med.* **78**, 850

Increase (haptoglobin is an acute phase protein)

- Carcinoma, especially with secondary deposits in bone.
- Inflammatory disease – may increase up to four times normal.
- Trauma, surgery.
- Collagen diseases.

Decrease

Haemolysis:

- Incompatible blood transfusion.
- Paroxysmal nocturnal haemoglobinuria.
- Sickle-cell anaemia.
- Thalassaemia major.
- March haemoglobinuria.
- Infections, including typhus, typhoid, meningococ-cal infection, glandular fever. Malaria–hypohap-toglobinaemia is easier to establish and monitor than blood parasite checks in malarial areas.

Reference
Rougemont, A., Dumbo, O., Bouvier, M. *et al.* (1988) *Lancet* **ii**, 709

- Pernicious anaemia.

In acute pancreatitis, pancreatic enzymes release hae-moglobin from haptoglobin, i.e. there is free circulating haemoglobin without complete saturation of hapto-globin.

Haemopexin

Haemopexin is a β-globulin with a molecular weight of 70 000 and is in the form of a single-chain poly-peptide. It is synthesized in the liver. Blood levels are low in the newborn infant, rising to adult levels of 500–1000 μg/ml plasma after the first year. Haemo-pexin has a great affinity for haem, and complexes with any free haem in the plasma, and these complexes are removed and catabolized by the hepatic paren-chymal cells. Because it has a greater affinity for haem

than does albumin, there is active transfer of haem bound to albumin.

Like haptoglobin, haemopexin has a normal half-clearance of about a day, which is reduced when haem is complexed. It is not an acute phase protein, and estimation of plasma haemopexin may therefore be useful in the detection of haemolysis.

Pathological

Increase

Increased plasma haemopexin has been found in diabetes mellitus, carcinoma and infection in rheuma-toid arthritis.

Decrease

- Thalassaemia major: virtually no haemopexin present in the plasma.
- Following cardiac surgery, results correlate in-versely with urine haemosiderin output and num-bers of circulating deformed red cells.

Reference
Hershko, C. (1975) *Br. J. Haematol.* **29**, 199

Plasma methaemalbumin

Methaemalbumin is haematin linked with plasma albumin or ferric compound of protoporphyrin linked with albumin.

Normally it is eliminated in the bile via the liver in the form of coproporphyrin III.

Intravascular haemolysis

The pigment is not normally detected in the serum, but appears after rapid intravascular haemolysis. During intravascular haemolysis free haemoglobin is first bound by haptoglobins in the α_2-globulin fraction. As more haemoglobin is liberated, it is taken up by the β_1-globulin fraction. Finally, when all the hapto-globin and β_1-globulin fraction are saturated, meth-aemalbumin is formed, and Schumm's test for meth-aemalbumin becomes positive.

If there is associated liver damage with intravascular haemolysis, the blood methaemalbumin level rises excessively, since the excretion of bile (and hence methaemalbumin) is reduced.

Acute haemorrhagic pancreatitis

Plasma methaemalbumin appears after 12h, reaching a peak in 4–5 days. It is thought to be due to high levels of pancreatic enzymes in the blood, and is associated with falling serum calcium and a higher mortality than in oedematous pancreatitis.

Small amounts of methaemalbumin may occur in some cases of Addisonian megaloblastic anaemia.

Note: Methaemalbumin does not appear in the serum in:

- Acholuric jaundice.
- Sickle-cell anaemia.
- Thalassaemia.

In these three conditions, haemolysis is not intravascular.

Reference
Winstone, N. E. (1965) *Br. J. Surg.* **52**, 804

Haemoglobinuria

When the plasma haemoglobin level exceeds about 30 mg/dl, some haemoglobin is excreted in the urine, one-third of the filtered haemoglobin being reabsorbed by the renal tubules. The plasma haemoglobin clearance rate is maximally 6 ml plasma/min per 1.73 m^2.

Haemoglobinuria may occur in the following conditions

Incompatible blood transfusion

Haemolysis
This is due to:

- Action of drugs and chemicals especially in subjects with low red cell glucose-6-phosphate dehydrogenase activity.
- Blackwater fever (malignant tertian malaria incompletely treated with quinine).
- Oroya fever (*Bartonella bacilliformis*).
- Severe burns: some red cells are destroyed at the time of the burn, other red cells are destroyed after a further 24 h.
- Intravascular haemolysis following snake or spider bites.
- Rarely in septicaemia, e.g. *Clostridium perfringens*, *Streptococcus haemolyticus*.
- Eclampsia (rarely).
- Aortic ball valve prosthesis.

Paroxysmal haemoglobinuria

- Paroxysmal nocturnal haemoglobinuria: the red cells are abnormally susceptible to normal serum factors in the presence of a fall in pH, and contain an amboceptor.
- Paroxysmal cold haemoglobinuria.
- Haemoglobinuria following severe exertion, e.g. karate exercises, long-distance running on metalled roads.

Note: In paroxysmal myoglobinuria the renal excretion of myoglobin is much more rapid than that of haemoglobin in haemoglobinuria.

Haemosiderin in urine

When free haemoglobin persists in the plasma and appears in the glomerular filtrate, haemosiderin can be detected in the urine. It is only found when there has been chronic haemoglobinaemia derived from intravascular haemolysis. In the early stages of a haemolytic anaemia with circulating free haemoglobinaemia the renal tubules reabsorb the haem pigment and haemosiderin does not appear in the urine.

The condition in which haemosiderinuria is best demonstrated is paroxysmal noctural haemoglobinuria, in which intravascular haemolysis is of long standing. As much as 15 mg of iron can be lost each day in the urine during an acute exacerbation.

Red cell osmotic fragility

This is a non-specific test of the red cell membrane, its sodium pump and ability to generate ATP. In a sufficiently hypotonic solution, normal red cells swell to +160% of their initial volume and then haemolyse. In the test, sample red cells are subjected to a gradient of successively more dilute saline solutions, and the degree of haemolysis at each saline dilution is measured. It is carried out in two stages, using (1) fresh blood and (2) blood incubated at 37°C for 24h under sterile conditions (when endogenous glucose has been used up, and sodium ions and water have leaked into the cells, and potassium has leaked out). The test is of greatest clinical use in the confirmation of hereditary spherocytosis.

It is important that buffered saline be used, as changes in pH greatly affect results. The red cells must be thoroughly oxygenated, as osmotic fragility increases with the carbon dioxide tension. The proportion of blood to saline should be such that there is not sufficient plasma to protect the red cells from saline action. For practical purposes, room temperature is adequate for the test.

Young red cells, cells with a low MCHC and older smaller cells from normal blood separated by differential centrifugation have a greater osmotic resistance, whilst larger red cells have a greater osmotic fragility.

Reference
Van der Vegt, S. G. L., Ruben, A. M. Th., Werte, J. M. *et al.* (1986) *Br. J. Haematol.* **61**, 405

Results

1. Decreased osmotic fragility in fresh blood

This is of little clinical value. Found in iron-deficiency anaemia, thalassaemia, sickle-cell anaemia, homozygous haemoglobin C disease and some cases with jaundice.

2. Increased osmotic fragility in fresh blood

- Hereditary spherocytosis.
- Stomatocytosis.
- Thermal injury to red cells.
- Red cells coated with immunoglobulin.
- Conditions with secondary haemolytic anaemia.

Normal values for saline osmotic fragility

Saline (g% NaCl)	Haemolysis (percentage)
0.3	97–100
0.35	90–99
0.40	50–95
0.45	5–45
0.50	0–5
0.55	0

- Normal onset of haemolysis at 0.45% (0.42–0.46%).
- Haemolysis, normally complete at 0.3% (0.28–0.32%).
- Mean corpuscular fragility (MCF), or the range for 50% haemolysis = 0.40–0.445% NaCl.

References
Dacie, J. V. (1960) *The Haemolytic Anaemias.* Part 1, 2nd ed. London: Churchill
Mortensen, E. (1963) *Acta. Med. Scand.* **174**, 289, 299

3. Increased osmotic fragility in incubated blood

- Hereditary spherocytosis.
- Some cases of elliptocytosis.
- Stomatocytosis.
- Congenital non-spherocytic haemolytic anaemia. The test may have been normal when fresh blood was tested:
  (a) glucose-6-phosphate dehydrogenase deficiency (variable);
  (b) glucose-phosphate isomerase deficiency [R];
  (c) hexokinase deficiency [R];
  (d) triose-phosphate isomerase deficiency [R]– flattened curve.
- Acquired haemolytic anaemia with spherocytosis.
- Haemolytic anaemia due to chemicals.
- Paroxysmal nocturnal haemoglobinuria.

The MCF after 24h of incubation (50% haemolysis = 0.465–0.590% NaCl).

Note: In all cases where the fragility increases on incubation for 24h there is increased autohaemolysis. Normally after 24h there is little or no haemolysis, and after 48h only small amounts are present. In paroxysmal nocturnal haemoglobinuria this autohaemolysis is frequently very marked.

Normal values for incubated osmotic fragility test

Saline (g% NaCl)	Haemolysis (percentage)
0.20	95–100
0.30	85–100
0.35	75–100
0.40	65–100
0.45	55–95
0.50	40–85
0.55	15–70
0.60	0–40
0.65	0–10
0.70	0–5
0.75	0
0.85	0

Autohaemolysis of red blood cells

Sterile defibrinated blood is incubated at 37°C for 24 h or 48 h. Then the amount of haemolysis which has occurred is measured. With normal red cells, there is less than 5% haemolysis. If glucose is added before incubation, haemolysis is reduced to less than 0.5%.

Two patterns of haemolysis were originally described: type I haemolysis (with increased haemolysis after incubation, reduced when glucose had been added beforehand) and type II haemolysis (with increased haemolysis after incubation, and either no improvement or increased haemolysis as a result of addition of glucose before incubation).

This was expanded by testing the effects of supplements of ATP added before incubation. With the development of specific enzyme estimation methods, it has been suggested that the autohaemolysis test is now obsolete. Hereditary spherocytosis can be detected by the presence of spherocytes in the blood film and the increased red cell osmotic fragility, and both elliptocytes and stomatocytes can also be seen in stained blood films. Of the non-spherocytic haemolytic anaemias, there are millions of sufferers with glucose-6-phosphate dehydrogenase deficiency, and moderate numbers with pyruvate kinase deficiency, the other enzyme deficiency states being exceedingly rare. The test is not of clinical value in acquired haemolytic anaemia.

Acid serum haemolysis test of Ham and Crosby

After incubation in acidified serum, red blood cells from cases of paroxysmal nocturnal haemoglobinuria (PNH) show marked haemolysis. The test is not specific, although it is usually performed to demonstrate PNH. Various controls must be set up to exclude other conditions.

The test has been modified by the addition of thrombin. This increases the degree of haemolysis of red cells in cases of PNH, as compared with other conditions. It has been suggested that this is due to the action of added properdin contaminating the thrombin preparation.

PNH red cells are very susceptible to haemolysis by high-titre 'cold' antibodies. In other conditions the presence of antibodies may be shown by use of Coombs test, which is negative in PNH.

References
Crosby, W. H. (1950) *Blood* **5**, 843
Crosby, W. H. and Damashek, W. (1950) *Blood* **5**, 822
Ham, T. H. (1939) *Arch. Med.* **64**, 1271

'Sugar-water' test for paroxysmal nocturnal haemoglobinuria

PNH red cells are lysed in this very simple test by incubation in a buffered sucrose solution. The test has been negative in other cases of haemolytic anaemia. It is thought that lysis occurs following complement damage to the PNH red cells.

Red cells from the following conditions are more sensitive than normal, but much less likely to haemolysis than PNH red cells: acute and chronic leukaemia; myeloproliferative disorders. Congenital dyserythropoietic anaemia, type II (HEMPAS)—positive Ham acid serum test, negative 'sugar-water' test.

References
Hartmann, R. C. and Jenkins, D. E. Jr. (1966) *N. Engl. J. Med.* **275**, 155
Stathakis, N., Arapakis, G., Kirtou, K. *et al.* (1970) *J. Clin. Pathol.* **25**, 452

Tests for paroxysmal nocturnal haemoglobinuria

Complement activated in fluid phase by
- Acidification of testing serum (Ham's test).
- Commercial bovine thrombin.
- Cobra venom factor.
- Inulin.
- Heating cells.

Specific antibodies

Used to activate complement on the erythrocyte surface, which can demonstrate two or three distinct subpopulations of erythrocytes circulating, each with abnormally increased sensitivity to complement.

Sucrose lysis test

Activation of complement in an isosmolar solution of reduced ionic strength, ?secondary to a conformational change in red cell membrane proteins induced by low ionic strength.

False positive results

If serum incompatible with the red cell blood group is used in the Ham test, false positive results may be obtained. The sucrose lysis test gives false positive results in the presence of immune haemolytic disease.

The most reliable results have been obtained in the detection of PNH, using complement lysis sensitivity test, but human anti-I serum with a high haemolytic activity is rare and difficult to obtain.

Rabbit antiserum prepared against human red cells can be substituted for human antiserum, but haemolytic titres are not proportional to agglutination titres.

Reference
Harruff, R. C. and Rohn, R. J. (1983) *Am. J. Clin. Pathol.* **80**, 152

Cold haemagglutinins

Normal cold autoagglutinins

Many samples of human sera can agglutinate red cells at 0°C. This phenomenon is reversible on warming, and has usually disappeared at 20°C or more. Although there appears to be no blood group specificity, and the agglutinins do not act preferentially on group O cells, it is possible that the titre is greater in groups A, B and AB, rather than group O subjects. Cold agglutinins are present in infants' cord blood if they are also present in maternal blood, but at a lower titre.

Normal titre: 1 in 16 to 1 in 32.

Incomplete cold antibodies

Red cells incubated in normal fresh human serum at 0–4°C for 2h or more, and then washed with saline to remove the serum, give a positive reaction with antiglobulin serum.

Heating the serum to 56°C inactivates the antibody. Heparin, oxalate and citrate all inhibit the reaction.

This normal incomplete cold antibody has anti-H specificity, i.e. it reacts more strongly using group O cells than with A_1 or B cells. The titre is unrelated to the titre of normal cold autoantibodies in the same sample of blood.

Cells of newborn infants contain little H substance. Therefore the presence of anti-H in their sera is unlikely to give false positive, direct Coombs' reactions.

Blood group antibodies which react at low temperature
- Naturally occurring anti-A and anti-B act better at 4°C than at 37°C (compare immune anti-A and anti-B which react better at 37°C).
- Anti-A_1 is occasionally found as a cold agglutinin in subjects of subgroups A_2 and A_2B.
- Anti-M, -N, -H, -O, -P, -Le^a, -Le^b, -A_1, all act more effectively at 4°C than at 37°C. Anti-Le^a and anti-Le^b have a wide thermal range of activity, as have anti-A and anti-B.

Cold agglutinins and surgery under deep hypothermia

Open heart surgery may be carried out with the patient's oesophageal and nasopharyngeal temperature at 25°C. When blood is cross-matched, it is tested at 12°C, 18°C, 25°C, 31°C and 37°C to detect the presence of cold agglutinins, in the donor blood and that of the recipient.

1. Clinically significant cold agglutinins

Haemolytic agglutinins:

- Almost always IgM.
- Act over a wide thermal range, from 4 to 32°C.
- They bind complement (hence haemolysis).
- Red cell agglutinates are irreversible, and therefore dangerous.
- Agglutination of red cells is enhanced when incubated at 30°C suspended in albumin. These are commonly associated with chronic cold agglutination disease, neoplasm of lymphoid origin and *Mycoplasma pneumoniae*.

2. Clinically insignificant

Cold agglutinins which are not associated with haemolysis. These do not involve any clinical risk.

Cold haemagglutinins occurring in disease

1. Paroxysmal cold haemoglobinuria

Serum contains a haemolysin which coats red cells in the cold, and then in the presence of complement, on warming, haemolyses the cells. This is the basis of the Donath–Landsteiner reaction (*see below*). The serum cold agglutinin titre is usually normal, and the Coombs' reaction is positive by the direct test. It is stated that in some cases which are non-syphilitic cold agglutinins are present which do not require complement to cause haemolysis.

2. Atypical virus pneumonia

High titres of cold haemagglutinins may be found.

3. Acquired haemolytic anaemia

This is frequently associated with very high titres of non-specific agglutinins. Binding of antibody to the red cells occurs at temperatures up to 30°C, but not at 37°C. A strong indirect positive Coombs' reaction is obtained at 20°C.

4. Cold haemagglutinins

These may be found in some cases of:

- Some apparently normal persons.
- Pregnancy.
- Cirrhosis of the liver.
- Leukaemia.
- Infectious mononucleosis.

- Myeloma.
- Tropical eosinophilia.
- Spirillosis.
- Malaria.
- Trypanosomiasis.

Donath–Landsteiner reaction

A cold autohaemolysin occurs in up to 10% of cases of late syphilis, and also in a proportion of non-syphilitics. The haemolysin becomes absorbed on red cells in the cold, and proceeds to lyse the red cells in the presence of complement when the system is warmed to 37°C. This reaction in vivo following exposure to cold leads to paroxysmal haemoglobinuria.

In vitro a simple qualitative test may be made by taking two samples of clotted blood from a patient. One sample is immediately placed in a water-bath at 37°C, and the other sample is placed on crushed ice at 0°C, for 30 min, after which the cooled specimen is placed in the water-bath at 37°C. In paroxysmal cold haemoglobinuria, haemolysis is evident in the serum of the cooled specimen but not in the other (compare, in paroxysmal nocturnal haemoglobinuria after prolonged incubation at 37°C haemolysis develops).

Using washed normal cells of group O and doubling dilutions of the patient's serum, incubated at 0°C for 30 min, and at 37°C for 1h, the Donath–Landsteiner antibodies, if present, can be titrated.

Note: For this latter test it is important that the blood immediately after collection is kept at 37°C until after the serum has been separated, otherwise the antibody is lost on the patient's cells, and a false negative result is obtained.

Red cell mechanical fragility

Spherocytes, agglutinated and sickled cells are more susceptible than normal cells to mechanical injury. This property is not necessarily directly related to the osmotic fragility. Red cells from newborn infants are more fragile than adult red cells, for the first few days of life. Ovalocytes are more mechanically fragile than normal cells.

The test for mechanical fragility is very difficult to standardize in vitro, and at present is not regarded as useful.

Note: Haemolysis is produced by forcing blood through:
- Gauge 24 needle (internal diameter = 0.55 mm) at more than 0.2 ml/s, i.e. ejecting a 5 ml blood sample in less than 25 s.
- Gauge 22 needle (internal diameter = 0.70 mm) at more than 1.2 ml/s, i.e. ejecting a 5 ml blood sample in less than 6 s.

It is not realized generally that it is important always to remove the needle from a syringe before ejecting a blood sample, or ejecting the blood *slowly* through the needle.

Reference
Macdonald, W. B. and Berg, R. B. (1959) *Pediatrics* **23**, 8

Antiglobulin test (Coombs' antihuman globulin test)

Antihuman globulin serum will agglutinate red cells which have been sensitized or coated with an antibody globulin. Normal uncoated red cells are not agglutinated by the serum.

Direct test

The patient's red blood cells are washed with saline to remove any traces of serum, and then treated with an antihuman globulin serum. The test can detect down to 500 IgG molecules bound to each red cell.

- Positive result

1. NEWBORN INFANT WITH RHESUS ANTIBODY HAEMOLYTIC DISEASE

The direct test is always positive, unless the baby has received blood transfusions while in utero. After in utero transfusion, the cord blood contains predominantly adult blood of the donor's blood group, and the test is weakly positive or negative.

Less commonly, haemolytic disease of the newborn may result from the action of antibodies against Kell, Kidd or Duffy blood groups, giving positive results. Rarely, the test may be weakly positive in ABO incompatibility, when the infant is group A or group B and the mother is group O.

2. WARM AUTOIMMUNE HAEMOLYTIC ANAEMIA

The direct test is positive in almost all cases, at least during active haemolysis, with negative results in less than 4%.

3. COLD HAEMAGGLUTININ DISEASE

The direct test is positive when blood is taken from the patient into a warm syringe and separated at 37°C, as complement components do not elute at 37°C.

4. PAROXYSMAL HAEMOGLOBINURIA

If red cells are taken from the patient during an attack or soon afterwards, when complement components are on the cells, the direct test is positive.

5. DRUG-INDUCED 'IMMUNE' HAEMOLYTIC ANAEMIA

Blood from most patients gives direct positive results, unless all sensitized cells have been destroyed. About 20% of patients treated with methyldopa develop IgG antibodies against red cells, but in most cases no haemolysis occurs. Procainamide commonly induces a positive direct result, but only rarely causes haemolytic anaemia.

References
Kelton, J. G. (1985) *N. Engl. J. Med.* **313**, 596
Kleinman, S., Nelson, R., Smith, L. *et al.* (1984) *N. Engl. J. Med.* **311**, 809

5. FAVISM

During haemolysis, the direct test is positive in 80% of cases.

Indirect test

Normal compatible red blood cells, after washing, are incubated with the patient's serum. If antibodies are present in the serum, they coat the red cells. After further washing, these coated red cells agglutinate when treated with antihuman globulin serum.

The test is used to detect and measure the titre of antibodies in maternal blood during pregnancy. It is also used during the cross-matching of blood prior to transfusion, to detect the presence of antibodies in the potential recipient's serum, which may have developed as a result of previous transfusion.

Reference
Worlledge, S. (revised by Jones, N. C. H. and Bain, B.) (1982) In *Blood and its Disorders.* Editors, Hardisty, R. M. and Weatherall, D. J. pp. 505–507. Oxford: Blackwell

Tests for antibodies using enzyme-treated red cells

Bromelin, ficin, papain and trypsin are used to partially digest the red cell surface to make it more sensitive to certain antibodies when they are present in the serum:

- Rh antibodies.
- Le^a antibodies.
- Anti-H antibodies.
- Anti-O antibodies.
- Anti-I antibodies.
- Anti-Jk^a antibodies.
- Antibodies in acquired haemolytic anaemia.
- Sensitivity to anti-P and anti-L^u is slightly enhanced.
- F^y, M, N and S binding sites are destroyed by enzyme treatment, and such treated red cells cannot be used for the detection of these corresponding antibodies.

Erythrophagocytosis

Erythrocytes may undergo phagocytosis by monocytes, and less commonly by neutrophils. This phenomenon may be seen more readily, when it is present, by incubating heparinized blood at 37°C for 1h. Those antibodies which produce haemolysis in the presence of complement, and agglutination of red cells in its absence, will produce erythrophagocytosis when red cells, white cells and serum (or plasma) are incubated together. The degree of phagocytosis is thought to correspond to the severity of the haemolysis. Probably it is a mechanism for the removal of damaged cells.

The condition may be demonstrated in peripheral blood in the following conditions.

Congenital red cell defect

Sickle-cell disease.

Acquired red cell defect

1. Secondary to chemicals
- Potassium chlorate.
- Naphthalene.
- Mushroom poisoning.
- Acquired sensitivity to quinine.

2. Secondary to infections

BACTERIA
- Subacute bacterial endocarditis.
- Typhoid fever.
- Tuberculosis.
- Streptococcal septicaemia.
- Meningococcal septicaemia.

PROTOZOA
- Malaria.
- Trypanosomiasis.

HOOKWORMS
- Ankylostomiasis.

3. Secondary to serum antibodies
- After incompatible blood transfusion.
- Erythroblastosis fetalis.
- Paroxysmal cold haemoglobinuria.
- Acquired haemolytic anaemia.

4. Symptomatic
- Leukaemia.

5. Idiopathic
- Lederer's acute haemolytic anaemia.

References
Cooper, M. B. (1950) Blood 5, 678
Zinkham, W. H. and Diamond, L. K. (1952) Blood 7, 592

Heinz body provocation test

Heparinized blood is incubated for 4h with a phosphate buffer (pH = 7.6), which contains 200 mg glucose and 100 mg acetylphenyl hydrazine per 100 ml. Wet preparations of the red cells are stained with crystal violet.

Pathological increase

Increased numbers of Heinz bodies are found in patient's red cells when compared with numbers in normal control red cells subjected to the same reagents:

- Glucose-6-phosphate dehydrogenase deficiency.
- 6-Phosphogluconate dehydrogenase deficiency [R].
- γ-glutamyl-cysteine synthase deficiency [R].
- Glutathione synthase deficiency [R].
- Glutathione reductase deficiency [R].
- Glutathione peroxidase deficiency [R].
- Adenosine triphosphatase deficiency [R].
- Ribose phosphate pyrophosphokinase deficiency [R].

Reference
Beutler, E., Dern, R. J. and Alving, A. S. (1955) J. Lab. Clin. Med. 45, 40

Pancytopenia

The peripheral blood count shows (1) anaemia, (2) leucopenia and (3) thrombocytopenia.

1. Leukaemia, especially in the elderly:
   (a) aleukaemic phase;
   (b) acute and subacute leukaemia;
   (c) the 'preleukaemic' phase.
2. Aplastic anaemia.
3. Bone-marrow damage:
   (a) Hodgkin's disease;
   (b) lymphoma and lymphosarcoma;
   (c) reticulum-cell sarcoma;
   (d) secondary carcinomatous invasion of bone marrow;
   (e) myelosclerosis;
   (f) multiple myeloma.
4. Hypersplenism.
5. Megaloblastic anaemia.
6. Disseminated lupus erythematosus.
7. Disseminated tuberculosis [R].
8. Associated with thymic tumours.
9. Disseminated anonymous mycobacterial infection.

Aplastic anaemia (see also p. 126)

The anaemia is usually normocytic or moderately macrocytic with associated leucopenia, thrombocytopenia and low reticulocyte count. No immature red cells or white cells are seen in the peripheral blood. The erythrocyte sedimentation rate is increased as the packed cell volume falls. Stem cells in the marrow are unable to proliferate. Prognosis is worse in cases with persistent thrombocytopenia. In some cases aplastic anaemia is primarily due to a sinusoidal microcirculation defect in the bone marrow. Once the supporting tissue in the marrow is damaged, e.g. by irradiation, erythropoiesis cannot restart and bone marrow grafts do not take.

References
Crosby, W. H. and Knospe, W. H. (1971) *Lancet* **i**, 20
Marsh, J. C. W. and Geary, C. G. (1991) *Brit. J. Haematol.* **77**, 447

In the human developing red cell the nuclear membrane is closely related to the endoplasmic reticulum (ER). The ER is the primary site for cell detoxication and metabolism. Since the red cell ER is relatively small, it is possible that the nuclear membrane has similar functions. Each individual chromosome is probably anchored at many points to the nuclear membrane, and chromatin fibres converge and attach to annuli of pores in the nuclear membrane. The nuclear membrane is associated with the activation of DNA synthesis and the nuclear pores regulate RNA efflux, only opening when adequate concentration is reached in the cell. Thus change in the endoplasmic reticulum, nuclear membrane or nuclear membrane pores may grossly interfere with red cell production.

Reference
Frisch, B., Lewis, S. M. and Sherman, D. (1975) *Br. J. Haematol.* **29**, 545

Patients with a total granulocyte count of $<0.5 \times 10^9/l$, platelets $<20 \times 10^9/l$, reticulocytes $<15 \times 10^9/l$ and non-myeloid marrow cellularity $>75\%$, have 100% mortality in 3 months. 20% of patients with 3 or less of these findings survive 3 months at least. The incidence of aplastic anaemia is less than 3 per million per year, suggesting that it is overestimated.

Reference
International Agranulocytosis and Aplastic Anaemia Study (1987) *Blood* **70**, 1718

Primary idiopathic aplastic anaemia

1. Due to unknown causes

2. Familial hypoplastic anaemia, without developmental anomalies

3. Fanconi's constitutional, familial aplastic anaemia

This condition is associated with growth retardation, skeletal abnormalities, skin pigmentation, urogenital abnormalities including male genital hypoplasia and cryptorchidism, increasing spontaneous chromosome damage and insidious pancytopenia.

It is thought that red cell precursors in Fanconi's anaemia may be defective in some aspect of DNA repair, with increased sensitivity to chromosomal damage, or inhibition of growth, by agents known to damage DNA.

Reference
Gordon-Smith, E. C. and Rutherford, T. R. (1989) In: Gordon-Smith, E. C., Ed. *Baillière's Clinical Haematology*, Vol. 2, No. 1, p. 139. London: Baillière Tindall

4. Pure red cell aplasia

Erythropoietin acts at the level of colony-forming units (CFU-E). Burst-forming unit (BFU-E) is regulated by cell-to-cell interactions.

- Diamond–Blackfan anaemia [R]

Congenital hypoplastic anaemia with an insidious onset at birth or in early infancy. The white cell and platelet counts are normal, but the red cells retain the fetal i-antigen, with fetal patterns of glycolytic and hexose monophosphate shunt enzymes, macrocytosis, raised haemoglobin F concentration and increased red cell adenosine deaminase activity which reflects perturbed erythroid stem cell function.

Corticosteroid therapy with maintenance on low doses of prednisolone results in correction of the anaemia in 70–80% of cases. It has been suggested that some patients have defective erythropoietin-insensitive propenitors, partially corrected by corticosteroids. In others, it is possible that progenitors are absent with failure of commitment of stem cells to erythroid differentiation.

Reference
Glader, B. E., and Becker, K. (1988) *Br. J. Haematol.* **68**, 165

- Acquired red cell aplasia in children [R]

- Transient erythroblastopenia of childhood.

This condition, in which red cells with fetal characteristics are absent, often follows acute virus infection. It has been found that serum from patients suppress both BFU-E and CFU-E (IgG antibody found in 8 of 12 cases, with no evidence of anti-erythropoietin activity).

- Pure red cell aplasia of adults [R]

This heterogeneous condition includes:

1. Self-limiting disease associated with infections, drugs etc.
2. Chronic disease:
   (a) associated with thymoma, lymphoproliferative disease, connective tissue disease;
   (b) idiopathic.

An IgG antibody has been demonstrated which interferes with erythroblast activity.

References
Krantz, S. B. (1974) *N. Engl. J. Med.* **291**, 345
Peschle, C., Marmont, A. M., Marone, G. *et al.* (1975) *Br. J. Haematol.* **30**, 411
Sief, C. (1983) *Br. J. Haematol.* **54**, 331

Secondary aplastic anaemia

Known bone-marrow depressants (dose-related)

Aminopterin, α-methopterin
Benzene
γ-benzene hexachloride
Busulphan
6-Mercaptopurine
Nitrogen mustards
Paraphenylenediamine
Triethylene melamine
Trinitrotoluene
Urethane

Drugs which may cause bone marrow depression (i.e. drugs to which a personal idiosyncrasy may develop)

Anti-epileptics

- Aloxidone.
- Methyl hydantoin.
- Paramethadione.
- Phenylacetylurea.
- Trimethyladione.

Antibiotics

- Chloramphenicol.
- Streptomycin.
- Sulphonamides.

Antirheumatics

- Gold salts.
- Phenylbutazone.

Other drugs

- Acetazolamide.
- Hydralazine.
- Mepacrine.
- Organic arsenicals.

Irradiation injury

Local irradiation exposure to 40–50 grays (Gy) results in marrow aplasia which resolves slowly, often incompletely, over several years. There was no increase in aplastic anaemia in the atomic bomb exposure survivors in Japan, whereas the incidence of aplastic anaemia is higher than in the general population, in ankylosing spondylitis patients treated with courses of irradiation and in radiologists.

Infections

1. Virus

HEPATITIS (usually non-A, non-B, = −C)

This occurs in 0.3–0.5% of cases, with a poor prognosis; 25% of patients with aplastic anaemia have abnormal liver function test results at diagnosis, suggesting subclinical infection or exposure to hepatotoxic agents.

Reference
Zeldis, J. B., Dienstag, J. C. and Gale, R. P. (1983) *Am. J. Med.* **74**, 64

HUMAN PARVOVIRUS (HPV)

This can cause acute red cell aplasia, which is not noticed in a normal individual, the normal red cell lifespan maintaining a satisfactory haemoglobin level during the acute interruption of red cell production. It is thought to be the causative agent of erythema infectiosum (fifth disease) in children. HPV aplastic crises are seen in homozygous sickle-cell disease, sometimes in hereditary spherocytosis, and a life-threatening outbreak has been described in patients with hereditary haemolytic anaemia in northern Ohio – all conditions with an abnormally short red cell lifespan.

References
Lefrere, J. J., Courouce, A-M., Girot, R. *et al.* (1986) *B. J. Haematol.* **62**, 653
Saarinen, U. M., Chorba, T. L., Tattersall, P. *et al.* (1986) *Blood* **67**, 1411

OTHER
- Infectious mononucleosis ⎫
- Dengue   ⎬ not common.
- Influenza   ⎭

2. Bacteria
- Tuberculosis and atypical mycobacterial infections.
- Brucellosis.

3. Parasitic diseases

Associated with peripheral cell destruction or hypersplenism.

4. Other conditions
- Paroxysmal nocturnal haemoglobinuria. Aplastic anaemia develops in up to 25% of cases; 5–10% of aplastic anaemia cases progress to paroxysmal nocturnal haemoglobinuria.
- Leukaemia: 1–5% of patients with aplastic anaemia have leukaemia. Rapid normalization of blood count following steroid therapy suggests underlying ALL rather than aplastic anaemia.
- Graft versus host disease: some cases progress to aplastic anaemia.

- Patients with primary or secondary cellular immune deficiency.
- Thymoma.
- X-linked lymphoproliferative system.
- Pre-ALL in childhood.
- Aplastic crises during sickle-cell disease, hereditary spherocytic anaemia, pyruvate kinase deficiency and thalassaemia intermedia are often associated with parvovirus infection.

Reference
Davis, L. R. (1983) *Br. J. Haematol.* **55**, 391

Treatment of aplastic anaemia

Eliminate exposure to any known cause.

Transfusion

- Washed red cells preferred to anaemia, to avoid antibody production.
- White cell transfusion—only useful if histocompatible, and only indicated in severe infections.
- Platelets—unnecessary if no overt bleeding. Preferably use single donor transfusions rather than pooled platelets (e.g. six different donors for six units of platelets) to avoid sensitization. ?Use white cell-poor platelets.

Steroids

Corticosteroid

?Improve capillary integrity, but they have undesirable side effects. Also ?prognosis of aplastic anaemia made worse by corticosteroid therapy.

Anabolic steroids

These may enhance red cell production, but are less effective in stimulating white cell and platelet production. They are not effective in severe aplastic anaemia.

Immunosuppressive treatment

Some cases benefit. In others, immunosuppression is used to prepare the patient for marrow transplanation. Patients with severe aplastic anaemia can be assessed for immunosuppressive therapy. Of those with pure red cell aplasia, perhaps 66% respond to immunosuppressive therapy and 56% respond to cytotoxics and steroids.

References
Clark. D. A., Dessypris, E. N. and Krantz, S. B. (1984) *Blood* **63**, 277
Torok-Storb, B., Doney, K., Brown, S. L. *et al.,* (1984) *Blood* **63**, 349
Gordon-Smith, E. C. (Ed.) 1989 Aplastic anaemia *Baillière's Clinical Haematology,* Vol. 2, No. 1. London: Baillière Tindall

Bone marrow transplantation

Reference
Camitta, B. M., Storb, R. and Thomas, E. D. (1982) *N. Engl. J. Med.* **306**, 645–712 (Review).

Drugs which may cause aplastic anaemia

The following drugs and chemicals are some of the substances which have been known to cause aplastic anaemia (not listed in order of severity or frequency of incidence). The incidence of aplastic anaemia due to drugs will obviosuly vary according to local prescription habits:

Apresoline
Arsenic, organic arsenicals, arsenobenzols
Benzene and volatile cellulose solvents

Note: commerical preparations of toluene and xylene may contain up to 20% of benzene. Pure preparations are probably not so dangerous.

Bismuth
Busulphan (Myleran)
Carbimazole (neo-mercazole)
Carbon tetrachloride
Chloramphenicol
Chlorophenothane (DDT)
Chlorpromazine
Chlortetracycline
Dinitrophenol
Gold and gold salts
Lead
Mepacrine
6-Mercaptopurines
Mercury
Methylmercaptoimidazole
Methylphenylethyl-hydantoin
Methylphenyl-hydantoin
Nitrogen mustards (also sulphur mustards)
Oxytetracyclines
Paraphenylenediamine hair dyes
Phenylbutazone (butazolidine)
Phosphorus
Pyribenzamine
Quinacrine (atebrine)
Silver, colloidal
Streptomycin
Sulphonamides
Thiosemicarbazones
Thorium dioxide
Triethylenemelamine (TEM)
Trimethadione
Trinitrotoluene
Troxidone
Urethane

In general, survival in aplastic anaemia is better in patients under 40 years old.
    Prognosis is worse:

- Over 40 years of age.

- Neutrophil count in peripheral blood less than $100 \times 10^6/l$.
- Pheripheral blood platelet count less than $20 \times 10^9/l$.
- High lymphocyte count in bone marrow.

Response to treatment with androgens or anabolic steroids takes at least 3 months of continuous treatment before it can be considered to have failed. A regenerative anaemia associated with hypercellular marrow shows a poor response to oxymethalone, and a high incidence of acute leukaemia.

Reference
Camitta, B. M., Storb, R. and Thomas, E. D. (1982) *N. Engl. J. Med.* **306**, 645, 712

Spleen

Splenic function

The blood flow through the spleen is at the rate of 150–200 ml/min. The splenic venules are surrounded by a cuff of predominantly T-lymphocytes, with an outer zone of predominantly B-lymphocytes in the germinal follicles. The blood flow through the spleen is divided into: less than 10% via the 'open' route through pulp cores where phagocytosis occurs, and more than 90% via the 'closed' route through the sinuses, where red cells have to undergo severe deformation to re-enter the circulation. The splenic tissue glucose is one-third of that existing in the peripheral blood, and any red cells with abnormalities of the enzyme systems, such that increased amounts of glucose are required for their survival, e.g. abnormalities of glycolytic enzymes, may be stressed to destruction. Similarly, the low oxygen tension in the splenic pulp stresses red cells sensitive to oxygen lack, e.g. sickle-cell disease. Red cells normally flow rapidly through the spleen, and red cell defects (e.g. spherocytosis) are of major importance in the severity of haemolysis due to splenic activity.

Reference
Ferrant, A., Leners, N., Michaux, J. L. *et al.*, (1987) *Br. J. Haematol.* **65**, 31

Reservoir

Normally about one-third of the total platelet mass is present in an exchangeable pool with the circulation. Only a relatively small number of red cells and neutrophils are sequestered in the spleen.

Phagocytosis

Macrophages in the pulp cords remove bacteria, especially pneumococci and bacteria with capsules, from the blood.

Red cells as they age expose surface antigens which indicate their senescence, and they are removed from the blood. Similarly, damaged red cells are removed.

The red cell membrane is repaired following the removal of:

- Red cell surface pits and craters.
- Howell–Jolly bodies.
- Heinz bodies.
- Pappenheimer bodies.
- Acanthrocytes.

In disease, the splenic reticuloendothelial cells remove:
- Spherocytes.
- Sickled cells.
- Haemoglobin C target cells.
- Antibody-coated red cells.
- Antibody-coated white blood cells.
- Antibody-coated platelets.

Splenic phagocytosis of red cells may occur in:

- Endocarditis.
- Infectious mononucleosis.
- Felty's syndrome.
- Portal hypertension.
- Chronic myeloid leukaemia.
- Myeloid metaplasia.
- Sarcoidosis.
- Amyloidosis.
- Gaucher's disease.
- Chronic lymphatic leukaemia.
- Lymphoma.

Immune response

Macrophages present bacteria and antigens to T-lymphocytes, which is turn stimulate B-lymphocytes to produce the necessary antibody to the invader. Blood borne antigen reaches the T-lymphocytes in the spleen and the same process occurs.

Haemopoiesis

The human fetal spleen is probably not a significant haemopoietic organ. In adult myelosclerosis, it has been suggested that primitive stem cells are reawakened in the spleen. In fact, findings in the fetal spleen suggest splenic trapping of normoblasts and rarely more primitive erythroid cells. This, in turn, suggests that haemopoietic cells are trapped in the spleen in myelosclerosis, rather than primarily multiplying there.

Reference
Wolf, B. C., Luevano, E. and Neiman, R. S. (1983) *Am. J. Clin. Pathol.* **80**, 140

Hypersplenism

For the diagnosis of hypersplenism to be made, the following criteria should be satisfied:

- Anaemia ⎫
- Neutropenia ⎬ Singly or in combination.
- Thrombocytopenia ⎭
- Active cellular marrow.
- Enlarged spleen.
- Demonstration of sequestration or pooling of red cells tagged with ^{51}Cr in the spleen.

Using a cell separator it may be possible to demonstrate that neutrophils labelled with ^{32}P-labelled di-isopropylfluorophosphate enter an enlarged splenic pool. Similarly platelets can be labelled, and an increase in the splenic platelet pool may be demonstrated.

- Return of the peripheral blood picture to normal after splenectomy.

Primary hypersplenism

Idiopathic; uncommon.

Secondary hypersplenism

Associated with red cell abnormality

Congenital

- Hereditary spherocytosis.
- Hereditary elliptocytosis.
- Pyruvate kinase deficiency.
- Thalassaemia.
- Haemoglobinopathies, e.g. sickle-cell disease.

Acquired

- Autoimmune haemolytic anaemia.
- Paroxysmal nocturnal haemoglobinuria.

Association with splenic abnormality

Chronic congestive splenomegaly

- Portal hypertension.
- Cirrhosis.

Lymphoma, lymphosarcoma, lymphadenoma (Hodgkin's disease), chronic lymphatic leukaemia

Myeloproliferative disorders

- Chronic myeloid leukaemia.
- Myelosclerosis.

Lipid storage diseases

- Gaucher's disease.
- Niemann–Pick disease.

- Hand–Schüller–Christian disease.
- Histiocytosis-X disease.

Infections

- Bacterial endocarditis.
- Brucellosis.
- Tuberculosis or syphilis, rarely.
- Malaria.
- Kala-azar.

Autoimmune

- Rheumatoid arthritis, Felty's syndrome, Still's disease.
- Systemic lupus erythematosus.

Other

Boeck's sarcoid.

Reference
Richards, J. D. (1976) *Hosp. Med.* **15**, 505

Postsplenectomy

Peripheral blood changes

The red cells have an increased surface area, MCV, mean surface area/MCV, osmotic resistance and reduced MCHC, compared with presplenectomy. They may contain Howell–Jolly bodies, increased stainable iron (siderocytes), target cells and occasional normoblasts, which would have been cleared by the spleen.

Neutrophilia develops after a few days, and may persist for months. The platelet count increases by the third to fourth day, with peak values (and risk of thrombosis) by the second week, falling slowly over months.

Reference
de Haan, L. D., Werre, J. M., Ruben, A. M. Th. *et al.* (1988) *Br. J. Haematol.* **69**, 71

Susceptibility to infection

Susceptibility to infection is increased, and serum from splenectomized patients may not promote normal phagocytosis and chemotaxis by neutrophils. Plasma IgM levels fall after splenectomy.

Overwhelming postsplenectomy infection (OPSI)

This may be due to *Streptococcus pneumoniae* (the most frequent), *Neisseria meningitidis*, *Escherichia coli* or *Haemophilus influenzae*, and children are particularly liable to fulminating septicaemia and meningitis. In malarial areas, infection with *Plasmodium falciparum* is very dangerous after splenectomy. Splenectomy in homozygous sickle disease in childhood requires preoperative 14-valent pneumococcal and *H*.

influenzae B vaccines, with long-term postoperative penicillin therapy.

References
Emond, A. N., Morais, P., Venugopal, S. *et al.* (1984) *Lancet* **i**, 88
Foster, P. N., Bolton, R. P., Cotter, K. L. and Losowsky, M. S. (1985) *J. Clin. Pathol.* **38**, 1175

Leucoerythroblastic (myelophthisic) anaemia

Immature red cells and white cells (normoblasts, myelocytes and myeloblasts) appear in the peripheral blood. The number of nucleated and red blood cells present is out of proportion to the degree of anaemia.

In about one-third of a series of cases the condition was associated with acute infection.

In a further one-third of the cases it was associated with myelofibrosis and malignant disease.

In the remaining one-third of the cases it was associated with haemolytic anaemia and miscellaneous conditions.

Leucoerythroblastic anaemia may be found in:

1. Metastatic carcinoma invading active bone marrow: leucoerythroblastic anaemia is said to be more common when the primary site is:
   (a) breast;
   (b) prostate;
   (c) lungs;
   (d) thyroid;
   (e) adrenal.

2. Acute leukaemia, and chronic leukaemia in relapse: in the lymphocytic varieties lymphoblasts are seen in the peripheral blood. Pancytopenia with small numbers of circulating 'blast' cells may indicate hypoplastic acute myelogenous leukaemia, which has a slow progressive course.
3. Aleukaemic leukaemia.
4. Erythraemic myelosis (Di Guglielmo's disease): the nucleated red cells resemble megaloblasts.
5. Myelosclerosis (agnogenic myeloid metaplasia).
6. Myelofibrosis.
7. Haemolytic disease of the newborn.
8. Marble-bone disease (Albers–Schönberg disease, osteopetrosis).
9. Myeloma (5% of cases).
10. Hodgkin's disease (some cases).
11. Thrombotic thrombocytopenic purpura.
12. Primary lipid storage disease:
    (a) Gaucher's disease;
    (b) Niemann–Pick disease;
    (c) Hand–Schüller–Christian disease.
13. Occasionally occurs:
    (a) after severe haemorrhage;
    (b) in some cases of severe sepsis;
    (c) after irradiation;
    (d) after poisoning with benzene, carbon tetrachloride, fluorine or phosphorus;
    (e) in some cases of disseminated tuberculosis.

References
Retief, F. P. (1964) *Lancet* **i**, 639
Weick, J. K., Hagedorn, A. B. and Linman, J. W. (1974) *Mayo Clin. Proc.* **49**, 110

Chapter 3

Haemoglobin and its disorders

Haemoglobin oxygen dissociation curve

(SI unit conversion factor = 0.133, i.e. 90–100 mmHg becomes 12–15 kPa)

The speed of reaction of uptake of oxygen or its release by haemoglobin is 0.07 second(s). Since blood is in the alveolar capillary for 0.5 s there is adequate time for oxygen uptake in the lungs, and similarly there is adequate time for release of oxygen to the tissues. Myoglobin, with a single molecule binding a single oxygen molecule, has a hyperbolic oxygen dissociation curve and a high affinity for oxygen. If the four molecules of oxygen carried by a haemoglobin tetramer were all bound equally, the curve would not change its shape. In fact, haemoglobin has a sigmoid oxygen dissociation curve. At the steepest slope of this S-shaped curve, a relatively small change in oxygen tension results in either rapid release or uptake of oxygen – i.e. rapid delivery of oxygen to the peripheral tissues where the oxygen tension is lower (PO_2 of 4–40 mmHg or 0.53–5.3 kPa) or rapid uptake of an equally large amount of oxygen in the lungs. Over this steep part of the curve, oxyhaemoglobin is very unstable. Haemoglobin operates by loading and unloading the β-chain, and affinity for oxygen increases with the level of oxygenation, oxygen being passed to the β-chain.

The change in the haem portion from oxy- to deoxy-, ready for more oxygen, takes less than 30 picoseconds.

The increase in the affinity of the available binding sites in the molecule by the binding of one oxygen molecule results in the sigmoid shape of the oxygen dissociation curve – in biochemistry, the so-called cooperative effect.

Various factors tend to shift the slope of the curve to the left or to the right, so that the steepest part of the slope moves into either a lower partial pressure of oxygen, or a higher one. It is normally kept in a fairly constant position by a balance of many factors.

A 'shift to the right' implies greater ease of release of oxygen to the tissues, but if the shift is excessive there is little effective oxygen transport by the blood at moderate PO_2 tension. Conversely, a 'shift to the left' of the curve implies a greater avidity in the red cells for oxygen, with no release of oxygen to the tissues until very low PO_2 values are reached.

Reference
Genberg, L., Richard, L., McLendon, G. and Miller, R. J. D. (1991) *Science* **251**, 1051

Introduction

In 1628, William Harvey described the unidirectional flow of blood in humans and, in 1674, Anthony Van Leewenhoek, using a simple microscope he had designed and made himself, was the first to describe red blood cells. It was not until 1865, however, that the content of red cells, haemoglobin, was described by Hoppe-Seyler and its fundamental importance in the transport of oxygen realized. In 1924, G. S. Adair calculated the molecular weight of haemoglobin as 68 000, comprising four subunits ($\alpha_2\beta_2$) of molecular weight 16 700 each. This was later confirmed by Svedberg. Since then the amino acid sequence of the protein chains that make up human haemoglobin have been established and Max Perutz, using X-ray crystallography, has described the shape and structure of the haemoglobin molecule.

Reference
Brzozowski, A., Derewenda, Z. Dodson E. *et al.* (1984) *Nature* **307**, 74.

Partial pressure of oxygen ($P_{50}\,O_2$)

The measurement of the partial pressure of oxygen at which there is 50% saturation of haemoglobin with oxygen can be used to demonstrate any shift to the left or right of the dissociation curve.

Normal $P_{50}\,O_2 = 27.0 \pm 1.2$ mmHg at pH 7.4 and 38°C.

'Shift to the right' of haemoglobin oxygen dissociation curve

- Carbon dioxide increase, e.g. chronic lung disease.
- Falling blood pH.
- Low oxygen tension, e.g. first 24 h at high altitude.
- Increased temperature.
- Hyperthyroidism, with high red cell 2,3-diphosphoglycerate (2,3-DPG).
- Anaemia of chronic renal failure.
- Pyruvate kinase deficiency (with high red cell 2,3-DPG and $P_{50} O_2$).
- Sickle-cell anaemia. Although HbS has a greater affinity for oxygen than HbA, red cell 2,3-DPG is high.

'Shift to the left' of haemoglobin oxygen dissociation curve

- Normal fetal haemoglobin: the oxygen affinity of HbF is higher than that of HbA, facilitating oxygen diffusion from mother to fetus across the placenta and delivery of oxygen to the fetal tissues at a low oxygen partial pressure. The $P_{50}O_2$ is lower in pre-term infants with a high concentration of HbF. In addition to increased oxygen avidity, HbF does not bind 2,3-DPG as much as does HbA.
- Abnormal haemoglobins (HbH, haemoglobin Bart's) have increased oxygen affinity.
- During hypothermia.
- Increased oxygen tension in the hyperbaric chamber. This is not important as oxygen is transported to the tissues adequately in the plasma.
- Anaemia.
- Inert haemoglobin pigments – carboxyhaemoglobin, methaemoglobin and sulphaemoglobin – in high enough concentrations cause tissue anoxia.
- Red cell hexokinase deficiency – low $P_{50} O_2$ with very low red cell 2,3-DPG concentration.
- Hypophosphataemia – resulting in low red cell 2,3-DPG in severe diabetic ketosis, with peripheral tissue anoxia.
- Hypothyroidism, with low red cell 2,3-DPG.
- Stored blood with low 2,3-DPG concentration if acid–citrate–glucose solution is used, Citrate–dextrose–phosphate solution helps to maintain red cell 2,3-DPG.

Reference
Holland, B. M., Jones, J. G. and Wardrop, C. A. J. (1987) In Oski, F. A. (Ed.) *Haematology/Oncology Clinics of North America*, vol. 1 No. 3, p. 355. New York: W. B. Saunders.

The red cell 2,3-diphosphoglycerate shunt

2,3-DPG is present in human red cells at the same molar concentration as haemoglobin. It is also present in high concentration in the red cells of horse, dog, rabbit, rat and guinea-pig, but only in low concentration in the red cells of sheep, goat, cow and cat. 2,3-DPG plays a very important part in human red cells in maintaining the sigmoid shape of the oxygen – haemoglobin dissociation curve, facilitating oxygen release to the tissues. The oxygen dissociation curve of a dialysed solution of haemoglobin is less sigmoid in shape than the curve obtained using intact red cells containing normal adult haemoglobin; it has a high oxygen affinity and does not release its oxygen easily as the partial pressure of oxygen falls. The higher the red cell 2,3-DPG concentration, the further the oxygen dissociation curve shifts to the right. For example, a 24% increase in red cell 2,3-DPG concentration above normal shifts the oxygen half-saturation point for haemoglobin upwards, so that there is an increase of 22% in oxygen release to the tissues. This is very important, as this is at about the partial pressure of oxygen found in the capillaries of the tissues.

The concentration of 2,3-DPG in the free unbound form is maintained by enzymatic action, and 2,3-DPG binds preferentially to deoxyhaemoglobin rather than to oxyhaemoglobin. In anaemia, the tissues remove relatively more oxygen from the circulating haemoglobin, and the increased concentration of deoxyhaemoglobin in the blood in the peripheral tissues binds the available free 2,3-DPG. The reduction in free 2,3-DPG results in increased formation of 2,3-DPG, increasing the total 2,3-DPG in the red cells in anaemia. This causes a tendency to a 'right shift' of the haemoglobin–oxygen dissociation curve, compensating the tendency to 'left shift' in anaemia.

Exercise, with a greater utilization of oxygen by the tissues, also results in increased red cell 2,3-DPG, which increases oxygen availability to the tissues per unit of blood. 2,3-DPG helps to reduce the post-exercise lactic acid concentration and oxygen consumption when exercise stops. An increase in red cell 2,3-DPG with a 'right shift' of the curve occurs in altitude acclimatization.

Fetal haemoglobin has evolved to pick up oxygen in the placenta and deliver it to the fetal tissues at lower partial pressures of oxygen than in the adult. Following normal birth, the oxygen dissociation curve shifts to the right as haemoglobin F is replaced by haemoglobin A, and red cell 2,3-DPG increases. Even though the haemoglobin level falls from about 17 g/dl to 11 g/dl during the first few months after birth, oxygen delivery to the tissues is better than at birth. In premature infants with a higher proportion of HbF and lower red cell 2,3-DPG, any respiratory distress results in a fall in pH, further reduction in 2,3-DPG and even less effective delivery of oxygen to the tissues, and HbF binds less 2,3-DPG anyway.

In patients with a low blood pH, there is a decreased affinity of haemoglobin for oxygen, the Bohr effect, resulting in low red cell 2,3-DPG. The low pH inhibits the mutase activity and stimulates the phosphatase activity. If severe metabolic acidosis with lactic acidosis is treated with sodium bicarbonate solution, the sudden increase in blood pH temporarily increases the red cell haemoglobin affinity for oxygen, exacerbating tissue hypoxia. When the glycolytic pathway is interfered with, in the rare haemolytic anaemia associated with hexokinase deficiency, 2,3-DPG is not formed in adequate amounts and there is a 'left shift' in the oxygen dissociation curve, with a greater tendency to tissue anoxia at any given reduced haemoglobin concentration, when compared with anaemia and normal red cells. By way of contrast, in the less rare haemolytic anaemia associated with pyruvate kinase deficiency, with a metabolic blockade below 2,3-DPG in the glycolytic pathway, the red cell 2,3-DPG is extremely high. This results in far greater toleration of relatively severe anaemia with adequate tissue oxygenation.

As would be expected, red cell 2,3-DPG concentration falls in stored blood, as the red cell glucose is used up.

2,3-DPG inhibits platelet aggregation, and probably therefore helps to protect against thrombosis in hypochromic anaemia, sickle-cell anaemia and chronic nephritis.

Increased red cell 2,3-DPG with reduced oxygen affinity of haemoglobin

- Pregnancy.
- Altitude hypoxia.
- Anaemia.
- Alkalosis.
- Hyperphosphataemia.
- Renal failure.
- Thyrotoxicosis.
- Cyanotic heart disease.
- Pyruvate kinase deficiency.
- Thalassaemia.
- Sickle-cell disease.

Decreased red cell 2,3-DPG with increased oxygen affinity of haemoglobin

- Following transfusion of stored blood.
- Hypophosphataemia, e.g. during diabetic ketoacidosis.
- Acidosis, e.g. lactic acidosis.
- Hypothyroidism.
- Severe septicaemia.
- Hexokinase deficiency.

Blood oxygen

One gram of haemoglobin, when fully converted to oxyhaemoglobin, has combined with 1.36 ml of oxygen at NTP (normal temperature and pressure). The oxygen capacity measures the total effective haemoglobin (oxyhaemoglobin and reduced haemoglobin), but not carboxyhaemoglobin, methaemoglobin or sulphaemoglobin. Normal arterial blood is not less than 94% saturated with oxygen, whilst normal venous blood averages 70–90% saturated. The oxygen carrying capacity of an infant's blood can be reduced by 15–31% by Rh antibodies, and this loss of efficiency is exaggerated by any associated anaemia.

Abnormal blood pigments

1. Methaemoglobin

Methaemoglobin, with the haem iron oxidized to the ferric state, is an inert non-toxic substance normally formed continuously in red cells during glycolysis. It cannot carry or deliver oxygen. The ferric iron is continuously reduced back to the ferrous state to restore normal haemoglobin, and NADH-linked methaemoglobin reductase I accounts for over 60% of this reconversion. NADH-methaemoglobin reductase II and NADPH-methaemoglobin reductase are minor pathways, as are the non-enzymatic activities of ascorbic acid and reduced glutathione. In the absence of the reductase system, methaemoglobin accumulates at 3% each day; normally methaemoglobin is kept below 1%. Both ascorbic acid and methylene blue are agents which can be used to reduce methaemoglobinaemia.

Methaemoglobinaemia

Methaemoglobin remains in the red cells during their life time, unless haemolysis releases the pigment into the plasma. As the methaemoglobin concentration rises in the blood, the oxygen dissociation curve is shifted to the left (as with carbon monoxide), limiting oxygen transfer to the tissues, and eventually causing tissue anoxia. Cyanosis is apparent when there is 1.5 g% of methaemoglobin (compare 5 g of deoxygenated haemoglobin which causes visible cyanosis). Levels of 10–20% cause dyspnoea and headache, unlike an equivalent drop in haemoglobin in anaemia.

Congenital

1. NADH-linked methaemoglobin reductase deficiency [R] [AR] – with 10–20% methaemoglobin in red cells from birth. Up to half the patients suffer

from mental handicap. The methaemoglobin increases with age, with a compensatory increase in the packed cell volume. The deficiency of enzyme activity is due to an abnormal enzyme structure in most cases, but rarely to a deficiency of the enzyme. Treatment with 300–500 mg ascorbic acid daily reduces the cyanosis. Heterozygotes are clinically normal, but they are abnormally susceptible to the effects of oxidant drugs, e.g. some antimalarials.
2. The newborn infant's red cells have a low NADH-linked methaemoglobin reductase activity, and very young infants are very susceptible to oxidant substances.
3. M-haemoglobins – various haemoglobinopathies in this group are associated with excessive methaemoglobinaemia and a compensatory increase in the packed cell volume. The abnormal α-chain type has obvious cyanosis from birth. In the abnormal β-chain type cyanosis appears after a few weeks, with reduction in haemoglobin F synthesis.

Acquired

1. Oxidant substances which may cause methaemoglobinaemia – especially in infants and heterozygotes for reductase deficiency: amyl nitrate and related substances in abnormally large doses, aniline dyes, antipyrine, chlorate, chromate, bivalent copper, dyes with a high oxidation–reduction potential, ferricyanide, lead, nitrates converted to nitrite in the gut, nitrite, nitrobenzene, phenacetin, phenylhydrazine, primaquine, quinones, sulphasalazine, sulphonamides, sulphone, vitamin K analogues in high dosage.
2. Methaemoglobinaemia with chronic intravascular haemolysis – prolonged exposure to aniline dyes, dapsone, sulphasalazine, phenacetin.
3. Methaemoglobinaemia with acute intravascular haemolysis – severe poisoning with chlorate or arsine gas, requiring urgent exchange transfusion. Methylene blue should not be used.

2. Sulphaemoglobin

The structure of sulphaemoglobin is not known. It is an inert non-toxic substance which cannot carry or deliver oxygen, does not alter the red cell lifespan, and remains in cells until they are removed from the circulation. Sulphaemoglobin only appears in the plasma after lysis of red cells containing the pigment. There are no genetic disorders which result in sulphaemoglobinaemia.

Sulphaemoglobinaemia [R]

This sometimes develops after phenacetin or sulphonamides. It has also been described as occurring rarely in chronic constipation and malabsorption, possibly resulting from hydrogen sulphide or related substances formed in the gut. Cyanosis is apparent when 3–5 g% of the total haemoglobin is in the form of sulphaemoglobin.

3. Carboxyhaemoglobin

The affinity of haemoglobin for carbon monoxide is over 200 times its affinity for oxygen. The higher the carboxyhaemoglobin concentration in the blood, the less haemoglobin will be available for oxygen carriage. Therefore anaemic patients will suffer from carbon monoxide poisoning sooner and more severely than normal people. Also, the haemoglobin–oxygen dissociation curve shifts to the left, and therefore oxygen release to the tissues is less effective in the presence of carboxyhaemoglobin.

Carbon monoxide in inspired air

- A concentration of 0.1% produces a blood carboxyhaemoglobin concentration of about 50% in 1h.
- A concentration of 0.2% will cause death within a few hours.
- A concentration of 0.4% is fatal in less than 1h.
- A concentration of 1.0% produces a lethal concentration in less than 10 min.

Blood–carboxyhaemoglobin concentrations

- Normal tobacco smoker – up to 5% carboxyhaemoglobin. This eventually results in an increased haematocrit (smoker's polycythaemia). The carboxyhaemoglobin concentration in a chain-smoker peaks late in the afternoon or evening, and the MCV is often increased (compare primary polycythaemia).
- Symptom free – up to 15–20% carboxyhaemoglobin.
- Nausea, weakness and dyspnoea – up to 50% carboxyhaemoglobin.
- Unconsciousness – 50–70% carboxyhaemoglobin.
- Rapid death – more than 80% carboxyhaemoglobin.
- Breathing air eliminates 50% of the carbon monoxide in the blood in 2–3h, compared with 15–30 min when pure oxygen is breathed. Hyperbaric oxygen is even more effective.

Note

- Carboxyhaemoglobin can only be detected by using a direct vision spectroscope when the blood concentration exceeds 30%.
- Rapid, accurate estimation of concentrations greater than 5–10% can be made using a reversion spectroscope.
- Following death at a fire, if concentration of carboxyhaemoglobin less than 10%, then probably death occurred before the fire.
- The rate of absorption of carbon monoxide is directly related to the degree of physical activity. When breathing air, carboxyhaemoglobin has a biological half-life of 250 min. This falls to 40 min if pure oxygen is breathed.

Myoglobin

Myoglobin is a ferrous–porphyrin complex with a molecular weight of 17 000 (one-quarter of haemoglobin). Each molecule contains one atom of ferrous iron, a fetal form preceding the adult form. It has a higher affinity for oxygen than haemoglobin, and acts as an oxygen store for muscle cells, releasing its oxygen to cytochrome oxidase when the oxygen supply is limited. Abnormal forms have been described in juvenile muscular dystrophy, some cases of myoglobinuria and some cases of dermatomyositis, but these do not cause defective muscle action.

Myoglobin in plasma and urine

Following release of myoglobin from muscle, it rapidly appears in the urine and disappears from the plasma, as its renal threshold is low, at about 15 mg/dl plasma.

Myoglobinuria

Myoglobin appears in the urine of both humans and horses after severe unaccustomed exercise.

Pathological

Rhabdomyolysis results from a massive release of calcium from the sarcoplastic reticulum in the cytosol, causing ATP breakdown, muscle contraction and necrosis.

- Rhabdomyolysis resulting in myoglobinuria occurs in men after severe unaccustomed exercise, especially following repeated eccentric contractions, for example, repeated 'press ups' by raw recruits in training, especially if dehydrated and hyperthermic.

- Trauma to muscle – including crush injury, muscle necrosis following thrombus in an artery supplying a large muscle mass, high-voltage electric shock, severe postural pressure after lying unconscious without movement for a long time.
- Following virus infection, including influenza, Coxsackie virus etc.
- Anoxia as a result of carbon monoxide poisoning, carbon monoxide replacing oxygen in the myoglobin molecule or anoxia in muscles following prolonged convulsions.
- Metabolic disturbances associated with alcohol or heroin abuse, hypersensitivity to ε-aminocaproic acid, severe hypokalaemia or hyperkalaemia, severe metabolic acidosis, heat stroke, acute hypophosphataemia, acute renal failure, anaesthetic agents including halothane, cyclopropane and other muscle relaxants; also disseminated intravascular coagulopathy.
- Inherited metabolic disorders including, malignant hyperpyrexia, McArdle's phosphorylase deficiency, Tarius's phosphofructokinase deficiency, idiopathic and familial paroxysmal myoglobinuria, mitochondrial inherited muscle disease.
- Hornet venom, and frequently after sea snake bite.

Haemoglobin synthesis

Regulation of haemoglobin synthesis

Nucleotide sequences which specify the structure of globins are encoded in discontinuous segments of DNA, flanked by portions of the gene that do not code for recognizable protein (introns).

Gene transcription occurs, and results in a longer nuclear RNA precursor that includes RNA transcripts of the intervening 'nonsense' sequences.

Nuclear RNA is processed to remove the intervening sequences, and the protein-coding segments (exons) are spliced together. A special cap structure is added, which ensures efficient translation, and a poly(A) tail is attached, which enhances the stability of mRNA.

Mature mRNA is translated on cytoplasmic polyribosomes with the aid of initiation and elongation factors and the transfer RNAs that convey the specified amino acids to the growing polypeptide chain. When the code for termination is translated, the globin chain production ceases in a chain length of: (1) 141 amino acid residues for α-like chains; (2) 146 amino acid residues for non-α-chains.

By 8–10 weeks in the fetus γ- and β-chain synthesis begins. γ-Chain synthesis is maximal by 30 weeks, and

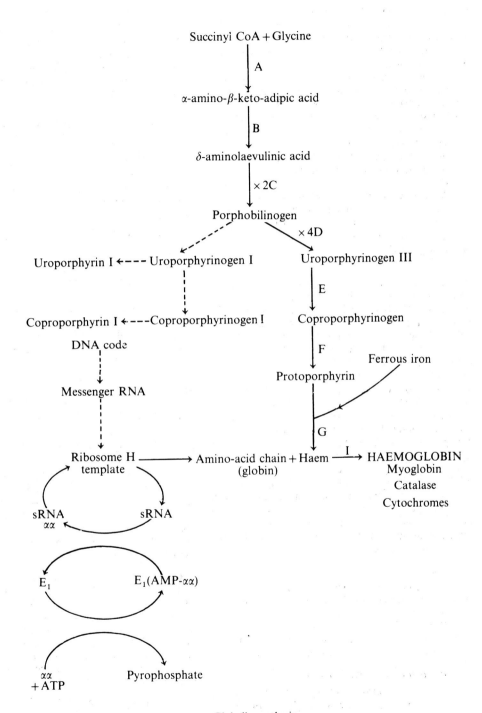

Globulin synthesis.

A = δ-aminolaevulinic synthetase. This reaction occurs in the mitochondria, depends on the presence of vitamin B_6, and is a rate controller of haemoglobin synthesis. It is inhibited by free haem.

B = decarboxylase.

C = δ-aminolaevulinic dehydrase.

D = porphobilinogen deaminase, followed by isomerase.

E = uroporphyringen decarboxylase.

F = corproporphyrinogen oxidase followed by protoporphyrinogen oxidase.

G = haem synthetase: in this reaction, ferrous iron is combined with protoporphyrin to form haem. The reaction is stimulated by the presence of free iron. It occurs in the mitochondria.

H = the complicated mechanism required for the synthesis of the globin chains. Globin synthesis is stimulated by the presence in the cell of free haem, and it is inhibited by low haem concentrations.

I = attachment of haem to globin chains, to form haemoglobin, myoglobin and haem-containing enzymes.

then declines, until at term, the proportions are 80% and 20%. The γ-chain synthesis is then switched off. δ-Chain synthesis starts just after birth and HbA_2 remains at about 2% of the total haemoglobin. γ-Chain synthesis is replaced by α-chain synthesis, such that total α-chain production balances $(\beta + \gamma + \delta)$ production.

Faults in haemoglobin production occur at various sites in the production chain and these include the thalassaemias.

Normal haemoglobin consists of two pairs of identical polypeptide chains, each chain carrying a haem group. The ferrous iron atom in each haem molecule is attached chemically to the proximal histidyl residue in the polypeptide chain, but not to the distal histidyl residue, and the amino acid residues lying in the loop between the proximal and distal histidyl residues form the so-called 'haem pocket'. Of all charged amino acids, histidine is the only one with fluctuation in the state of ionization of the imidazole group within the physiological pH range.

α-CHAINS

These consist of 141 amino acid residues, with histidyl residues at positions no. 87 (proximal) and 58 (distal).

β-, δ- AND γ-CHAINS

These consist of 146 amino acid residues, with histidyl residues at positions no. 92 (proximal) and 63 (distal).

Classification of disorders of haemoglobin synthesis

1. (a) Failure of normal switch from fetal to adult haemoglobin synthesis, e.g. haemoglobin F persistence.
   (b) Thalassaemia:

(i) α-thalassaemia;
(ii) β-thalassaemia.

2. Inherited abnormality of haemoglobin structure which may result in:
   (a) Increased tendency to haemolysis, due to inherent instability in the haemoglobin molecule.
   (b) Abnormality in oxygen transport:
      (i) increased oxygen affinity, with associated polycythaemia;
      (ii) decreased oxygen affinity.
   (c) Deficient rate of formation of haemoglobin, e.g. haemoglobin Lepore, especially in association with another haemoglobin abnormality.

3. Abnormalities in the rates of haemoglobin synthesis, e.g. thalassaemia.

Haemoglobins

Haemoglobin Gower 1 and 2: $\alpha_2\varepsilon_2$ occurs in the fetus before 10 weeks.

Reference
Lorkin P. A. (1973) *J. Med. Genet.* **10**, 50.

- Hb Gower 1 $\zeta_2\varepsilon_2$.
- Hb Gower 2 probably $\alpha_2\varepsilon_2$.
- Hb Gower 3 $\zeta_2\gamma_2$.

Normal adult haemoglobin (haemoglobin F): $\alpha_2\gamma_2$.
Normal adult haemoglobin (haemoglobin A): $\alpha_2\beta_2$.
Normal adult haemoglobin variant (haemoglobin A_2): $\alpha_2\delta_2$.

Reference
Fantoni, A., Ferace, M. G. and Gambari, R. (1981) *Blood* **57**, 623.

HAEMOGLOBIN F $(\alpha_2\gamma_2)$

In 20–25% of normal pregnant women there is a temporary increase in HbF of maternal origin, suggesting that a factor is synthesized in early pregnancy, which is capable of inducing HbF synthesis. Fifty-five to 98% of the infant's haemoglobin at birth is of the fetal type (haemoglobin F). No fetal haemoglobin is detectable in the normal infant's blood at the end of the first year, and most of the fetal haemoglobin has been replaced by adult haemoglobin (haemoglobin A) by the third month.

Normal newborn: $71 \pm 7.7\%$ haemoglobin F.
Pre-term infant: $81 \pm 4.7\%$ haemoglobin F.
Post-term infant: may be as low as 55% haemoglobin F.
Normal adult: not more than 2% as haemoglobin F.
HbF exists as two molecular species, $\alpha_2\gamma_2^{136gly}$ and $\alpha_2\gamma_2^{136ala}$ in a ratio of 3:1 in cord blood and 2:3 in adult blood.

Abnormal persistence of haemoglobin F

1. Absence of activity of both β- and δ-chain messenger RNA:

(a) West African variety:
   homozygote haemoglobin F = 60–90%;
   heterozygote haemoglobin F = 25%;
(b) *Greek variety*: heterozygote haemoglobin F = 10–20%. Haemoglobin A_2 is not reduced, and haemoglobin F is distributed evenly through the red cells;
(c) *Swiss variety*: haemoglobin F 1–2%. Haemoglobin A_2 levels are normal (These subjects are otherwise clinically normal, and they are usually detected during screening programmes for haemoglobinopathies);
(d) Negro or Greek persistent HbF + heterozygote β-thalassaemia;
(e) British hereditary persistence of HbF. HbF 20% in homozygotes, otherwise normal haematological findings.

References
Weatherall, D. J. and Clegg J. B. (1975) *Br. J. Haematol.* **29**, 191
Wood, W. G. Clegg, J. B. and Weatherall, D. J. (1979) *Br. J. Haematol.* **43**, 509

2. Associated with haemoglobinopathies:
   (a) β-thalassaemia;
   (b) *sickle-cell anaemia*: Shia Arabs with sickle-cell disease;
   (c) *Haemoglobin Lepore disease*.
3. Hypoplastic and aplastic anaemias:
   (a) *Fanconi's aplastic anaemia*;
   (b) Other aplastic anaemias in young children. In those cases which respond to treatment with anabolic steroids those with up to 10% HbF survive longer.
4. D_1 trisomy syndrome.
5. Juvenile chronic myeloid leukaemia. HbF 20–60%.
6. Myeloblastic and myelomonocytic leukaemia in children. HbF up to 6%.
7. Mean HbF and number of HbF-containing red cells greater than normal in untreated hyperthyroidism, returning to normal on treatment.

Reference
Davidson, R. J., How, J., Bewsher, P. D. *et al.* (1981) *Scand. J. Haematol.* **27**, 130.

8. Occasionally:
   (a) megaloblastic anaemia;
   (b) polycythaemia vera;
   (c) haemolytic anaemia;
   (d) aplastic anaemia;
   (e) macroglobulinaemia;
   (f) metastatic bone marrow carcinoma;
   (g) fetal bleed into the maternal circulation;
   (h) some leukaemia cases.

HbF is the predominant haemoglobin in early erythroblasts in pernicious anaemia, and in both early and late erythroid elements in erythroleukaemia and erythremic myelosis.

Reference
Forni, M., Meyer, P. R., Levy, N. B. *et al.* (1983) *Am. J. Clin. Pathol.* **80**, 145

Tests for the presence of haemoglobin F

1. Paper, starch gel or cellulose acetate electrophoresis.
2. Alkali denaturation test: fetal haemoglobin (and also haemoglobin Barts – γ_4), when treated with alkali, is more slowly converted to alkaline haematin than is adult haemoglobin. This delay in conversion is used to detect and estimate the percentage of fetal haemoglobin present in a given blood sample. The test is of particular use in the detection of fetal bleeding in utero, revealed by the presence of fetal haemoglobin in vaginal bleeding in the mother, or in circulating fetal haemoglobin in the maternal circulation.
   Because of the relative insensitivity of the method of estimation, results showing less than 2% of fetal haemoglobin may be regarded as normal.

Reference
Singer, K., Chernoff, A. I. and Singer, L. (1951) *Blood* **6**, 413

3. Detection of fetal red cells: fetal erythrocytes can be differentially stained in the presence of adult red cells. The detection of fetal red cells in the maternal circulation is important when a severe loss has occurred from the fetus, but also when there is a serious risk of the mother becoming immunized against the fetal red cell blood groups.

Reference
Zipursky, A., Hull, A., White, F. D. *et al.* (1959) *Lancet* **i**, 451

HAEMOGLOBIN A_2 $(\alpha_2\delta_2)$

Normal cord blood: 0.05–0.45%
Normal adult blood: 1.5–3%

Pathological increase

β-Thalassaemia, both homozygote and heterozygote.
Megaloblastic anaemia.
Unstable haemoglobin disease.

Pathological decrease

β-δ-Thalassaemia.
Haemoglobin Lepore.
HbH disease.
Severe iron deficiency anaemia.
Some sideroblastic anaemias.
Hereditary persistence of HbF.

Haemoglobin abnormalities

Haemoglobin abnormalities may be congenital or acquired. In this section, we shall consider congenital abnormalities of globin chains.

Congenital chain abnormalities

These can be qualitative, e.g. sickle-cell disease, where there is synthesis of an abnormal globin chain, or quantitative, e.g. β-thalassaemia, where there is absent or reduced synthesis of an otherwise normal globin chain.

Qualitative abnormalities

Virtually all known clinically significant changes affect the β-chain. The gene for the β-chain is found on chromosome 11, closely associated with the genes for δ-chain and γ-chain;

Chromosome 11

5'----[ ]----[ ]--------[ ]----[ ]----3'
      Gγ Aγ δ β

The β-gene region has been completely mapped.

Reference
Sander-Haigh, L., Anderson, W. F. and Franke, U. (1980) *Nature* **283**, 683–686

Sickle-cell disease (HbS)

First described by Herrick in Chicago during 1910, this life-threatening disorder is caused by a point mutation in the β-gene. A codon change from -GAG- to -GUG- means that glutamic acid is changed to valine at position 6 of the β-chain. This simple substitution brings about the synthesis of HbS.

If a single βS-gene is inherited then the heterozygous or carrier state will be seen clinically, which is associated with normal quality of life. Both HbA and HbS will be found in red blood cells. When two βS-genes are inherited, then the red cells contain more than 90% HbS and the patient suffers from sickle-cell disease.

The fundamental problem is that HbS is unstable when deoxygenated and will precipitate to form a gel, as oxygen leaves the red blood cell in the peripheral circulation. The precipitation and gel formation causes marked changes in the shape of the red blood cell with membrane projections and damage. Many cells take on the characteristic 'sickle' shape that gives the disease its name. Ultimately, these sickle-shaped red blood cells are unable to regain their original shape even when HbS becomes reoxygenated. Such 'fixed sickle cells' are rapidly removed from the circulation by the spleen. Some undergo intravascular haemolysis. Clearly this results in a chronic haemolytic anaemia.

However, the major clinical problem in sickle-cell disease is not haemolysis, but vasocclusion. This latter occurs because, following 'gel formation', the altered red blood cells may become rigid and unable to squeeze through the capillaries. Whether the capillaries become blocked or not depends on:

1. The time to gel formation – which may be 1–15 seconds.
2. The capillary transit time.

If (2) is longer than (1), the red blood cell will become rigid and may block the capillary. Gel formation time is affected by the following:

1. Rate of oxygen extraction.
2. pH.
3. HbS concentration.
4. The presence of other haemoglobins – HbF, HbA, HbC Harlem and Hb Memphis reduce gel formation (i.e. reduce sickling): HbO Arab, HbD Punjab and both variants at β 121 promote gel formation (i.e. increase sickling).

Vasocclusion, causing severe pain and damage to tissues, is responsible for the serious, life-threatening pathology of sickle-cell disease.

• World distribution

The sickle-cell gene is found right across Central Africa. It was originally thought to have arisen by mutation in West Africa and spread by population movements. However, recent DNA analysis suggests that the gene has appeared independently in West Africa, East Africa, central India and perhaps northern Greece. The gene has been spread in recent centuries by the slave trade to the West Indies and the Americas. Immigration from the West Indies to the UK has further distributed the gene and, of course, the disorder.

• Clinical problems

The diagnosis of sickle-cell disease is a simple matter. Patients have a haemoglobin of between 6 to 10 g/dl in the stable state and the blood film shows a variable number of elongated 'sickle'-shaped red blood cells. There may be target cells. Haemoglobin electrophoresis, on cellulose acetate at pH 8.2, shows an abnormal band, HbS, running separately from a control HbA band.

A small amount of HbA_2 (2–5%) and a variable amount of HbF (2–40%) make up the rest of the haemoglobin. Persistent high levels of HbF protect against sickling and give rise to a mild clinical picture. This is clearly seen in Arabia where high HbF levels (4–40%) in patients with sickle-cell disease often means a benign clinical course. West African patients, however, with HbF levels at 2–16% nearly always have severe disease.

Haemoglobin electrophoresis must always be carried out to confirm the diagnosis. When a diagnosis of sickle-cell disease has been made, family studies should be completed. Family members who are heterozygous will have two bands on electrophoresis: HbA, 60%; HbS, 40%. Those people with sickle-cell trait lead a normal life, their red blood cells do not sickle under physiological conditions. There have been cases of splenic infarct at high altitude and they do occasionally develop haematuria, due to papillary necrosis.

At birth, babies with sickle-cell disease are normal as most haemoglobin is still HbF. By 6 months, however, when the β-chain production is in full swing and HbS levels rise, the first vasocclusive crisis will occur. There is early damage to the spleen causing hyposplenism and life-threatening infections with *Streptococcus pneumoniae* and *Haemophilus influenzae*.

Bony infarction, particularly of hands and feet, will cause painful swellings and ultimately unequal growth of digits. Osteomyelitis may also follow with staphylococcal or salmonella infection. Splenic sequestration with rapid reduction of circulating blood volume can cause sudden death in young children. It must be treated promptly with blood transfusion, so parents must be taught to recognize the signs and bring their child immediately to hospital. Splenectomy should be considered to prevent further attacks. Aplastic crisis following infection with parvovirus B19 requires blood transfusion support until the marrow recovers. All organs can be affected by vasocclusion, renal damage can lead to a failure to concentrate urine, and hence patients very easily become dehydrated.

- Management

The earlier active management is started, the better will be the survival and quality of life for patients with sickle-cell disease. Screening programmes for at-risk groups are all important. Newborn babies in such groups need electrophoresis, using alkaline cellulose acetate and acid–citrate agar. Other methods of screening are being developed, e.g.

1. Isoelectric focusing: better resolution by a single procedure but more costly.
2. High performance liquid chromatography (HPLC): highly sensitive and still being evaluated.

Babies and children should be immunized; prophylactic penicillin will also help reduce levels of infection.

Parents must be warned about the danger of fever and dehydration.

Vasocclusive crisis needs to be treated aggressively with:

1. Fluids.
2. Antibiotics.
3. Adequate analgesia.
4. Oxygen – particularly with pulmonary infarction or infection.

If they do not settle quickly, then blood transfusion or even exchange transfusion must be used. The latter will rapidly reduce levels of HbS and hence prevent further sickling. Exchange transfusion is the only effective way to treat priapism – a common, distressing problem in males, with a high incidence of impotence.

- 'Anti-sickling' drugs

Many attempts have been made to prevent sickling using a whole variety of drugs – none is currently in routine clinical use!

1. Carbon monoxide ⎫
2. Sodium nitrate ⎬ have no effect.
3. Urea ⎭
4. Potassium cyanate – prevents sickling in vitro, but too toxic for clinical use.
5. Sodium cyanate – has been used in clinical trials, where it improved red blood cell survival, but caused peripheral neuropathy!
6. Hydroxyurea ⎫ increase HbF levels, reduce
7. 5-Azacytidine ⎬ sickling, but are
   ⎭ both marrow toxic.
8. Pentoxyfylline – increases red blood cell deformability, and hence reduces blood viscosity; still under investigation.
9. Ceteidil – reports of clinical improvement.

- Prenatal diagnosis

Prenatal diagnosis of sickle-cell anaemia, with abortion of the affected fetus, is one way to reduce the morbidity and mortality from this disease. When both parents are heterozygous, they can now be offered:

1. Either amniocentesis at 16–18 weeks with DNA analysis.
2. Or, preferably, chorionic villous biopsy at 9–11 weeks with DNA analysis.

The abnormal gene can be identified directly using the restriction enzyme MstII. The technique is sensitive and very accurate.

- Future prospects

BONE MARROW TRANSPLANTATION

There is the prospect that bone marrow transplantation will cure sickle-cell disease. However, at present there are certain problems:

1. Availability of suitable donor.
2. Morbidity and mortality of the procedure.

Thus the risks have to be balanced against each patient's quality and expectation of life. In the future, however, bone marrow transplantation may become more feasible.

GENE INSERTION

To change the base mutation in the βS-gene is not yet practical, but to insert an extra, normal β-gene is! This would have the effect of reducing HbS concentrations.

References
Alavi, J. B. (1984) Med. Clin. North Am. **68**, 545
Blacklock, H. A. and Mortimer, P. P. (1984) Clin. Haematol. **13**, 679
Charache, S. (1986) Hosp. Pract. **15**, 173
Eaton, W. A. and Hofrichter, J. (1987) Blood **70**, 1245
Galloway, S. J. and Harwood-Nuss, A. L. (1988) J. Emerg. Med. **6**, 213
Newborn Screening in Sickle Cell Disease (1987) National Health Institute Health **6**, no. 9
Onwubalili, J. K. (1983) J. Infect. **7**, 2
Serjeant, G. R. (1988) Trans. R. Soc. Trop. Med. Hyg. **82**, 177

Haemoglobin C

In the most common form of HbC disease, lysine replaces the glutamyl residue at the sixth position from the NH_2 terminal on each β-chain.

Homozygous condition

There is usually moderate anaemia with reduced osmotic fragility of the red cells. Blood films show many target cells, with anisocytosis, poikilcytosis and microspherocytes. Haemoglobin synthesis is two to three times as fast as normal.

Heterozygous condition

HbC makes up 28–44% of the haemoglobin, the residue being HbA. There is usually no anaemia, but osmotic fragility of the red cells is reduced, and target cells are seen in blood films.

HbC is found in about 2% of US Blacks, and is most common in Nigeria.

Haemoglobin D and haemoglobin E

Heterozygotes are asymptomatic and clinically normal but with moderate microcytosis. Homozygotes suffer from a mild haemolytic anaemia. The osmotic fragility of the red cells is reduced and stained blood films show target cells, microcytes and spherocytes. HbE is commonest in S.E. Asia.

Reference
Fairbanks V. F., Gilchrist G. S., Brimpall, B. et al. (1979) Blood **53**, 109

Haemoglobin M

The abnormality results from substitution of either proximal or distal histidyl residues in either the α- or the β-chains by other amino acid residues or of mutations altering the amino acid residues in the haem pocket between the two histidyl residues in either chain. The ferrous iron in the haem molecule is abnormally easily oxidized to ferric iron, resulting in methaemoglobinaemia. In addition, these haemoglobins have either abnormally high or abnormally low affinity for oxygen, with associated instability of the pigment.

At least five different HbM varieties are known. At least 50 varieties of unstable abnormal haemoglobin have been described.

1. Distal histidyl substitution

- Haemoglobin M$_{Boston}$ – α-chain substitution.
- Haemoglobin M$_{Saskatoon}$ – β-chain substitution.
- Haemoglobin M$_{Zurich}$ – β-chain substitution.

These patients are liable to develop haemolysis following primaquine.

2. Proximal histidyl substitution

- Haemoglobin M$_{Iwate}$ – α-chain substitution.

3. Haem pocket substitution

- Haemoglobin M$_{Milwaukee}$ – β-chain substitution.

The thalassaemias

First described by Cooley in 1925 the thalassaemias affect, in varying ways, millions of people world wide. Thalassaemias are caused by reduced or absent β- or α-chain synthesis. Changes in δ- or γ-chain synthesis are of no known clinical significance.

β-Thalassaemia

The single β-gene is found on each chromosome 11, closely associated with the δ-gene.

$\gamma\delta\beta$- Gene complex

Chromosome 11

```
         E          Gγ    Aγ          δ    β
5'---[]------[] []------[]--[]---3'
```

Each gene complex consists of initiating and promoting sequences, exons, introns and terminating sequences. The β-gene has been extensively investigated at the molecular level; there are 54 known alleles of the β-gene causing thalassaemia, of which 20 account for 90% of β-thalassaemia world wide.

β = Normal β-chain gene.
β^+ = Denotes partial production of β-chain.
β^0 = No β-chain production.

Deletion of the β-gene is a rare cause of β-thalassaemia. Small or part deletions have been reported – they do not remove the entire gene, just enough to inactivate it.

Mutations in the gene promotor

The promotor region lies 5' to the structural gene; mutation here may increase or decrease transcription. A mutation has been described in one of the promotor 'boxes' causing reduced transcription and hence synthesis of β-chain. A β^+-thal gene!

Reference
Antonarakis, S. E., Irkin, S. H., Cheng, T. C. et al. (1984) Proc. Natl. Acad. Sci. USA **81**, 1154–1158

It is of interest to note that the δ-gene lacks a 'CCAAT' box promotor which may account for the lack of transcription of the δ-gene and its 'thalassaemia-like' quality!

Reference
Ross J. and Pizarro A. (1983) J. Mol. Biol. **167**, 607–617

Mutations affecting mRNA splicing

There are key nucleotides at the 5'-donor, 3'-acceptor splice junction.

1. Mutation may affect splice junction.
2. Mutation may mimic splice junction elsewhere.

Thus, although the structural gene is apparently 'normal' no β-chain is produced. A β^0-thal gene.

Mutation affecting gene termination

If there is a fault in termination, elongated, unstable mRNA will be produced. This will in turn lead to reduced β-chain production. A β^+-thal gene.

Nonsense mutations (e.g. a mutation that causes a termination codon in the middle of the 'chain').

A nonsense codon at position 39 of the β-globin gene is one of the most common causes of β-thalassaemia in the Mediterranean: a β^0-thal gene. There are now at least 45 molecular defects known to cause β-thalassaemia: they are mainly point mutations in critical regions.

Common examples in the Italian population

β^0 39	=	C – T Substitution at codon 39 (nonsense mutation)
β^+ IVS-1 nt 110	=	G – A Substitution at nucleotide 110 of the first intervening sequence
β^+ IVS-1 nt 6	=	T – C Substitution at position 6 of the first intervening sequence
β^0 IVS-1 nt 1	=	G – A Substitution at position 1 of the first intervening sequence

Reference
Cao, A., Pirasto, M., Ristaldi, M. S. et al. (1988) Haematologica **73**, 331

DNA technology has shown the remarkable heterogenicity of β-thalassaemia. Each ethnic population has its own specific alleles, and there is good evidence that, even when alleles in different populations are the same, they arose independently.

Heterozygotes (e.g. $\beta\beta$ or $\beta\beta+$ (β-thalassaemia trait or β-thalassaemia minor).

There is reduced but adequate β-chain production. The haemoglobin level will be normal or only slightly reduced. The blood film shows a microcytic hypochromic picture with an inappropriately low MCV. Haemoglobin electrophoresis gives a raised haemoglobin A_2 (>3.5%), but is otherwise normal. Serum ferritin must be measured to exclude iron deficiency: these patients lead an entirely normal life, it is important to identify them for counselling.

Homozygotes

- (e.g. β^0 β^0 or β^+ β^+ and β^0 β^+ (the latter homozygous for abnormality))
- β^+ β^+ and β^0 β^+ or β-thalassaemia intermedia

These patients have inadequate β-chain production and suffer variable anaemia. They have a microcytic hypochromic blood film and raised haemoglobin A^2 levels. The bone marrow shows marked expansion of erythropoiesis which is ineffective. Many, however, have a stable chronic haemolytic anaemia and do not require blood transfusion. They should be carefully followed from childhood for proper growth and absence of bone deformity (due to marrow expansion). If worried, blood transfusion should be instigated, with chelation therapy. Even when not, transfused iron overload can occur due to increased gut absorption. Patients should receive regular folate supplements.

At the molecular level they are often associated with mutations in the promotor region, e.g. TATA box -29(A – G) American blacks 25% β-chain; TATA box -31 (A – G) Japanese; IVS- 1 T – C mild disease found in Mediterranean Portuguese.

Reference
Wainscoat, J. S., Thein, L. S. and Weatherall, D. J. (1987) *Blood Reviews* 1(4), 273

● β^0 β^0: β-thalassaemia major

Total lack of β-chain production gives rise to a severe clinical syndrome characterized by chronic progressive anaemia, pronounced erythroblastosis, characteristic facies, splenomegaly, familial incidence and leads to early death in untreated cases.

The fetus is relatively unaffected in utero due to normal γ-chain synthesis. However, by 6 months, and certainly at 1 year, babies will have become anaemic and show 'failure to thrive'. There is unbalanced α-chain production with free α-chains, which aggregate to form insoluble inclusions. These may be so great that many cells are destroyed in the bone marrow. It is estimated that only 15–30% of red cells escape into the circulation. A profound haemolytic anaemia results.

Haemoglobin values can be as low as 2–3 g/dl. The blood film shows gross anisocytosis, poikilocytosis, microcytosis and hypochromia. There will also be polychromasia, nucleated red cells and target cells. Gross splenomegaly with hypersplenism and pancytopenia may follow. Bone changes due to massive hypertrophy of marrow are seen particularly in maxillary and frontal bones. Skull X-rays show typical 'hair on end' appearance. There is failure of growth and sexual development.

In an attempt to overcome the poor prognosis (natural history is death by 5 years) blood transfusion therapy was introduced in the 1930s. Haemoglobin was kept at around 7.5 g/dl, which improved general well-being but not growth or sexual development. A much better quality of life is achieved by increasing transfusion to keep haemoglobin at or above 10 g/dl. This does not appear to increase iron overload because gut absorption is reduced. Recently 'super transfusion' with fresh blood or neocytes has been used in an attempt to reduce transfusion rate; haemoglobin is kept at 12 g/dl.

Problems with transfusion therapy

1. Antibody formation.
2. Viral transmission.
3. Iron overload.

Iron overload is the major cause of death in treated thalassaemia. Iron at 0.7 g/kg will cause organ damage especially to the heart and liver. At an iron level of 1 g/kg most patients die of cardiac failure, usually in their late teens.

Further treatment

Splenectomy may be required if the spleen becomes very large or if hypersplenism develops causing increased transfusion requirements.

Iron chelation therapy is now widely used to reduce or prevent iron overload. Desferrioxamine, given as a daily 12-hour subcutaneous infusion, can bring about a negative iron balance. The 12-hour infusion will chelate iron, with subsequent excretion in the urine and faeces. Between 50 and 150 mg desferrioxamine in each 12-hour infusion is used. Unfortunately, desferrioxamine is not effective orally and compliance with the subcutaneous regimen is often poor, requiring a high level of commitment from patients or parents. Although it is possible to extend life in countries with well-developed health care services, subcutaneous desferrioxamine is not a satisfactory treatment world wide. Clinical trials are under way with an orally effective chelating agent (1,2-dimethyl-3-hydroxypyridone), which is equally as effective as desferrioxamine although it does appear to chelate out zinc. An oral agent would be a great step forward in management.

Reference
Kontoghiorghes, G. J., Aldouri, M. A., Sheppard, L. *et al.* (1987) *Lancet* i, 1294–1295

Bone marrow transplantation (BMT) – because severe β-thalassaemia is not curable or even easily manageable with conventional therapy, many centres have been turning to BMT as a means of cure. At present, cure rates of 60–70% are reported. The major problems of engraftment, graft versus host disease (GVHD) and postgraft infection are being overcome. BMT will become an increasingly viable alternative for treating severe β-thalassaemia in the future.

Reference
Slavin, S. and Rachmilewitz, E. A. (1986) *Bone Marrow Transpl.* 1, 11–15

Prenatal diagnosis of β-thalassaemia

Even with good iron chelation patients only seem to survive 25–30 years. BMT is still hazardous, and thus prevention by accurate prenatal diagnosis with abortion of the severely affected fetus would seem a sensible alternative.

It is possible to obtain adequate amounts of DNA by chorionic villous biopsy at 9–11 weeks' gestation using various techniques such as direct restriction endonuclease analysis or indirectly with restriction length polymorphism linkage analysis. This DNA can be very accurately assessed for the presence of different β-gene alleles. If only β^0-genes are found, termination of pregnancy can be offered. This approach has brought about a dramatic reduction in the incidence of severe β-thalassaemia in Sardinia.

References
Cao, A. (1987) *Blood Reviews*, 1, 169
WHO (1985) Report of WHO working group for hereditary anaemia. Unpublished WHO document Hmg/WG/85.8

α-Thalassaemia

α-Thalassaemia does not present the same clinical problems that are seen in β-thalassaemia: it is mainly caused by gene deletion. The α-gene complex is found on chromosome 16; nearby is the gene for an embryonic α-like chain, and the recently discovered O-gene, again producing a chain found in fetal tissue.

Chromosome 16

```
        T
        J           O           α₂  α₁
5'----[]-------[]-------[ ]-[ ]----3'
```

There are two α-genes on each chromosome 16 producing identical protein chains. They are designated $\alpha_2 : \alpha_1$ in the 5'–3' direction. The α_2-gene produces three times the protein of α_1.

References
Hsu, S. L., Marks, L., Shaw, J. P. *et al.* (1988) *Nature* **331**, 94–96
Liebhaber, S. A., Goossens, M. J. and Kan, Y. W. (1980) *Proc. Natl Acad. Sci. USA* **77**, 2054

Deletions may remove one or both α-genes from chromosome 16. The frequency of single gene deletions has reached 80% in some populations.

The single gene deletion

```
α⁺ --------[]---,
α  --[]----[]----)
```

is most commonly seen in Africa but also found in the Mediterranean, Middle East, south-east Asia and the Pacific Islands.

The double gene deletion (α^0 ---------) is seen in Mediterranean Island people but most commonly in south-east Asia.

The α^+ or single gene deletion can be of two types:

```
       α₁   4.2
------[]---
```
Where there is a 4.2 kb deletion removing the α_2 gene. This is uncommon and found in south-east Asia.

or

```
--[------]---
```
Where there is a 3.7 kb deletion, removing part of α_1 and part of α_2 by crossover and the formation of a single fusion gene. This is much more prevalent and found in the Mediterranean, Africa and Asia.

Thus the following phenotypes have been identified:

Silent carrier ($\alpha\alpha^+$)
```
------[]---
--[]------[]--
```
No clinical symptoms, only identified by family studies.

'African trait' ($\alpha^+\alpha^+$)
```
------[]--
-------[]--
```
There is a microcytic hypochromic picture with or without mild anaemia. The red cell count is increased but the haemoglobin is low. Serum ferritin levels are normal, globin chain synthesis shows reduced α-chain synthesis. Haemoglobin Barts (γ_4) may be found in cord blood.

'Asian trait' ($\alpha\alpha^0$)
```
-------------
--[]-----[]---
```
These patients lead a normal life.

Haemoglobin H disease ($\alpha\alpha^+$)
```
-----------
------[]---
```
There is a microcytic hypochromic anaemia with haemoglobin values of 7–12 g/dl. Incubation with cresyl blue causes precipitate of haemoglobin H (β_4) in the cell. There may be hepatosplenomegaly, but this is variable. Haemoglobin H levels are between 2.5 and 25%. Small amounts of haemoglobin Barts (γ_4) are also found. Most patients never require blood transfusion, yet in those studied at post mortem moderate to severe iron overload was found, presumably due to increased gut absorption. In one study, two or three patients who died with haemoglobin H disease died of iron overload. However, most patients seem to lead a normal life; the age range in 107 cases reported in Hawaii is from newborn to 83 years.

Hydrops fetalis ($\alpha^0\alpha^0$)
```
----------
----------
```
No α-chain produced: only γ_4, β_4 found in fetus. Stillborn or intrauterine death. Found almost exclusively where the double gene deletion is most common, i.e. south-east Asia.

Reference:
Jim, R. T. S. (1988) *Hawaii Med J.* **47** (8), 374

Haemoglobin abnormalities and the 'malaria hypothesis'

The distribution and high incidence of the genes for haemoglobins S, C, E and the thalassaemias strongly suggests a selective advantage for the carrier status of these disorders:

- Haemoglobin S: West and Central Africa, but also East Africa, Arabia, North Greece, India

- Haemoglobin C: West Africa
- Haemoglobin E: South-east Asia
- β-Thalassaemia: Mediterranean, but also Middle East, India, South-east Asia
- α-Thalassaemia: South-east Asia, but also West Africa, Mediterranean

β-Gene abnormalities tend not to be found together to any great extent. Gene mutations have arisen in different populations independently and reached high incidence by natural selection. Their distribution matches past and present distributions of the malaria parasite, for example, haemoglobin S trait can be shown to be protection against falciparum malaria.

Heterozygous combinations of abnormal haemoglobins and defective haemoglobin synthesis

- Sickle-cell-thalassaemia
  Mild to severe anaemia.
- Sickle-cell-haemoglobin C
  Moderate anaemia.
- Sickle-cell-haemoglobin D
- Sickle-cell-haemoglobin E
- Thalassaemia-haemoglobin C
- Thalassaemia-haemoglobin D
- Thalassaemia-haemoglobin E

Chapter 4

Peripheral white blood cells

Total white cell count

(S. I. unit conversion factor = 10^6, i.e. 4000–10 000/mm^3 becomes 4.0–10.0 × 10^9/l)

- Infants (full term at birth)

  Range: 10–25 × 10^9/l

For the first 24 h the differential count shows a preponderance of neutrophils. During the first 3 days the majority of new white cells are immature myeloid cells. From the fourth to seventh days labelled lymphoid cells increase without concomitant increase in the total number of lymphocytes, i.e. manifestation of cellular immunity, probably representing immunological response to antigenic challenge in extrauterine life. By the third to fourth day the total count has fallen to 9–15 × 10^9/l. The absolute neutrophil count is not very useful in the detection of infection. The absolute 'band' or 'stab' cell count is more useful. By the third to fourth week, the relative percentage of neutrophils to lymphocytes has reversed, and the relative lymphocytosis persists until about the fourth year.

Reference
Weitzman, M. (1975) *Am. J. Dis. Child.* **129**, 1183

- Infant (1 year)

  Range: 6–18 × 10^9/l (approximately 60% lymphocytes)

- Childhood (4–7 years)

  Range: 6–15 × 10^9/l

- Childhood (8–12 years)

  Range: 4.5–13.5 × 10^9/l

- Adults

  Range: 4–10 × 10^9/l

Counts in adult females lower on average than in adult males, and counts in adult Negroes lower than in White adults.

It is possible that no. 21 chromosome controls total white cell count since:

- Cases with trisomy of this chromosome have abnormally high white cell counts.
- Cases of myeloid leukaemia with abnormally small no. 21 chromosome have low white cell counts.

References
Allan, R. N. and Alexander, M. K. (1968) *J. Clin. Pathol.* **21**, 691
Karayalcin, G., Rosner F. and Sawitsky A. (1972) *Lancet* **i**, 387
Lalla, M. (1975) *Acta Haematol.* **53**, 129
O'Sullivan, M. A. and Pryles C. V. (1963) *N. Engl. J. Med.* **268**, 1168

Differential white cell count

The *adult differential count* is attained at about puberty:

Neutrophils	40–75%	2.5–7.5 × 10^9/l
Lymphocytes	20–50%	1.5–3.5 × 10^9/l
Monocytes	2–10%	0.2–0.8 × 10^9/l
Eosinophils	1–6%	0.04–0.44 × 10^9/
Basophils	<1%	0.015–0.1 × 10^9/l

Note: Although the differential count (expressed as a percentage) may be useful, the most valuable figures in a white cell count are the total white cell count and the differential count in absolute figures.

The total white cell count

This may be:

- Normal.
- Below the lower limit of normal (leucopenia).
- Above the upper limit of normal (leucocytosis).

The differential count in absolute figures

It is possible for the total white cell count to be normal, but for the differential count to be grossly abnormal, e.g. acute leukaemia. Also the total white cell count may be increased above normal, but the relative counts may appear to be normal when expressed as percentages, e.g. acute infections. The total white cell count may be above normal, and the differential count may also be abnormal, e.g. chronic myeloid leukaemia. Finally, the total white cell count may be reduced below normal, with an apparently normal differential count, expressed as percentages, e.g. aplastic anaemia; or in addition to a reduced total white cell count, the differential may be grossly abnormal, e.g. aleukaemia phase of leukaemia.

There is a linear relationship between the logarithms of the meridians of circulating neutrophils plus metamyelocytes and of monocytes in:

- Normal adult males, normal pregnant females.
- Persistent leucocytosis.
- Polycythaemia vera.
- Myelofibrosis.
- Essential thrombocythaemia.

A different relationship exists in chronic myeloid leukaemia.

References
Bain, B. J. and Wickramasinghe, S. N. (1976) *Acta Haematol.* **55**, 89
England, J. M. and Bain, B. J. (1976) *Br. J. Haematol.* **33**, 1

For convenience, each of the cell types found normally in the circulating peripheral blood is considered in detail in the following pages.

Neutrophil chemistry

- Leucocyte sodium 15.7 ± 5.0 mmol.
- Leucocyte potassium 120 ± 7.0 mmol.

There is a marked change in cation fluxes with temperature, probably explaining previous very wide ranges of results reported.

Reference
Cividalli, G. and Nathan, D. G. (1974) *Blood* **43**, 861

Peripheral blood neutrophils

Normal range: $2.5–7.5 \times 10^9/l$

This makes up 40–75% of the total normal white cell count. The level in any one normal person varies throughout the 24 h, and is affected by such factors as:

- Moderate exercise.
- Emotion.
- Changes in external temperature.
- Ingestion of food.

Thus for comparable results on a person over a period, the counts should be taken at the same time each day, under similar conditions.

The bone marrow contains 11 days' supply of myelocytes, metamyelocytes, 'stab' cells and neutrophils ($\equiv 2000 \times 10^7$ cells/kg body weight).

Total blood neutrophils $= 70 \times 10^7/kg$ body weight.
Blood pool turnover $= 2–3$ times daily.

Neutrophils circulate in the blood for only about 10 h. Neutrophils leave the circulating blood in a random exponential fashion, with a half-disappearance time of 4–10 h. Following large doses of steroids, the neutrophil count rises because of an increased inflow of neutrophils and a decreased rate of egress from the circulation.

Reference
Karle, H. and Hansen, N. E. (1975) *Scand. J. Haematol.* **14**, 190

There is an inverse relationship between the percentage of granulocyte progenitor cells in the S-phase (cells in the DNA-synthesis phase of the cell cycle) and the peripheral blood neutrophil count, i.e. suggesting a negative feedback regulation of granulopoiesis.

Reference
Greenberg, P. L. and Schrier, S. L. (1973) *Blood* **41**, 753

Increase in total neutrophil count

Physiological

1. Severe exercise: neutrophilia greater in unconditioned subjects.
2. Late in normal pregnancy (during the last 2 months).

Reference
McCarthy, D. A., Perry, J. D., Melson, R. D. and Dale M. M. (1987) *Br. Med. J.* **295**, 636

3. During labour, as a result of:
   (a) severe exertion;
   (b) haemorrhage;
   (c) tissue damage;
   (d) great excitement.
4. Normal in the newborn infant.
5. Chronic 'normal' idiopathic leucocytosis, with total WBC persistently $10–20 \times 10^9/l$ and no other abnormal findings.

Pathological

1. Infections

This applies especially to coccal infections. Following phagocytosis of bacteria, presence of 'phlogistic' agents, and products of antigen-sensitized lymphocytes, endogenous pyrogens (EP) are released, which result in release of leucocyte endogenous mediator (LEM), which in turn causes increased release of granulocytes from the bone marrow, as well as uptake of iron, zinc and amino acids from the plasma by the liver. Increased synthesis of acute-phase glycoproteins and decreased albumin synthesis by the liver, follows. LEM is a heat-labile, trypsin-sensitive protein with a molecular weight of 10 000–30 000. In infections in the newborn infant, the neutrophil count very frequently exceeds $7 \times 10^9/l$.

2. Non-infective tissue damage
- Coronary thrombosis.
- Pulmonary infarctions and other infarctions.
- Crush injury.
- Burns.
- Rapidly growing neoplasia.
- Poisoning with carbon monoxide, lead etc.
- Anergy: leucocytosis may reflect an acute deficit in lymphocyte function rather than a transient depression of inflammatory response.

3. Metabolic disorders
- Eclampsia.
- Diabetic ketosis.
- Acute gout.
- Uraemia.
- Cushing's syndrome: neutrophils frequently make up more than 80% of the differential count.

4. Leukaemia
- Chronic myeloid leukaemia
The total neutrophil count is usually greater than $100 \times 10^9/l$ in untreated cases, and counts of up to $1000 \times 10^9/l$ may be found.

- Acute myeloblastic leukaemia
The total white cell count ranges between $20 \times 10^9/l$ and $50 \times 10^9/l$ and consists of up to 90% myeloblasts or myelocytes.

- Polycythaemia vera
Moderate increases in the neutrophil count to $20-40 \times 10^9/l$ may be found.

- Erythraemic myelosis (Di Guglielmo's disease)
Moderate increases, with many primitive myeloid cells (e.g. myeloblasts and myelocytes).

- Myelosclerosis
Variable results may be obtained. Counts of $20-30 \times 10^9/l$ are not uncommon.

5. Others
- Heavy smoking.
- Oral contraceptives – increase in 14% reported.
- Obesity – tendency to increase reported.
- Neutrophilia is a marker for myocardial infarction risk and for reinfarction risk.

References
Ernst, E., Hammerschmidt, D. E., Bagge, V. et al. (1987) J. Am. Med. Assoc. 257, 2318
Lowe, G. D. O., Machado, S. G., Krol, W. F. et al. (1985) Thrombos. Haemostas. 54, 700

Decrease in total neutrophil count

Physiological

Neutrophil counts fall in normal subjects with no social contacts, and hence antigen deprivation (e.g. Polar-base).

Pathological

- Depressed as part of a syndrome of pancytopenia (*see* 'Pancytopenia').
- Depressed as part of a syndrome of aplastic anaemia (*see* 'Aplastic anaemia').
- Depression of neutrophils (moderate = neutropenia, severe = agranulocytosis).

Bone marrow damage

1. X-ray irradiation.
2. Poisoning with benzene, urethane, gold etc.
3. Busulphan (Myleran), 6-mercaptopurine, triethylene melamine etc. The fall in the white cell count is predictable, and proportional to the dosage. (L-Cystine will tend to prevent this fall following dosage with nitrogen mustards.)
4. Severe infections:
   (a) disseminated tuberculosis;
   (b) severe osteomyelitis;
   (c) septicaemia: in overwhelming infection in the newborn infant there may be a massive fall in the neutrophil count with eosinopenia. The presence of 'stab cells' and 'toxic granulation' are useful indications of infection.
5. Chronic alcoholics:
   (a) associated with cirrhosis and hypersplenism;
   (b) acute intoxication and bacterial infection:
   (c) megaloblastosis with folate deficiency;
   (d) myelopoiesis directly suppressed by large continuing doses of alcohol;
6. Acute malaria: infections with *P. vivax* and *P. falciparum* commonly have a neutropenia with a reduction in neutrophil lobe count ('left shift').

Bone marrow obliteration

1. Osteosclerosis.
2. Myelofibrosis.
3. Neoplastic infiltration:
   (a) carcinoma:
   (b) sarcoma;
   (c) myeloma;
   (d) leukaemia: lymphocytic leukaemia, monocytic leukaemia or aleukaemia phase of myeloid leukaemia;
   (e) malignant myelosclerosis: anaemia, leucopenia, thrombocytopenia, peripheral blood myeloblasts, marrow aspirate 'dry tap';

Reference
Chan, W. C., Brynes, R. K., Kim, T. H. et al. (1983) Blood 62, 92

   (f) lymphoma;
   (g) lymphadenoma.

Immune antibodies due to drug sensitivities
(i.e. circulating leucoagglutinins and leucolysins)

- Amidopyrine: the incidence rate is low. The onset is rapid. Very small doses of the drug cause a second attack. The onset is unpredictable.
- Chlorpromazine: agranulocytosis due to chlorpromazine may be due to an immunological reaction, or due to direct toxic action on the marrow.
- Hydantoin.
- Sulphonamides etc.
- Thiouracils.
- Phenothiazines: heavy dosage leads to a fall in the neutrophil count before the tenth day, and the development of agranulocytosis is relatively gradual, as compared with other drugs.

Other immune bodies

- Primary atypical pneumonia.
- Infectious mononucleosis.
- Virus agranulocytosis.
- Felty's syndrome: there is excessive margination of neutrophils, and one-third of cases have subnormal neutrophil production.
- Disseminated lupus erythematosus: antineutrophil antibody-mediated activation of complement.

Reference
Rustagi, P. K., Currie, M. S. and Logue, G. L. (1985) Am. J. Med. 78, 971

- Chronic neutropenia in children.
- Raised leucoagglutinin titre.
- Some 'idiopathic' neutropenias are autoimmune, with antibodies promoting neutrophil decrease by mononuclear macrophages.
- Prolonged agranulocytopenia may follow incompatible platelet transfusion.
- Isoimmune neonatal neutropenia: maternal IgG antibodies against fetal leucocytes cross the placenta and cause transient neonatal neutropenia which may be associated with neonatal infections, especially skin infections and uncommonly respiratory tract and urinary tract infections or septicaemia. The neutropenia lasts 2–17 weeks.

Due to deficiencies:

- Vitamin B_{12} deficiency.
- Folate deficiency: in pregnancy folate deficiency may be associated with leucopenia.
- Hypopituitarism.
- Hypoadrenalism.

Other conditions

- Familial cyclical neutropenia
Episodic with fever and oral ulcers, anaemia, thrombocytopenia, neutropenia and eosinophilia. Autosomal dominant inheritance.

- Benign familial neutropenia

No anaemia, no thrombocytopenia, constant neutropenia. Autosomal dominant inheritance. In the genetic neutropenia affecting some Africans and some Yemenite Jews, there is no deficiency in granulocyte colony-forming cells. The defect is in the release of cells from the bone marrow into the peripheral blood.

Reference
Zucker-Franklin, D., L'Esperance, P. and Good, R. A. (1977) Blood 49, 425

- Chronic benign granulocytopenia
Limited duration of 10–18 months.

- Infantile genetic agranulocytosis of Kostmann
Autosomal recessive inheritance. The bone marrow is deficient in mature granulocytes, rich in promyelocytes. There is an intrinsic neutrophil defect which allows normal proliferation of precursor cells, but abnormal granulogenesis and apparent inability to form secondary granules.

- Familial granulocytopenia with reduced serum γ-globulin

Recurrent attacks of infection with neutropenia, anaemia and bone marrow maturation arrest.

- Chronic idiopathic neutropenia
No anaemia, no thrombocytopenia, but no response to steroids and duration of 1–19 years.

- Chédiak-Higashi–Steinbrinck anomaly
Neutropenia with increased granulocyte turnover.

- Fanconi's pancytopenia
- During renal dialysis in patients with chronic renal failure

During haemodialysis there is a rapid fall in white cells in the first half-hour with a more gradual fall between 1 and 6h, due to leucocytes adhering to the membrane.

Granulocyte transfusions

Early reports suggested a reduction in mortality in neutropenic patients receiving granulocyte transfusions during febrile periods. There appears to be no evidence of improvement, and transfusion of large numbers of irradiated granulocytes from patients with chronic myeloid leukaemia only reduces fever temporarily in neutropenic recipients. Recipients have included:

- Patients with acute leukaemia during induction, or in relapse.
- Very severe Gram-negative septicaemia with marrow depression.
- Infected patients with underlying malignancy.
- Infected patients with aplastic anaemia.

Reverse barrier nursing is indicated, as are suitable antibiotics.

Suitable donors are normal volunteers or patients with chronic myeloid leukaemia.

Ideally the donors and recipient should be HLA-A and HLA-B compatible (as these two HLA groups are expressed in the granulocytes, and ABO-compatible, since it is inevitable that some red cells will be transfused with the white cells).

In neutropenia with severe bacterial infection, phagocytic function measured before and after granulocyte infusion in ALL, AML and chronic granulomatous disease, resulted in a very poor increase in phagocytic activity.

Acetanilide
Acetazolamide (Diamox)
Amidopyrine
Amodiaquine
Antimony, organic compounds
Antipyrine
Arsenic, organic compounds
Barbiturates
Bismuth
Busulphan (Myleran)
Benzene
Carbimazole (Neo-Mercazole)
Carbutamide
Chloramphenicol
Chlorophenothane (DDT)
Chlorothiazide
Chlorpromazine
Cinchopen
Diethazine hydrochloride (Diparcol)
Dinitrophenol
Diphenylhydantoin sodium
Dipyrone
Gold, and its salts
Imipramine
Iodolysin
Isoniazid
Mepazine
Meprobamate
Mepyramine
Mercurial diuretics

Reference
Tono-Aka, T., Matsumoto, T. and Matsumoto, S. (1983) *N. Engl. J. Med.* **309**, 245

Agranulocytosis due to drugs

The following drugs and chemicals are some of the substances which have been known to cause agranulocytosis. They are not listed in order of severity or frequency of incidence. It will be seen that many of them, in certain cases, may severely affect the bone marrow as a whole, causing aplastic anaemia. The incidence of drug-induced agranulocytosis will obviously depend on local prescription habits. Drug-induced blood disorders, other than those caused by anti-tumour drugs, are rare and reversible in most cases.

Reference
Danielson, D. A., Douglas, S. W., Herzog, P. *et al.* (1984) *J. Am. Med. Assoc.* **252**, 3257

6-Mercaptopurines
Mesantoin (Methoin)
Methaphenilene (Diatrin)
Methimazole
Mustard gas
Nitrogen mustards
Nitrous oxide anaesthesia
Perphenazine
Phenacetamide
Phenacetin
Phenothiazine
Phenylbutazone (Butazolidine)
Phenylindanedione (Dindevan)
Phosphorus
Plasmoquine
Procainamide
Prochlorperazine
Promazine
Promethazone
Pyribenzamine
Pyrithyldione
Quinine
Sulphanilamide and sulphonamides
Thiantoin
Thioglycollates ('cold' hair waves)
Thiosemicarbazone
Thiourea and thiouracils
Tolbutamide
Trifluoroperazine
Trimethadione (Troxidone)
Trinitrotoluene
Urethane

Release of mature neutrophils from the bone marrow is a function of the rate of loss from the blood and proceeds normally even when the marrow granulocyte reserve is partially depleted (this may explain the sudden onset of neutropenia in many cases). In drug-induced agranulocytosis, marrow aspirates showing an increased number of promyelocytes and myelocytes with few 'stab' cells and polymorphonuclear leucocytes are not representing 'maturation arrest', but rather intense granulocyte proliferative activity, i.e. encouraging observations.

The real incidence of drug-induced neutropenia greatly exceeds the reported incidence, since only fatal cases tend to get reported.

Reference
Arneborn, P. and Palmblad, J. (1982) *Acta Med. Scand.* **212**, 289

Neutrophil segmentation

The degree of lobulation of neutrophil polymorphs is not a measure of the age of the cells. Thus, where there are predominantly immature cells with one or two nuclei, there is said to be a 'shift to the left'. Conversely, where most of the cells have four nuclei or more, there is said to be a 'shift to the right'. Neutrophil lobulation varies in different animal species. Various methods have been used to assess this degree of maturity:

- *Arneth count*, and Cooke's modification of Arneth's count, involve a lobe count.
- *Von Bonsdorff* included a count of myelocytes, metamyelocytes, and 'stab' cells as well, which gives a better indication of cell maturity and formation.

Nowadays detailed lobe counts are not often performed. Bone-marrow biopsy gives a much more accurate assessment of white cell production. As a rough working rule 40–50% of the neutrophils have three lobes, 20–40% have two lobes and 15–25% have four lobes. The finding of more than three five-lobed cells per 100 white blood cells, or even one with more than five lobes in the peripheral blood, suggests the possibility of incipient megaloblastic anaemia.

'Shift to the left'

- Infections.
- Toxaemias.
- Haemorrhage.
- Chronic neutropenia in children.

Normal lobe count = on average three lobes per cell.

Hypersegmentation

1. Megaloblastic anaemia:
   (a) vitamin B_{12} deficiency;
   (b) Folate deficiency.

Reference
Bills, T. and Spatz, L. (1977) *Am. J. Clin. Pathol.* **68**, 263

   (c) (a) + (b).
2. Liver disease.
3. In some cases of sepsis (increased stab cell and myelocyte count with fall in average lobe count is more common).
4. Heat-stroke.

Reference
Friedman, E. W., Williams, J. C. and Prendergast, E. (1982) *Br. J. Haematol.* **50**, 163

5. Hereditary hypersegmentation: this harmless anomaly is inherited as a dominant character.
6. Iron deficiency: present in many cases in the absence of either vitamin B_{12} or folate deficiency.

Disturbances of neutrophil function

Opsonins, which are probably antibodies, are activated by complement and alter the surfaces of bacteria to encourage their phagocytosis by neutrophils. Following migration of neutrophils, which results from the action of chemotactic substances derived from bacteria, damaged tissues and/or damaged neutrophils, plus probably the C5, C6, C7, components of complement, a particle due to be phagocytosed is surrounded by pseudopodia from a neutrophil. The pseudopodia meet round the particle, and the cell membranes fuse. The particle or bacteria is intracellular, but is separated by a membrane from the neutrophil cytoplasm. The neutrophil cytoplasmic granules consist of *primary granules* which contain acid phosphatase, β-glucuronidase, aryl sulphatase, 5'-nucleotidase, and myeloperoxidase, *secondary granules* which contain alkaline phosphatase and *tertiary granules*, which develop later and which contain acid phosphatase.

These membrane-bound organelles are lysosomes, and, by a process of fusion of membranes of the granules with the membrane surrounding the particle or bacteria, their contents are released into the phagosome (phagocytic vacuole containing the bacteria or particle) to act on the bacteria. Hydrogen peroxide is produced by glucose oxidation through the hexose-monophosphate shunt, and it plays a very important part in the killing of ingested bacteria.

Similarly, iodination of bacteria is involved in the bactericidal peroxide–peroxidase system.

Since many steps are involved in the ingestion and killing of bacteria and yeasts, it follows that many different abnormalities have been discovered, related to specific deficiencies.

Many extrinsic factors interfere with neutrophil function, while intrinsic neutrophil defects are uncommon. Neutrophil function tests are not often requested in routine laboratories.

References
Goldstein I. M. (1979) Role of the plasma membrane. In: Piomelli, S. and Yachmin S., Ed *Current Topics in Haematology*, 2. pp 145–202 New York: Alan R. Liss Inc
Karnovsky, M. L. (1983) *N. Engl. J. Med.* **308**, 274
Tauber, A. I. (1981) *Am. J. Med.* **70**, 1237

Plasma factors

1. Activated trimolecular complex for chemotaxis

- C5, C6, C7, components of complement.
- Plasmin-split C3 fragment of complement (molecular weight 6000).
- Chemotactically active fragments found following cleavage of C3 component of complement by tissue protease.
- Bacterial chemotactic factors.

2. Opsonization
- IgG and IgM antibodies, preferentially IgG1 and IgG3.
- Complement components (C1, C4, C2, C3).
- Basic polypeptides.

Defective opsonization of yeast for phagocytosis is fairly common in association with bacterial infection, and is possibly evidence of dominant inheritance of a specific plasma factor.

Reference
Soothill, J. F. and Harvey, B. A. M. (1976) *Arch. Dis. Child.* **51**, 91

3. Inherited C3 deficiency

Pneumococci poorly phagocytosed, due to serum deficiency.

4. Pseudoglobulin deficiency

Deficiency of a pseudoglobin distinct from complement, but interacting with complement, results in poor ingestion of pneumococci, even if the type-specific antibody to the organism is present in the serum (it is possible that the pseudoglobulin is an inhibitor of protease which acts on C3).

5. Lack of a serum factor

There is an increased susceptibility to pyogenic infection, with decreased phagocytosis of yeasts. This condition is from the two deficiencies mentioned above.

Neutrophil factors

1. Marrow neutrophils

Some morphologically mature neutrophils are also functionally mature, but a proportion of normal morphologically mature neutrophils in the bone marrow are inactive and not capable of phagocytosis.

Reference
Altaman, A. J. and Stossel, T. P. (1974) *Br. J. Haematol.* **27**, 241

2. 'Lazy leucocyte' syndrome

Neutrophils are present in the marrow in normal numbers, but are not mobilized into the circulation in response to infection. Although neutrophil chemotaxis is poor, phagocytosed bacteria are killed normally. Random mobility is also abnormally reduced.

Reference
Miller, M. E., Oski, F. A. and Harris, M. B. (1971) *Lancet* **i**, 665

3. Circulating leucocyte

The normal neutrophil is capable of *random movement*. There is a leucocyte migration-enhancing protein in the plasma (mol. wt = 160 000) associated with inflammatory response. Excess of this protein has been reported, with increased inflammatory response and inappropriately exuberant leucocyte exudation in response to trivial stimuli, resulting in skin and joint damage (pyoderma gangrenosa and hypertrophic erosive arthritis).

Reference
Jacobs, J. C. and Goetzl, E. J. (1975) *Pediatrics, Springfield* **56**, 570

4. Chemotaxis

During active bacterial infection there is an increase in leucotactic activity in neutrophils, aiding localization of invading bacteria.

References
Gillin, J. I., Clarke, R. A. and Kimball, H. R. (1973) *J. Immunol.* **110**, 233
Hill, H. C., Gerrard, J. M., Hogan, A. *et al.* (1974). *J. Clin. Invest.* **53**, 996

Cases have been described in which the leucocytes exhibit normal random mobility but abnormally reduced chemotaxic response. In 'Job's syndrome' there is a severe defect in neutrophil chemotaxis with marked increase in plasma IgE levels, and recurrent staphylococcal abscesses and chronic eczema.

References
Hill, M. R., Quie, P. G., Pabst, H. F. *et al.* (1974) *Lancet* **ii**, 617
Miller, M. F., Norman, M. E., Koblenzer, P. J. *et al.* (1973) *J. Lab. Clin. Med.* **82**, 1

A serum chemotaxis-inhibiting factor has been described in alcoholic liver disease.

Reference
Van Epps, D. E., Strickland, R. G. and Williams, R. C. Jr (1974) *Am. J. Med.* **59**, 200

5. Recognition

Immune adherence involves antigen–antibody–complement complexes including C$\overline{3}$, before these complexes adhere to the leucocyte surface, prior to phagocytosis. Neutrophil adherence is reduced in alcoholic liver disease, and during treatment with prednisone or aspirin.

6. Phagocytosis

Capsulated bacteria are phagocytosed more easily and rapidly after fixation of complement. Bacteria without capsules are more easily attacked by lysozyme and lysed after fixation of complement in the cell wall. Antigen–antibody complexes require chemotaxic activity in the presence of complement (1–7 components). Some bacteria can be phagocytosed without the presence of antibodies or even serum factors. Other highly pathogenic bacteria require the presence of both antibodies and complement before phagocytosis will occur.

Phagocytosis is reduced during tetracycline therapy. An abnormality of neutrophil phagocytosis due to failure of the actin microfilaments to polymerize reversibly – essential for the generation of pseudopodia for ingestion and locomotion, has been reported.

References
Boxer, L. A., Hedley-Whyte, E. T. and Stossel, T. P. (1974) *N. Engl. J. Med.* **291**, 1093
Root, R. K., Ellman, L. and Frank, M. M. (1972) *J. Immunol.* **109**, 477

7. Neutrophil granule activities

Azurophil granules formed during the promyelocyte stage contain peroxidase. Specific granules formed during the myelocyte stage are peroxidase negative. Metamyelocytes and 'band' forms are both non-secretory and non-proliferating, and at these stages 33% of granules are peroxidase positive and 67% are peroxidase negative.

When micro-organisms are engulfed both granules discharge into the enclosing vacuole (specific granule contents preceding azurophil granule contents). The pH in the phagocytic vacuole rapidly falls from a neutral value to pH 4 within 7–15 min.

GRANULE CONTENTS

- Peroxidase (+ hydrogen peroxide and halide): antibacterial, virucidal and fungicidal. There is a close relationship between H_2O_2 formation and the rate of phagocytosis by human granulcoytes.
- Lysosmal acid hydrolases, causing lysis at acid pH.
- Phagocytin and cationic proteins present in the cell are antibacterial, with chymotrypsin-like protease activity.
- Lysozyme is an aminopolysaccharidase which degrades bacterial cell walls and lyses some bacterial species.
- Lactoferrin chelates both copper and iron ions, and increases the effectiveness of lysozyme activity on bacteria.
- Collagenase acts on non-denatured collagen fibres in micro-organisms.

References
Bainton, D. F. (1975) *Br. J. Haematol.* **29**, 17
Odeberg H. and Olsson, I. (1975) *J. Clin Invest.* **56**, 1118
Root, R. K., Metcalf, J., Oshino, N. *et al.* (1975) *J. Clin. Invest.* **55**, 945

There is simultaneous activation of myeloperoxidase activity and disposal of peroxide. Superoxide dismutase present in neutrophils protects the phagocytic cell against autodamage during destruction of organisms.

References
De Chatelet, L. R., McCall, C. E., McPhail L. C. *et al.* (1974) *J. Clin. Invest.* **53**, 1197
Root, R. K. and Stossel, T. P. (1974) *J. Chin. Invest.* **53**, 1207

DISORDERS OF DEGRANULATION

1. Reduction in number of granules.
2. Reduction in enzyme activities in granules:
    (a) X-linked chronic granulomatous disease, with no increase in oxygen or glucose utilization after phagocytosis, no production of hydrogen peroxide or superoxide, and failure to reduce nitroblue tetrazolium;
    (b) glucose-6-phosphate dehydrogenase deficiency in males and females;
    (c) glucose-6-phosphate dehydrogenase instability in males;
    (d) reduced NADH oxidase deficiency in males and females;
    (e) glutathione peroxidase deficiency in females;
    (f) Job's syndrome;
    (g) lipochrome histiocytosis;
    (h) pyruvate kinase deficiency.

Reference
Burge, P. S., Johnson, W. S. and Hayward, A. R. (1976) *Br. Med. J.* **1**, 742

3. Granules fail to secrete into phagosomes.

DISORDERS OF PEROXIDATION

- *Lack of myeloperoxidase:* lack of myeloperoxidase (granule-associated) is associated with neutrophils incapable of killing some organisms after ingestion, but capable of killing *Staphylococcus pyogenes* slowly.

References
Klebanoff, S. J. (1970) *Science N Y* **169**, 1095
Olsson, I., Oloffson, T. and Odeberg, H. (1972) *Scand. J. Haematol.* **9**, 483

- Selective deficiency of myeloperoxidase, resulting in impaired ability to fix iodine. This is not important unless the patient is also suffering from other disorders including: allergy; dermatoses; surgical trauma.

Reference
Stendahl, O. and Lindgren, S. (1976) *Scand. J. Haematol.* **16**, 144

- Defect in superoxide production in chronic granulomatous disease.

Reference
Curnutte, J. T., Kippes, R. S. and Babior, B. M. (1975) *N. Engl. J. Med.* **293**, 628

- Total glucose-6-phosphate dehydrogenase deficiency.

8. Intracellular killing

The pH drops in the normal phagocyte vacuole down to pH 3.0, partly due to lactate formation. Some bacteria, such as *Strep. pneumococci*, are killed by low pH. Both lysosomal acid hydrolases and the myeloperoxidase-mediated systems are favoured by low pH.

DEFECTS IN KILLING

1. Chédiak–Higashi–Steinbrinck: there is abnormal degranulation and lysosomal function, with lack of enzymes necessary for effective function of activated halide complexes. Both staphylococci and streptococci can be killed.

Reference
Salmon. S. E., Cline, M. J., Schultz, J. *et al.* (1970) *N. Engl. J. Med.* **282**, 259

2. Inadequate amounts of hydrogen peroxide generated to allow normal halide utilization.

Reference
Baehner, R. L., Nathan D. G. and Karnovsky, M. L. (1970) *J. Clin. Invest.* **49**, 865

3. Acute myeloid leukaemia. The granulocytes are less effective in ingesting and killing *Candida albicans* in vitro. Both cell and plasma factors are involved.

Reference
Wilkinson P. M. (1975) *Br. J. Haematol.* **30**, 128

4. Chronic granulomatous disease. In chronic granulomatous disease neutrophils can kill bacteria which produce hydrogen peroxide, e.g. lactobacilli, streptococci, and are thought to lack diaphorase activity of NADH oxidase in the region of the phagocytic vacuole:
   (a) typical: sex-linked recessive inheritance, with normal or elevated immunoglobulin levels;
   (b) atypical:
      (i) sex-linked inheritance, with associated selective immunoglobulin deficiencies,
      (ii) non-familial inheritance,
      (iii) familial, non-sex-linked 'Job syndrome'.

The neutrophils in chronic granulomatous disease kill streptococci, but not staphylococci. There may be a defective triggering to degranulation. Neutrophils must adhere to the phagocytic stimulator for degranulation to occur.

Reference
Gold. S. B., Hanes D. M., Stiles, D. P. *et al.* (1974) *N. Engl. J. Med.* **291**, 332

It has been found that Kx, the antigen necessary for proper expression of Kell in red cells, may be absent from leucocytes, and is associated with a transmembrane transport defect for cell metabolites which inactivate ingested bacteria.

Reference
Marsh, W. L. (1975) *Med. Lab. Technol.* **32**, 1

NEUTROPHIL BACTERICIDAL CAPACITY
This can be measured.

References
Mickenberg, I D., Root R. K. and Wolff, S. M. (1970) *J. Clin. Invest.* **49**, 1528
Stossel, T. P. (1974) *N. Engl. J. Med.* **390**, 717, 774, 833

Nitroblue tetrazolium test

The rate of reduction of nitroblue tetrazolium (NBT) is stimulated by normal phagocytosis of bacteria. In chronic granulomatous disease the rate of reduction of NBT is reduced markedly in affected homozygotes, and moderately reduced in carrier heterozygotes due to a genetic fault in oxidase activity. Neutrophils from patients can kill bacteria which produce hydrogen peroxide, e.g. lactobacilli, streptococci, and there is a lack in diaphorase activity of NADH oxidase in the region of the phagocytic vacuole.

Pathological

1. Test results inappropriately normal, or reduced activity:

- Chronic granulomatous disease of childhood.
- Congenital or acquired agammaglobulinaemia.
- Nephrosis.
- Myeloperoxidase deficiency.
- Glucose-6-phosphate dehydrogenase deficiency in neutrophils.
- Kwashiorkor.
- In acute tissue rejection the NBT result is normal, whereas in acute infection to a transplanted patient the NBT score is high.

Reference
Gordon, A. M., Briggs, J. D. and Bell, P. R. F. (1974) *J. Clin. Pathol.* **27**, 734

- Reduced levels of activity in iron deficiency.

2. Test results increased activity:

- Untreated bacterial infection.
- Miliary tuberculosis.
- Systemic fungus infection.
- Malaria.
- Normal newborn infant with lower levels of NBT + ve cells in low-birth-weight infants.

Reference
Goel, K. M. and Vowels, M. R. (1974) *Acta Paediatr. Scand.* **63**, 122

- Lobar pneumonia (not raised in pulmonary thromboembolism).

Reference
Rowan, R. M., Gordon, A. M., Chandhuri, A. K. R. *et al.* (1974) *Br. Med. J.* **3**, 317

Corticosteroids do not produce a reduction in normal response. Also there is no correlation between NBT activity and:

- Total white blood cell count.
- Differential white blood cell count.
- Vacuolation of neutrophil cytoplasm.
- Presence of 'toxic granulation'.

References
Editorial (1971) *N. Engl. J. Med.* **285**, 347
Feigin, R. D., Shackelford, P. G. and Choi, S. (1971) *J. Pediatr.* **79**, 170
Lace, J. K., Tan, J. S. and Watanakunakorn, C. (1975) *Am. J. Med.* **58**, 685

Neutrophil mobilization

Normally 50% of the neutrophils in the vasculature are stuck to the vessel endothelial linings, i.e. marginated, and can release and recirculate in the blood. Margination is a function of cell stickiness, requiring active cell metabolism, divalent cation and a heat-labile plasma component.

Decrease in margination

1. Physiological

- Exercise.
- Adrenaline (epinephrine).

2. Pathological
- Alcohol
- Prednisone therapy ⎫ Neutrophils less sticky.
- Acute and chronic ⎬ Greater tendency to lung myeloid leukaemia ⎭ infection.

Excessive deposition of neutrophils in lungs

- Shock

Massive irreversible pooling in the lung vasculature.

- Pneumonia

Deposition of most of the marrow neutrophil reserves in the lung vasculature.

References
MacGregor, R. R., Spagnuolo, P. J. and Centnek, A. L. (1974) *N. Engl. J. Med.* **291**, 642
Miller, M. E., Norman, M. E., Koblenzer, P. J. *et al.* (1973) *J. Lab. Clin. Med.* **82**, 1

Neutrophil anomalies and inclusion bodies

'Toxic' granulations

Large numbers of purple granules appear in the neutrophil cytoplasm on staining with Romanowsky stains:

- Infections, especially in the presence of toxaemia.
- After X-ray irradiation.
- Toxaemia of pregnancy.
- Liver disease.

The 'granules' probably represent a disturbance of granule formation resulting in decreased intraneutrophilic lysozyme content.

Cytoplasmic vacuolation of neutrophils in the peripheral blood

- Acute alcoholism.
- Infection, especially septicaemia, but it is not specific evidence of bacteraemia.

Reference
Malcolm, I. D. and Flegel, K. M. (1975) *Arch. Intern. Med.* **139**, 675

- Ketoacidosis in diabetes mellitus.
- Progressive muscular dystrophy.
- Blood standing in sample tube at room temperature for a few hours before the blood film is prepared, i.e. artefact.

Pelger-Hüet anomaly

The neutrophil polymorphs never have more than two lobes per nucleus, and about 30% of the neutrophils are band forms. Deficiency of nuclear segmentation is associated with a defect in chromatin synthesis.

1. Primary: inherited [AD]

The homozygous state is lethal in humans, whereas the heterozygous state is benign. Phagocytosis is normal, but affected subjects suffer from more local infections than normal.

2. Secondary

This has been described in myxoedema, acute enteritis, multiple myeloma, chronic lymphatic leukaemia, drug reactions and severe infections.

Reference
Savage, P. J., Dellinger, R. P. and Barnes, J. V. (1984) *Chest* **85**, 131

Alder's anomaly

This rare condition is inherited by means of a dominant gene and may be associated with skeletal abnormalities. The neutrophils, basophils and eosinophils contain profuse dark azurophilic granules. The same findings have been described in gargoylism.

Chédiak–Higashi–Steinbrinck anomaly

The neutrophil nuclei are only rarely completely segmented. The neutrophil cytoplasm contains coarse triangular indented clumps of deeply red-blue (Giemsa) material. The lymphocyte cytoplasm contains azurophilic granules up to 3 μm in diameter. These changes are also found in the myeloblasts. The majority of cases are partial albinos. The children suffer from repeated infections and die by 7 years of age. There is a profound decrease in natural killer cell activity.

Döhle (Amato) bodies

These are small elliptical bodies found in the cytoplasm of neutrophils and eosinophils, about 5 μm long and 1–2 μm thick. With Romanowsky stains they appear bright blue.

- May–Hegglin anomaly: a constitutional disorder of maturation of the granulocytes, it is associated with the occurrence of Döhle bodies, thrombocytopenia, purpura, peripheral giant platelets and coarsely granular megakaryocytes in the bone marrow. The inclusions develop in immature granulocytes in the bone marrow. They resemble depolymerized ribosomes.
- Scarlet fever ⎫
- Other specific fevers ⎬ some cases.
- Coccal infections ⎭
- After burns: during the first few days, in some cases.
- Normal pregnancy: oxidase-positive granules are found in: granulocytes; myelocytes; myeloblasts (if not too primitive).

Monocytes and promonocytes often contain a few faintly positive granules, which may be remains of ingested granulocytes.

In myeloid leukaemia and in some infections, the peroxidase staining reaction in the granulocytes shows an inverse relationship with the alkaline phosphate reaction.

Auer bodies, which may be found in myeloblasts, monoblasts and monocytes, give a positive oxidase reaction.

Lymphoblasts and lymphocytes give a negative oxidase reaction.

Jordan's anomaly

Vacuoles (lipid) are found in the neutrophils, monocytes and occasional lymphocytes in association with ichthyosis in this familial condition.

Neutrophil 'R' anomaly

Two cases have been described in which mature neutrophils had round nuclei.

Neutrophil pseudoplatelets

Neutrophils in acute infections or myeloid leukaemia may shed nuclear remnants which are platelet sized, but contain myeloperoxidase.

Reference
Hanker, J. S. and Giammara, B. L. (1983) *Science* **220**, 415

Peroxidase reaction

Peroxidase-positive granules are present in normal developing and adult granulocytes. Small numbers of peroxidase-positive granules are present in promonocytes and monocytes. Lymphocytes do not contain these granules, and early myeloblasts also give negative results.

The peroxidase-positive granules probably coincide with the positive sudanophilic granules, and with the Romanowsky-positive specific granules. Auer bodies are peroxidase positive.

Abnormal increase in reaction

Relapse in myeloid leukaemia (inversely proportional to alkaline phosphatase content).

Abnormal decrease in reaction

1. Many infections.
2. Vitamin B_1 deficiency (beri-beri).
3. Brain lesions in the region of the corpus striatum.
4. Idiopathic familial absence of peroxidase:
   (a) in neutrophils ⎫
   (b) in eosinophils ⎬ harmless.
5. Some cases of leukaemia during cytotoxic drug therapy.

This stain is most useful in the differentiation of early myelocytes and late myeloblasts from lymphocytes and lymphoblasts in leukaemia. It also distinguishes monocytes from lymphocytes.

References
Grignaschi, V. J., Sperperato, A. M., Etcheverry, M. J. *et al.* (1962) *Revta Asoc. Med. Argent.* **77**, 218
Presentey, B. (1969) *Am. Clin. Pathol.* **51**, 451, 458
van der Schoot, C. Ellen, Daams, G. Marjolein, Pinkster, Janita, *et al.* (1990) *Br. J. Haematol.* **74**, 173

Sudan black reactions

Now that the peroxidase reaction is proscribed because of its use of carcinogenic substances, the staining reactions with Sudan black have been found to offer satisfactory alternative results:

Positive staining

- Myeloblasts: numerous positively stained granules.
- Monoblasts: a few positively stained granules.

Negative results
- Proerythroblast.
- Lymphoblast.

Reference
Coeur, P., Charrin, C., Germain, D. *et al.* (1969) *Nouv. Rev. Fr. Hematol.* **9**, 703

Neutrophil alkaline phosphatase activity

The specific granules present in promyelocytes, myelocytes, metamyelocytes, stab cells and adult neutrophils give a positive test for the presence of alkaline phosphatase. No relationship has yet been demonstrated between the serum alkaline phosphatase level and the leucocyte alkaline phosphatase activity. It has been suggested that leucocyte alkaline phosphatase is an inducible enzyme dependent on *de novo* protein synthesis, possibly controlled by group 21–22 chromosomes. Alkaline phosphatase activity is highest in the youngest circulating neutrophils. Only immature forms can synthesize alkaline phosphatase.

Reference
Williams D. M. (1975) *Br. J. Haematol.* **31**, 371

Alkaline phosphatase activity is absent from monocytes, lymphocytes, eyrthrocytes and platelets in all species. Neutrophil alkaline phosphatase is present in the horse, cow, sheep, goat, pig, rabbit and monkey, and is absent in the cat and the dog.

References
Jain, N. C. (1968) *Acta Haematol.* **39**, 51
Macaraeg, P. V. Jr., Conell, E. and Biachine, J. R. (1968) *Arch. Intern. Med.* **122**, 412
Wiltshaw, E. and Moloney, W. C. (1955) *Blood* **10**, 1120

Normal activity or moderate increase

- Normal cases.
- Normal pregnancy: there is an increase in activity after the third month, with return to normal in the puerperium.
- Oral contraceptives.
- Down's syndrome.
- Secondary polycythaemia.
- Neutrophilia following infections etc.
- Essential thrombocythaemia.
- Myeloid metaplastic (depressed levels of activity in some cases).
- Myelosclerosis.
- Kwashiorkor. *Note:* low serum alkaline phosphatase).
- Active Hodgkin's disease.

Increased activity

- Polycythaemia vera. The marked increase seen in many cases is not affected by treatment with radioactive phosphorus (^{32}P).
- Leukaemoid reactions.
- Cushing's syndrome (direct correlation with urine 17-hydroxycorticosteroid output).

Decreased activity

- Myeloid leukaemia: following splenectomy in chronic myeloid leukaemia neutrophil alkaline phosphatase activity returns to normal. The explanation for this is not known. Only after a prolonged remission produced by busulphan does the alkaline phosphatase activity approach normal. Occasionally in relapse with an outpouring of myeloblasts the leucocytes may contain alkaline phosphatase.

- Rickets.
- Congenital hypophosphatasaemia: alkaline phosphatase activity is absent from the neutrophils.
- Familial myeloproliferative disease: low neutrophil phosphatase in cases and in many relatives, with anaemia, thrombocytopenia and white cell counts up to $128 \times 10^9/l$.
- Some cases of paroxysmal nocturnal haemoglobinuria.
- Some cases of infectious mononucleosis.
- Some cases of pernicious anaemia in relapse.
- Some cases of myelosclerosis.

References
Hayhoe, F. G. J. and Quaglino, D. (1958) *Br. J. Haematol.* **4**, 375;
Ozsoyhu, S. (1969) *N. Engl. J. Med.* **280**, 1221
Perry, S. (1966) *J. Am. Med. Assoc.* **190**, 918

Peripheral blood eosinophils

Normal peripheral blood count

This is 0.04–$0.4 \times 10^9/l$.

Diurnal variation

- Highest count at night during sleep.
- Lowest count in the morning.
- Count rises by mid-afternoon.

(The rhythm is reversed in night workers.)

Formation and function

The majority of eosinophils are produced in the bone marrow, differentiation being apparent at the myelocyte stage, and their production is under separate genetic control distinct from that of the neutrophil polymorph.

On electron microscopy, the granules in eosinophilic myelocytes are large spherical and homogeneous. In eosinophilic polymorphs the granules are small and irregular.

Eosinophils migrate to areas exposed to the external environment:

- Skin, connective tissue immediately below the epithelial layer.
- Bronchial mucosa.
- Gastrointestinal tract.
- Lactating mammary gland.
- Vagina and walls of the uterus.

Less than 1% of the body's eosinophils are circulating in the blood stream. In the vascular compartment half are marginated. Eventually eosinophils enter lymphatic channels and are destroyed by the reticuloendothelial system. They appear to have a role in the defence of the body against attack by foreign materials. Eosinophilia of parasitic infection is associated with generalized mast cell degranulation.

Eosinophils can neutralize 5-hydroxytryptamine and histamine, and they carry profibrinolysin from the bone marrow to parts of the body. Antigen–antibody complexes give chemotactic stimuli for their phagocytosis by eosinophils, with subsequent release of substances stimulating mucus secretion. A proportion of eosinophils have receptors for IgG1 and IgG3 and complement receptors. They contain a variety of hydrolytic enzymes (peroxidase, aryl sulphatase, phospholipase and acid phosphatase). Prostaglandins may be released in allergic reactions.

Lifespan

This may be up to 12 days.

Reference
Bass, D. A. (1979) *Ann. Intern. Med.* **91**, 120

Pathological

INCREASE

- Allergic conditions

1. Angioneurotic oedema
2. Asthma: in steroid-dependent asthmas the total eosinophil count rises in activity and falls with steroid therapy. The counts are inversely proportional to specific airway conductance, and are useful in the regulation of steroid dosage and in the early detection of exacerbation.

Reference
Horn, B. R., Robin, E. D., Theodore, J. *et al.* (1975) *N. Engl. J. Med.* **292**, 1152

3. Food sensitivity.
4. Drug sensitivity:
    (a) chlorpromazine jaundice;
    (b) liver extracts;
    (c) penicillin;
    (d) streptomycin;
    (e) viomycin.
5. Hay fever.
6. Serum sickness.
7. Urticaria.

(The total eosinophil count is useful both in diagnosis and response to treatment in atopic subjects.) Lymphoid and myeloid cells may be integrated with eosinophilia in certain types of immune response.

Reference
Editorial (1971) *Lancet* **ii**, 1187
Lowell, F. C. (1967) *JAMA* **202**, 875

- Parasites

(Eosinophilia probably induced by allergic reaction.) Eosinophil granules contain at least four basic proteins toxic to some parasites.

Reference
Spry, C. J. F. (1985) *J. R. Soc. Med.* **78**, 845

1. Bilharzia
2. Filaria.
3. Hookworm.
4. Hydatid.
5. Loeffler's syndrome (endomyocardial disease and eosinophilia).

Reference
Oakley, C. M. and Olsen, E. G. J. (1977) *Br. Heart J.* **39**, 233

- Malaria (occasionally).
6. Roundworm (*Ascaris, Strongyloides and Anklylostoma spp., Toxocara canis, T. cati*).
7. Trichiniasis.
8. Tropical eosinophilia, ?mites primary or secondary lung invaders.

Reference
Roberts, W. C., Liegler, D. G. and Carbone, P. P. (1969) *Am. J. Med.* **46**, 28

- Skin diseases (accompanied by variable eosinophilia)

1. Dermatitis herpetiformis.
2. Eczema.
3. Exfoliative dermatitis.
4. Pemphigus.
5. Psoriasis.
6. Prurigo.
7. Scabies.

INFECTIONS

8. Scarlet fever, in the early stages, and again in the convalescence at about 6 weeks.
9. ?Some cases of chorea.
10. ?Some cases of erythema multiforme.
11. *Aspergillus fumigatus* lung infection in grain handlers.

- Malignant conditions

1. Myeloid leukaemia. In chronic myeloid leukaemia the total eosinophil count is usually above the normal limit.
2. Eosinophilic leukaemia: the occurrence of this condition as a distinct entity is in doubt.
3. Association with acute lymphoblastic leukaemia in childhood.

References
Evans, T. S. and Nesbit, R. R. (1949) *Blood* **4**, 603 (review of 18 cases in the literature and description of one further case)
Weinger, R. S., André-Schwarz J., Desforges, J. F. *et al.* (1975) *Br. J. Haematol.* **30**, 65

4. Hodgkin's disease: about 10% of cases may show an eosinophilia in the peripheral blood. It is interesting that about 50% of cases show an increase in lymph gland eosinophils.

- Eosinophilia associated with chemicals

1. Nickel, causing dermatitis.
2. Penicillin.
3. P-Aminosalicylic acid.
4. Hydralazine.
5. Nitrofurantoin.
6. Mecamylamine.
7. Mephenesin.
8. Sulphonamides.
9. Many cases of non-tropical eosinophilic pneumonia with cause unknown, and good prognosis.

- Rarities

1. Eosinophilic granulomatosis.
2. Familial eosinophilia – a hereditary autosomal dominant condition. A benign anomaly diagnosed by exclusion of other causes, and demonstration on other members of the family.
3. Hand–Schüller–Christian disease.
4. Letterer–Siwe disease.
5. Disseminated eosinophilic collagen disease.
6. Eosinophilic gastroenteritis.
7. Hypereosinophilic syndrome: affecting more men than women, especially in the fourth decade:
   (a) angio-oedema with high serum IgE levels: responds well to steroids;
   (b) eosinophilic endomyocardial disease and/or neurological defects: poor prognosis;
   (c) myeloproliferative disorder with cytogenic abnormalities in the eosinophil precursors.

References
Spry, C. J. F., Davies, J., Tai P. C. et al. (1983) Q. J. Med. **52**, 1
Editorial (1983) Lancet **i** 1417

DECREASE

1. After ACTH, adrenocortical steroids, adrenaline, ephedrine or insulin.
2. After stress:
   (a) acute severe infection;
   (b) trauma;
   (c) burns;
   (d) postoperation;
   (e) for a few hours after electroconvulsive therapy;
   (f) after excessive exercise.
3. Cushing's syndrome: many cases have counts of less than 0.04×10^9/l.
4. Acromegaly.
5. Disseminated lupus erythematosus.

References
Editorial (1969) Lancet **ii**, 1237
Hardy, W. R. and Anderson, R. E. (1968) Ann. Intern. Med. **68**, 1920

- Eosinophils in pleural fluid

Found in idiopathic effusions and in effusions due to benign asbestosis. Eosinophilia in pleural fluid is rare in malignancy and in tuberculous effusions.

Reference
Adelman, M., Albelda, S. M., Gottlieb, J. et al. (1984) Am. J. Med. **77**, 915

Peripheral blood basophils

Normal peripheral blood count ($<0.1 \times 10^9$/l)

Function

All of the blood histamine is carried by the basophils confined to the specific cytoplasmic granules. The large basophilic granules, which are peroxidase negative, contain a substance very similar to, or identical with, heparin. It has been found that disodium cromoglycate indirectly inhibits most cell degranulation. IgE can activate C3 by means of an alternative pathway (i.e. not when reacted with antigen). IgE binds to the basophil cell surface and, in atopic subjects, all IgE binding sites on the basophils are nearly saturated. Basophils and mast cells are found in areas of local inflammation during healing.

Reference
Orr, T. S. C. and Cox, J. S. G. (1969) Nature **223**, 197

Pathological

INCREASE

Occurs in some cases of the following conditions:

- Chronic myeloid leukaemia: up to 80% of the total white cells may on occasion consist of basophils ?A sudden increase in basophil polymorphs heralds a 'blastic' crisis. The existence of pure basophil-cell leukaemia is in doubt.

Reference
Quattrin, N., Dini, E. and Palumbo E. (1959a) Blut **5**, 166 (reviews 76 cases in literature and 10 cases of their own)
Quattrin, N., Dini, E. and Palumbo, E. (1959b) Schweiz. Med. Wochenschr. **89**, 1045 (review of varieties of basophilic leukaemia, with 32 cases from literature, and 8 cases of their own)

- Recovery from infection
- Hypothyroidism
- Erythraemic myelosis (Di Guglielmo's disease)
- Polycythaemia vera
- Hodgkin's disease
- Cirrhosis of the liver
- Chronic haemolytic anaemia
- Following splenectomy
- Chronic inflammation
- Chickenpox
- Smallpox

} uncommon.

DECREASE

May occur in some cases of the following conditions:

1. More commonly in children:
   (a) acute rheumatic fever;
   (b) acute lobar pneumonia;
   (c) anaphylactoid purpura.
2. Non-leukaemic leucocytosis.
3. Following steroid therapy with concurrent fall in blood histamine levels.
4. Chronic myeloid leukaemia following treatment with X-rays or busulphan, with remission.
5. Thyrotoxicosis
6. Stress: in general, the accurate assessment of stress by means of the basophil count is not possible.
7. Urticaria: the low initial basophil count rises following antihistamine therapy.

References
Fredericks, R. E. and Moloney, W. C. (1959) *Blood* **14**, 571
Hofer, R. and Thumb, N. (1968) *Blut* **16**, 342

Peripheral blood lymphocytes

Normal peripheral blood lymphocyte count

At birth the lymphocyte count is $3.5-8.5 \times 10^9/l$, although at the end of the first week after birth the count may reach $12 \times 10^9/l$. The upper limit of normal during the first 6 years is about $5.5 \times 10^9/l$, averaging about $4 \times 10^9/l$, approximating to the neutrophil count at 4 years of age. The normal adult range of $1.5-3.5 \times 10^9/l$ is reached by about 12 years of age. During normal pregnancy $0.1-0.5\%$ of the circulating lymphocytes are fetal in origin.

Pathological

INCREASE

This especially in young children.

- Specific fevers

1. Measles.
2. German measles.
3. Mumps.
4. Whooping-cough (lymphocytosis very common).
5. Later stages of smallpox.
6. Later stages of chickenpox.
7. Typhoid and paratyphoid fever.
8. *Brucella melitensis* and *Br. abortus*.
9. Typhus.
10. Tularaemia
11. Dengue.

- Other infections

1. Influenza (the lymphocytosis may persist for weeks).
2. Benign lymphocytic meningitis.
3. Infective hepatitis
4. Infectious mononucleosis (after neutropenia or neutrophilia).
5. Healing stage of chronic tuberculosis.
6. Acute infective lymphocytosis in children:
   (a) very young children;
   (b) abdominal pain, diarrhoea and vomiting;
   (c) fever;
   (d) cough;
   (e) absolute lymphocytosis for 2-3 weeks: in one series, counts of $26-98 \times 10^9/l$ lymphocytes and an untyped enterovirus with neutralizing antibodies were found;
   (f) eosinophilia common.
7. Congenital syphilis.
8. Reports of lymphocytosis in hyperthyroidism do not appear to be very reliable.

So-called 'virocytic' lymphocytes occur in infectious mononucleosis, acute viral hepatitis, viral pneumonitis, herpes zoster, herpes simplex, roseola infantum and viral upper respiratory infections.

- Leukaemia

1. Acute lymphatic leukaemia.
2. Chronic lymphatic leukaemia.

LYMPHOID MYELOFIBROSIS

Reference
Duhamel, G. (1971) *Acta Haematol.* **45**, 112

DECREASE

1. After ACTH there is a fall in circulating lymphocytes maximal at 4–6 h, returning to normal by 6–8 h.
2. After burns and trauma, i.e. stress reaction.
3. Disseminated lupus erythematosus (some cases).
4. Hodgkin's disease (some cases).
5. Acute uraemia: in acute uraemia, there is lymphocytopenia associated with neutrophilia. The neutrophil nuclei tend to be hypersegmented, irrespective of the presence or absence or infection. The bone marrow shows myeloid hyperplasia.
6. Chronic uraemia: lymphocytopenia is also found, which correlates with the elevation of the blood urea.
7. In 178 cases out of 7350 differential lymphocyte count was less than 15% of total, or total lymphocyte count was less than $1 \times 10^9/l$. Diagnosis in 42.7% of cases was malignancy, and in 22.5% no abnormality was detected clinically.

References
Horowitz M. S. and Moore, G. T. (1968) *N. Engl. J. Med.* **279**, 399
Jensson, O. (1958) *Br. J. Haematol.* **4**, 422
Zacharski, L. R. (1971) *Mayo Clin. Proc.* **46**, 168

Lymphocyte development

Lymphocytes are the main cellular constituent of lymph nodes, spleen and Peyer's patches. They occur in small follicles throughout the bone marrow and the intestinal mucosa; and are found in the lymphoid tissue in bone marrow, thymus and spleen. The small lymphocytes, in a 'resting state', circulate continuously between the blood stream and the lymphatic system, entering lymphoid tissue where they leave the vascular space, entering the substance of the lymph nodes. After a time, they pass into the efferent lymphatics and eventually reach the thoracic duct, which drains into the main venous return to the heart. The lifespan of the small lymphocyte is uncertain, but may be some years.

Some lymphocytes from the bone marrow pass through the thymus, where they are processed by the presence of thymosin, becoming effective or immunologically competent T-lymphocytes, with acquisition of new surface antigens.

T-LYMPHOCYTES (T-CELLS)

In humans, T-cells are capable of delayed hypersensitivity reactions, graft rejection and graft-versus-host reaction. They migrate rapidly in response to stimuli. They have no surface immunoglobulin or complement receptors, and form spontaneous rosettes with sheep red blood cells, and they transform rapidly in response to non-specific mitogens. In all, they normally make up 40–80% of the total circulating lymphocyte population. Using T-lymphocyte surface antigens, it has been possible to generate specific antibodies with which it is possible to divide the T-cells into:

1. Regulatory cells

- Helper cells: assist B-cells in IgG production (T_H).
- Suppressor cells: suppress response of other lymphocytes (T_S).

2. Effector cells
1. Cytolytic.
2. Produce factors other than antibody:
   (a) direct mediator factor;
   (b) activate certain macrophages.

3. *K-cells* (killer cells)

Lymphocytes which destroy cells via IgG antibody.

4. *NK-cells* (natural killer cells)

Lymphocytes with spontaneous cytolytic activity against certain types of cell. Lymphocytes gain and lose various cell membrane activities, T6, T9 and T10 antigens, as they differentiate and mature. These markers may be used to examine T-cell maturation in cases of immunodeficiency and to classify T-cell malignancies, influencing form of treatment given and assessment of patient prognosis.

Mature T-cells in the peripheral blood possess T1 and T3 antigens. In addition, T4 antigen is expressed in 60% and T8 in 20% of peripheral blood lymphocytes.

- *T3*: mature peripheral blood lymphocyte.
- *T4*: helper/inducer cell, assisting B-cells in antibody production, and involved in delayed hypersensitivity. T-cells with receptors of IgM (T) provide 'help' in B-cell proliferation and subsequent differentiation into plasma cells.
- *T8*: cytotoxic/suppressor cells, which inhibit T-cell and B-cell function. T-cells with receptors of IgG (Tγ) suppress B-cell proliferation that may be induced by other T-cells. Cytotoxic T-cells possess an antigen-specific receptor.

Maturation of T-cells

- The first enzyme to develop is acid phosphatase.
- Followed by β-glucuronidase.
- Followed by α-naphthyl acetate acid esterase.
- Followed by n-acetyl-β-glucosaminidase, α-naphthyl acetate esterase, and α-naphthyl butyrate esterase.
- Final maturation to normal T-cell.

This approach may be useful eventually in the study of leukaemia, but otherwise the separation of T-lymphocytes by antibody reaction is the more promising.

Reference
Reinherz, E. L. and Schlossman, S. F. (1980) *Cell* **19**, 821

T-cell receptor structure (review).

Reference
Marx, J. L. (1983) *Science NY* **221**, 444

B-LYMPHOCYTES (B-CELLS)

B-lymphocytes (originally named B-cells in birds, as they originated from the bursa of Fabricius) originate in humans in the bone marrow. They have surface immunoglobulin and complement receptors, but do not form spontaneous rosettes with sheep red blood cells. When they are exposed to foreign antigen, they synthesize RNA and differentiate into plasma cells which produce antibodies (IgG immunoglobulins), a single clone or group of plasma cells all producing the same antibody against a single antigen.

In humans they normally make up 10–30% of the total circulating lymphocyte population.

NON T, NON-B-CELLS

Normally in humans 2–10% of the circulating lymphocytes are non-T-, non-B-cells. With increasing age the peripheral blood T-lymphocyte count falls and there is impairment of activation by T-cell mitogens and PPD antigens. This results in a relative and absolute increase in blood non-T-cells, and IgG-F_c + C3-receptor carrying cells. There is also increased sensitivity in lymphocytes from older subjects to the effects of radiation, and a reduced capacity to repair DNA damage. Perturbation of the cell cycle is progressively induced by [^{3}H]thymidine incorporation.

References

Staiano-Coico, L., Darzynkiewicz, Z., Hefton, J. M. *et al.* (1983) *Science NY* **219**, 1335

Wedelin, C., Bjokholm, M., Holm, G. *et al.* (1982) *Scand. J. Haematol.* **28**, 45

Following splenectomy, the lymphocytosis is due to increase in both T- and B-cells. T-cells with receptor for F^c of IgG are significantly increased (the group which includes T-suppressor cells).

T-cells

INCREASED

- Active Graves' disease.
- Hashimoto's thyroiditis.
- In salivary glands in Sjögren's syndrome.
- In synovial fluid in rheumatoid arthritis.

DECREASED

- Low-birth-weight infants.
- Severe protein–energy malnutrition.
- Severe viral infections.
- Metastatic and advanced malignancy.
- DiGeorge's syndrome.
- Nezelof's syndrome.
- Ataxia telangiectasia (also with B-cells reduced).
- Wiskott–Aldrich syndrome.
- Cell-mediated lymphocytolysis.
- Orotic aciduria: profound impairment of T-cells [R].
- Nucleoside phosphorylase deficiency [R].
- Adenosine deaminase deficiency [R] with reduction in B-cells.

MONOCLONAL T-CELL MALIGNANCIES

- Sézary's syndrome.
- Lymphatic leukaemia with erythroderma and lymphoid infiltration of the skin.
- Some acute lymphoblastic leukaemias.

INDIVIDUAL T-CELL PHENOTYPE VARIATIONS

Multiple sclerosis: T4 cells are actively involved in extension of the lesions, with I_a + cells associated with demyelination.

Reference

Traugott, V., Reinherz, E. L. and Raine, C. S. (1983) *Science NY* **219**, 308

Low helpers/suppressor ratio occurs in haemophiliacs. ?Related to susceptibility to AIDS.

B-cells

NORMAL OR INCREASED

- Common variable immunodeficiencies.
- Transient hypogammaglobulinaemia of infancy.
- X-linked immunodeficiency with hyper-IgM and selective IgA deficiency.

DECREASED

- X-linked agammaglobulinaemia.
- Some acquired agammaglobulinaemia.
- Some severe combined immunodeficiencies.

B-CELL MALIGNANCIES

- Lymphosarcoma.
- Burkitt's lymphoma.
- Waldenström's macroglobulinaemia.
- Myelomatosis.
- Occasional acute lymphoid leukaemia (ALL).

Lymphocyte function

Lymphocytes circulate continuously in the blood, entering the tissues and returning via the lymphatics to the blood stream, detecting foreign material directly or via contact with macrophages which have ingested material, in the lymph nodes and spleen. When immunologically competent T-cells meet foreign antigenic material they undergo blast transformation, and numerous lymphocytes are produced with specific receptors for that antigen on their surface. When these activated T-cells migrate to the site of the foreign antigen, and encounter the antigen, they release *lymphokines* which:

- Are factors for chemotaxis of macrophages to the site.
- Are lymphotoxic, and kill foreign cells.
- Produce interferon, which inactivates viruses.

T-cells

- Cell-mediated immunity.
- Graft rejection, tumour immunity – cytotoxic T-cells, mediate graft-versus-host reaction (GVHR) (killer T-cells).
- Correlate delayed hypersensitivity – T-cells release soluble factor which inhibits migration of macrophages away from the antigen, acts as transfer factor to transform other lymphocytes, and is lymphotoxic.
- Immunological memory – T-cells divide to form a population of antigen-sensitive cells with a long lifespan, triggered by later exposure to the same antigen.

- Cooperate with B-cells ('helper' T-cells). A hapten reacts with B-cell, but the carrier reacts with T-cells to yield antibody production response.
- 'Suppressor T-cells – T-cells inhibit B-cells antibody formation (immune tolerance and autoimmune phenomenon), modifying the immunological response.
- Non-specific response to mitogens, e.g. phytohaemagglutinin, or concavalin A.
- Viral infection can generate a population of 'killer T-cells' which are specifically cytotoxic for host cells infected with that virus. Similarly killer T-cells can be generated against an allogeneic graft.

B-cells

When B-cells are exposed to foreign antigen, they synthesize RNA and differentiate into plasma cells to produce immunoglobulins (antibodies). A group of plasma cells produces antibodies against one antigen, and are then known as a clone. ?Tonsils, appendix and intestinal lymphoid tissue correspond to, and act in the same way as, the bursa of Fabricius in fowls.

B-cells have a short lifespan (days–weeks). Some large lymphocytes can revert to become small B-cells to acts as 'memory cells'. Attachment of antigen to IgG, or antigen–antibody complex to the F_c receptor on the immunoglobulin molecule stimulates B-cell proliferation and 'blast cell transformation'.

In the presence of some large polymers (e.g. mucopolysaccharide of pneumococcus capsule or high-molecular weight dextran), B-cells are stimulated directly to produce antibody without T-cell assistance.

Acquired immune deficiency syndrome (AIDS)

In the early 1980s a new disease was described, initially in the homosexual population of the USA. It has since become apparent that this sexually and blood transmitted disease is caused by a small retrovirus, the immunodeficiency virus (HIV), first discovered in France in 1983. The virus, which has a reverse transcriptase, attacks and kills specific lymphocytes, and T4 helper/inducer cells, thus causing immune deficiency. HIV infection has been classified into the following stages:

1. The initial infection which may be associated with rash, fever, myalgia, arthralgia, headache, sore throat, diarrhoea.
2. Chronic asymptomatic carrier – may or may not have laboratory abnormalities, e.g. reduced T4 levels.
3. Persistent generalized lymphadenopathy – may or may not have laboratory abnormalities.
4. Serious clinical disease:
   (a) constitutional disease – fever, weight loss, diarrhoea;
   (b) neurological disease.
   (c) infectious disease – Pneumocystis carinii, candidiasis, cytomegalovirus (CMV), cryptococcosis, mycobacteria, herpes simplex;
   (d) malignancy – Kaposi's sarcoma, non-Hodgkin's lymphoma.

Progression to stage (4) is associated with serious illness, poor quality of life and short survival. However, progression is variable being anything from 6 months to 10 years or more, although it does seem to be inevitable.

In the USA today at least one million people are affected by HIV and there are certainly many millions world wide.

Groups infected in the USA and Europe include homosexuals (by sexual transmission), intravenous drug abusers (by blood contaminated needles) and haemophiliacs (from infected blood products, e.g. factor VIII).

However, in Africa the virus is found throughout the heterosexual population and there are no well-defined 'high-risk' groups. This could happen in the USA and Europe also. It has to be hoped that better education about sexual activities, the use of condoms and safer blood products for blood transfusion may help to slow down the spread of the disease. Rather worryingly, a second virus – HIV-2 – is increasingly being reported, especially from Africa!

PREDICTION OF PROGRESSION TO STAGE 4

1. Clinical: herpes zoster, thrush, lymphoma-like symptoms (e.g. weight loss, night sweats, fever).
2. Laboratory:
   (a) T4 levels (normal $0.8–0.9 \times 10^9$/l);
   (b) T4 < 200, progression 87% at 3 years;
   (c) T4 > 400, progression 16% at 3 years;
   (d) serum β_2-microglobulin (normal 1.7 mg/l);
   (e) β_2 > 5, progression 69% at 3 years;
   (f) β_2 < 3, progression 12% at 3 years.

MANAGEMENT
Support care with counselling and active treatment of opportunistic infections was the only initial help in this disease. Anaemia and even pancytopenia due to direct viral action in the bone marrow is also now well recognized and, where possible, treated.

Recently, the drug zidovudine (originally called azidothymidine or AZT), which inhibits the viral reverse transcriptase, has been used to treat AIDS and as prophylaxis in HIV-positive patients in an attempt to prevent progression to stage 4. Its use is still being evaluated although results look promising both in treatment and prophylaxis. There are side effects, however, particularly bone marrow failure.

References
Mindel, A. (1987) *Br. Med. J.* **294**, 1214–1218
Morris, A. R. and Bacchetti, P. (1989) *AIDS* **3**, 55–61
Moss, A. R. (1988) *Br. Med. J.* **297**, 1067–1068
Pedersen, C., Lindhardt, B. O., Jensen, B. L. *et al.* (1989) *Br. Med. J.* **299**, 154–157

Factors affecting lymphocyte populations in the peripheral blood

Physiological

● Diurnal rhythm

There is a diurnal rhythm in the total number of circulating lymphocytes, T-cells, inducer/helper cells, suppressor/cytotoxic cells, Ia-positive cells and B-cells, lowest at 09:00 h and highest at 21:00 h, the inverse of the plasma cortisol concentration.

References
Bertouch, J. V., Roberts-Thompson, P. J. and Bradley, J. (1983) *Br. Med. J.* **286**, 1171
Ritchie, A. W. S., Oswall I., Mieklem, H. S. *et al.* (1983) *Br. Med. J.* **286**, 1773

● Fasting

There is an increase in bactericidal activity and killer cell cytolytic activity, with increases in plasma IgG, IgA and IgM. Peripheral blood neutrophils, T- and B-cells do not change significantly.

Reference
Wing, E. J., Stanko, R. T., Winkelstein, A. *et al.* (1983) *Am. J. Med.* **75**, 91

Pathological

● Surgical Operation

Natural killer cell cytolytic activity in the peripheral blood increases after premedication, is increased during general anaesthesia during major surgery, and falls to low levels postoperatively for at least 5 days (in parallel with the fall in the numbers of circulating T- and B-cells in the peripheral blood).

Reference
Tonnesen, E., Mickley, H. and Grunnet, N. (1983) *Acta Anaesthesiol. Scand.* **27**, 238

● Steroid therapy

Following treatment with glucocorticoids, the peripheral blood lymphocyte count falls, with selective depletion of T-cells, which are sequestered in the bone marrow. This results in the diminishing probability of lymphocyte–antigen interaction. Lymphoid cell proliferation is slowed down, and consequently antibody production is reduced.

● Haemophilia

Male patients with classic haemophilia, treated with lyophilized clotting factor concentrates, are at risk for contracting AIDS (acquired immune deficiency syndrome). Initially serum levels of human leucocyte or α-interferon are nil, but rise over a period of time. The helper/suppressor T-cell ratio is reduced.

● Promiscuous homosexual males

Homosexual males with lymphadenopathy, or with Kaposi's sarcoma, have reduced helper/suppressor T-cell ratios in the peripheral blood, and increasing titres of human leucocytes of α-interferon.

Reference
Eyster, E. E., Goedert, J. J., Poon, M-C. *et al.* (1983) *N. Engl. J. Med.* **309**, 583

In their lymph nodes there were numerous suppressor/cytotoxic phenotypes in the germinal centres and mantle zone (in comparison in control lymphoid tissue there were only B-cells and a subpopulation of helper/inducer cells present).

● Virus infections

Reduced peripheral helper/suppressor T-cell ratio.

● Sarcoidosis

Reduced peripheral blood helper/suppressor T-cell ratio, due to sequestration of helper T-cells at the sites of disease activity, and the ratio of helper/suppressor T-cells was increased in the lymph glands (the reverse of homosexual males).

● Liver disease

In primary biliary cirrhosis there is abnormal impaired suppressor cell function, and this was also found in some first-degree relatives. There is similar defect in suppressor cell function in chronic active hepatitis, and in both conditions there is negligible alteration in the proportion of suppressor cells. Suppressor cell function is defective in both HBsAg-positive liver disease and in some alcoholic liver disease.

References
Alexander, G. J. M., Nouri-Aria, K. T., Eddleston, A. L. W. F. *et al.* (1983) *Lancet* **i**, 1291
Miller, K. B., Sepersky, R. A., Brown, K. M. *et al.* (1983) *Am. J. Med.* **75**, 75

● Orotic aciduria

Decreased total T-cell population with profound impairment of cell-mediated lymphocytosis.

● Leprosy

● Tuberculoid leprosy: a substantial population of T4+ cells in infiltrates.

● Lepromatous leprosy: a much higher proportion of T8+ cells.

- Gut mucosa

An excess of T8-positive cells in the intestinal mucosa in coeliac disease. In regional ileitis and ulcerative colitis the T4 and T8 cell numbers are normal with T8 predominantly in the epithelial layer and T4 cells in the lamina propria in the intestinal mucosa.

- Opportunistic infection following renal transplanta- tion

The helper/suppressor ratio falls.

Note: It is important that blood samples are dealt with rapidly. Overnight storage reduces the number of cells, distorting the helper/suppressor ratio.

Reference
Weiblen B. J., Debell, K. and Valeri, C. R. (1983) *N. Engl. J. Med.* **309**, 793

Lymphocyte anomalies and inclusion bodies

Atypical lymphocytes

There is a non-specific antigenic response by cells in the phase of DNA synthesis, which are removed from the circulation before dividing.

1. More than 20% atypical

- Infectious mononucleosis (probably due to Epstein-Barr virus).
- Cytomegalovirus infection.
- Toxoplasmosis.
- Infective hepatitis.
- Post-transfusion hepatitis ('serum jaundice').
- Hypersensitivity to certain drugs, e.g. *p*-aminosalicylic acid, Dilantin, Mesantoin.

2. Less than 20% atypical

- Virus infections, including mumps, varicella, rubella, herpes simplex, influenza, roseola infantum.
- Rickettsial infections.
- Tuberculosis.
- Post-irradiation.
- Letterer–Siwe disease.
- Agranulocytosis.
- Lead poisoning.
- ?Stress.
- Blood transfusion: atypical lymphocytes occur normally at 6–7 days after blood transfusion. At least some of these are activated recipient cells.

References
Hutchinson, R. M., Fraser, I. D., Sejeny, S. A. *et al.* (1975) *Br. J. Haematol* **30**, 128
Wood T. A. and Frenkel E. P. (1967) *Am. J. Med.* **42**, 923

3. Lymphocyte vacuolation

- Infectious mononucleosis.
- Viral infections.
- Some lipid storage diseases.

- Mucopolysaccharidoses.

Inclusion bodies
- Alder–Reilly bodies in gargoylism.
- Azurophilic cytoplasmic inclusion bodies in Chèdiak–Higashi–Steinbrinck disease.
- Various virus inclusions have been described.
- Rheumatoid arthritis with leucopenia: cytoplasmic inclusion bodies which did not contain either DNA or RNA, but which probably consisted of phospholipids, have been described.

Reference
Hovig, T., Jeremic, M. and Stavem, P. (1968) *Scand. J. Haematol.* **5**, 81

Peripheral blood lymphoblasts

Normally no lymphoblasts are seen either in the peripheral blood or in the bone marrow. They appear in the peripheral blood in the following conditions:

- Acute lymphoblastic leukaemia.
- Chronic lymphatic leukaemia.
- Lymphosarcoma.
- Lymphoblastic lymphoma.

Notes: In some cases of infectious mononucleosis cells resembling lymphoblasts may appear in the peripheral blood. The clinical course, the absence of anaemia and the absence of thrombocytopenia distinguish this condition from the malignant conditions. The Feulgen reaction may be useful where many of the cells appear to contain nucleoli.

Peripheral blood monocytes

Formation and function

Monocytes are derived from bone marrow promonocytes. They enter the blood stream, circulate and reach the tissues as mature macrophages. They are present in connective tissue, but concentrate especially in:

- Lung – alveolar macrophages.
- Liver – Kupffer cells.
- Spleen – lining the sinusoids.
- Lymph nodes – in the medullary sinuses.

They also occur in specialized forms, as mesangial cells of the glomerulus, brain microglia and osteoclasts in bone.

The monocytes and macrophages are long-lived, and act as a defence against bacteria, viruses and protozoa capable of living in the host's cells. Destructive macrophages are present in the lymph node cortex and in the skin. Lymphokines from stimulated sensitized lymphocytes act on macrophages:

- MCF – macrophage chemotactic factor, which attracts macrophages to the site.
- MIF – migration inhibition factor, which discourages macrophages from leaving the site.
- MAF – macrophage activating factor, which alters the monocyte surface and increases the ability of the cell to kill ingested intracellular organisms. Macrophages ingest viruses non-specifically, and either kill them, or the virus multiples in the cell. This latter happening results either in a lethal infection or a persistent infection. Macrophages prevent the passing of virus from one cell to another across the intercellular junction, macrophages being attracted to the site by chemotactic factor from T-cells.

Monocytes and macrophages bind IgG1 and IgG3 readily to their surface; they trap and concentrate antigen at the cell surface for presentation to lymphocytes. Antigen–antibody complex is trapped for antigen-specific B-cells to generate B-cell memory.

Macrophages and monocytes pick up antigen, present it to T-lymphocytes which, in turn, stimulate the macrophages to ingest and destroy the antigen after ingestion, and stimulate B-cells to produce specific antibody against the antigen.

Monocyte adherence leads to the development of procoagulant activity, possibly a factor in disseminated intravascular coagulation.

Normal peripheral blood count

- From birth for the first week, the normal upper limit may be as high as $4 \times 10^9/l$.
- After the first week of life it is $0.2–0.8 \times 10^9/l$, varying with both time of day and site of collection.

Automatic counting by different machines gives different results. The visual method is cumbersome.

Reference
Goossens, W., Van Hove, L. and Verwilghen, R. L. (1991) *J. Clin. Pathol.* **44**, 224

Pathological

Increase

BACTERIAL INFECTIONS

- Tuberculosis
- Subacute bacterial endocarditis
- Brucellosis
- Typhoid and paratyphoid fever
- During recovery from acute infection.

} variable counts.

PROTOZOAL INFECTIONS

- Kala-azar
- Malaria
- Trypanosomiasis

} especially in chronic infections.

VIRUS INFECTIONS
Infectious mononucleosis (some cases).

MALIGNANT CONDITIONS

- Monocytic leukaemia.
- Hodgkin's disease (some cases).
- Myeloma.
- Malignant tumours: many young monocytes with cytoplasmic vacuoles may be found with increased disease activity.

Reference
Barrett O'N. (1970) *Ann. Intern. Med.* **73**, 991

OTHER

- Collagen disease.
- Chronic ulcerative colitis.
- Regional enteritis.

(It is thought probable that blood monocytes originate in the bone marrow from promyelocytes, and that they migrate from blood vessels to become macrophages.)

References
Leder L.-D. (1967) *Blut* **16**, 86
Maldonado, J. E. and Hanlon, D. G. (1965) *Mayo Clin. Proc.* **40**, 248
Schmalzl, F. and Braunsteiner, H. (1967) *Wien. Z. Inn. Med.* **48**, 409

Peripheral blood plasma cells

Normally only occasional plasma cells are seen in the peripheral blood. B-lymphocytes develop into the plasma cell series, following activation by T-lymphocytes, and the mature plasma cell actively synthesizes and secretes antibody. Plasma cells contain IgG, IgA, IgM and IgD, usually only one immunoglobulin being present in a cell. They are normally present in interstitial tissues of various organs, and make up to 2.5% of the nucleated cell population of the bone marrow.

Increased peripheral blood plasma cells

1. Some myeloma cases.
2. Plasma cell leukaemia [R].
3. Extramedullary plasmacytoma [R], when there are metastases.
4. Post-irradiation damage.
5. Serum reactions, e.g. serum sickness.
6. Rarely in infections:
   (a) rubella;
   (b) scarlet fever;
   (c) measles;

(d) chickenpox;
(e) benign lymphocytic meningitis;
(f) infectious mononucleosis.
7. Carcinomatosis [R].

Plasma cell abnormalities

Russell bodies

These are granular and hyaline bodies occurring in the cytoplasm of plasma cells in myeloma and plasma cell leukaemia. They stain red with Romanowsky stains, and contain non-immunoglobulin molecules, byproducts of immunoglobulin synthesis and altered forms of immunoglobulin no longer recognized by anti-immunoglobulin antibody.

Reference
Hsu, S. M., Hsu, P.-L., McMillan, P. N. *et al.* (1982) *Am. J. Clin. Pathol.* **77**, 26

Snapper–Schneid inclusion bodies

These are basophilic granules which consist of amidine and ribonucleic acid, which appear in plasma cells during treatment with stilbamidine or pentamidine.

Peripheral blood megakaryocytes

Megakaryocytes may appear in the peripheral blood, in some cases, in the following conditions:

* Leucoerythroblastic anaemia.
* Myeloid leukaemia (chronic).
* Polycythaemia vera.
* Hodgkin's disease.
* Severe lobar pneumonia (the lungs are believed to be a major site of platelet formation).
* Rarely in cases of severe untreated pernicious anaemia.
* Rarely in lead poisoning.
* In some cases of sudden death (either traumatic or natural).

There appears to be a diurnal variation in circulating megakaryocytes in the blood with increased counts in the evening. These cells have been mistaken for cancer cells in some cases.

Megakaryocytes may be found in the lungs, spleen, kidney, liver and heart.

Reference
Hume, R., West, J. T., Malmgren, R. A. *et al.* (1964) *N. Engl. J. Med.* **270**, 111

The presence of megakaryocytes in serous fluids signifies an advanced haemopoietic malignancy.

Reference
Kumar, N. B. and Nagler, B. (1980) *J. Clin. Pathol.* **33**, 1153

Leukaemoid reactions

The peripheral blood picture may suggest a diagnosis of leukaemia, e.g. a gross increase in either the lymphocytic or myeloid series of cells, possibly with immature cells of the particular series and even nucleated red cells present:

Resembling lymphatic leukaemia

1. Virus infections
* Measles.
* Chickenpox.
* Infectious mononucleosis.
* Acute viral lymphocytosis (counts up to 90×10^9/l.).

Reference
Shipp, J. C. and Baden, H. (1959) *Arch. Intern. Med.* **104**, 619 (description of a case)

2. Bacterial infections
* Whooping cough.
* Pertussis vaccination.
* Disseminated acute tuberculosis (uncommon).

3. Neoplasia
* Lymphocytic and lymphoblastic lymphomas (some cases).
* Follicular lymphomas (some cases).
* Carcinoma of the stomach (rare).

4. Dermatitis herpetiformis

Reference
Even-Paz, Z. and Sagher, F. (1959) *Br. J. Dermatol.* **71**, 325

Resembling myeloid leukaemia

1. Severe bacterial infections, e.g. meningococcal septicaemia.
2. Severe burns.
3. After severe haemorrhages and after acute haemolysis, especially in young children.
4. Eclampsia (some cases).
5. Reaction to chemicals:
   (a) mercury poisoning;
   (b) mustard-gas poisoning;
   (c) benzene poisoning (before the stage of marrow aplasia is reached);
   (d) sulphonamides (some cases);
   (e) bone-marrow recovery following severe drug-induced marrow depression, e.g. butazolidine, etc.
6. Pernicious anaemia: during a remission or after specific treatment (especially after treatment with liver extract).

Reference
Strauss, M. B., Brokaw, R. and Chapman, C. B. (1952) *Am. J. Med. Sci.* **223**, 54

7. Megaloblastic anaemia of pregnancy: after specific treatment with folic acid.
8. Agranulocytosis: in cases associated with a maturation arrest, in the recovery phase a leukaemoid reaction is often found.
9. Hodgkin's disease (some cases).
10. Thalassaemia major (some cases).
11. Acute disseminated non-reactive tuberculosis (some cases).
12. Gastric carcinoma with secondary deposits in bone.
13. Myeloma (rarely).
14. Postsplenectomy (especially after splenectomy in idiopathic thrombocytopenic purpura).
15. Polyarteritis nodosa (rarely).
16. Myelosclerosis.(*Note:* cases may convert to frank myeloid leukaemia.)
17. Occasionally in rheumatoid arthritis in young children.
18. Phocomelia with congenital hypoplastic thrombocytopenia.
19. Familial myeloproliferative disease, with anaemia, thrombocytopenia, marrow granulocytic hyperplasia and low neutrophil alkaline phosphatase score.

References
Dignan, P. St J., Mauer, A. M. and Frantz, C. (1967) *J. Pediatr.* **70**, 561
Holland, P. and Mauer, A. M. (1967) *Am. J. Dis. Child.* **105**, 568
Tsuchiya, K., Kitamura, S. and Ouchi, S. (1958) *Fukushima J. Med. Sci.* **5**, 1 (13 cases described)

Resembling 'eosinophilic leukaemia'

● Thyroid adenocarcinoma (some cases).
● *Strongyloides stercoralis* infestation of gut.
● Disseminated eosinophilic collagen disease.
● Disseminated malignant melanomatosis (?'leuco-virus' active in debilitated patients).

References
Moore, G. E. and Pickren, J. W. (1967) *Lab. Invest.* **16**, 882
Odeberg, B. (1969) *Acta Med. Scand.* **177**, 129

Human leucocyte antigen, HLA (major histocompatibility complex, MHC)

The ABO system is a major histocompatability complex, and the human leucocyte antigen (HLA) is also an MHC which is built into the surface membrane of most cells. Each person carries 6 antigens from this system, a pair from each of HLA–A, –B, and –C, and they are controlled by genes on chromosome 6 from each parent. Neutrophils carry HLA-antigens plus neutrophil-specific antigen, and platelets carry HLA-antigens plus platelet-specific antigen, while adult red cells carry ABO-antigen but no HLA-antigen.

The HLA system is important in tissue transplantation (as it can facilitate acute graft rejection), platelet and granulocyte transfusion outcome, problems of parentage and identity, and susceptibility to certain diseases, e.g. HLA B27 is positive in 90% of cases of ankylosing spondylitis, only 5–10% of normal subjects being positive.

Chapter 5

Bone marrow

General

Development

The bone marrow is the site of erythropoiesis by 20 weeks, with an increase in activity during the third trimester of pregnancy. At birth, haemopoietic cells occupy all the bone marrow space. During childhood, there is gradual replacement with yellow fatty marrow, until red marrow is confined to the pelvis, cranium, ribs, vertebrae and sternum in the adult. In the adult, when there is continuous increased haemopoietic demand, the marrow throughout the body may become red and active once more.

Structure

The red marrow consists of a system of sinusoids lined by endothelial cells in a matrix of fat cells, reticulum cells, mast cells, plasma cells and developing haemopoietic cells.

Mature erythrocytes are able to deform sufficiently to pass through pores in the sinusoid wall to enter the circulation.

Formation and release of blood cells

The pluripotent haemopoietic stem cell (PSC)

The PSC is the most primitive cell capable of extensive replication, giving rise to all the haemopoietic progenitor elements. The mechanisms whereby cells derived from stem cells become committed to a particular cell line are not known. Nor are the mechanisms known whereby the numbers of stem cells are kept constant, with regulation of interconversion between active and resting modes. The control of maturation and eventual release of the different cell lines are also only incompletely understood. It has been suggested that the differential potentials of these early cells may be successively restricted.

Reference
Nicola, N. A. and Johnson, G. R. (1982) *Blood* **60**, 1019
The study of the various factors involved and their actions has developed as a result of the many attempts to determine the causes of the various types of leukaemia and of aplastic anaemia, and the attempts to improve treatment. The PSC has different committed lineage daughter cells:

BFU-E

Erythroid burst-forming cell, which can produce the CFU-E, or erythroid colony-forming unit, which eventually results in the formation of erythrocytes in response to erythropoietin.

Human bone marrow fibroblasts produce a factor which acts on human myeloid progenitor cells more primitive than BFU-E or CFU-E.

Reference
Blackburn, M. J. and Goldman, J. M. (1981) *Br. J. Haematol.* **48**, 117
CFU-C

This is the colony-forming unit committed to granulocyte/macrophage differentiation. The number of these colony-forming units in frozen bone marrow has been found to be useful in the prediction of its abilit to repopulate bone marrow in vivo.

CF-EO

Eosinophil-committed colony-forming unit.

CFU-MEGA

Megakaryocyte-committed colony-forming unit, leading eventually to the production of platelets. *Thrombopoietin* has been shown to increase ploidy in megakaryocytes and an increase in peripheral blood platelets in mice.

Reference
Levin, J., Levin, F. C., Hull, D. F. *et al.* (1982) *Blood* **60**, 989
LYMPHOID PSC

The lymphoid pluripotential stem cell.

GM-CSA

Granulocyte/macrophage colony-stimulating activity, necessary for proliferation and maturation of CFU-C in culture. This substance is increased in some cases of carcinoma with high peripheral blood white counts. Unfortunately, CSA increases cell proliferation in

AML (acute myeloid leukaemia), but does not favour cell differentiation. Lymphoid monocytic cells from peripheral blood and marrow provide CSF-GM necessary for granulocyte/macrocyte progenitor cells (CFU-GM) to undergo proliferation and differentiation in vitro.

CSF

Colony-stimulating factor has been identified as a glycoprotein. It stimulates production of granulocytes and macrophages from immature precursor cells in vitro.

LACTOFERRIN

This cation-binding protein has a molecular weight of 77 000 and is found in specific granules in neutrophils. It is a potent inhibitor of CSF activity in vitro and ? in vivo. This inhibitory activity requires the presence of T-lymphocytes and mononuclear phagocytes.

T-CELL GROWTH FACTOR (TCGF)

This substance is released by a subset of mature T-cells following lectin–antigen activation, resulting in T-cell subsets that have developed specific receptors for TCGF, essential for clonal expansion of all activated T-cells. Neoplastic T-cells respond directly to TCGF and do not require prior activation – this obviously has significance in both leukaemia and lymphoma. It is thought that glucocorticoids and cyclosporin A disrupt the interaction between T-cells and TCGF.

Normal value

Approximately, there are 0.56 g of marrow per 1 g of blood. The bone marrow represents about 3.4–5.9% of the total body weight, i.e. it occupies about 70 ml at birth and about 4000 ml in an adult.

Activity

In an infant 100% of the bone marrow is red and active. On the other hand, in the adult only about 50% is active, 50% being yellow inactive marrow. This yellow marrow can become active if necessary, and therefore adults have a large reserve available. Red cell formation can be increased until the apparent red cell life is about 20 days (i.e. marrow activity six times normal) before the haemoglobin level falls due to blood loss. (This is assuming that there are adequate supplies of protein, iron, vitamin B_{12}, folic acid etc.)

Because the infant's marrow is normally all active, this means that the infant's blood regenerating reserve is very small and therefore the infant rapidly becomes anaemic following blood loss. When the marrow in infants and young children becomes hyperactive, the bone cortex is thinned as the marrow expands (e.g. in thalassaemia major and sickle-cell disease).

Normal infant bone marrow values:

Reference
Rosse, C., Kraemer, M. J., Dillon, T. L. et al. (1977) *J. Lab. Clin. Med.* **89**, 1225

There are intrinsic differences between the stroma of red and yellow marrows. Blood cells require a framework on which to grow in red marrow. If this framework is destroyed by X-rays, no haemopoiesis can occur.

Reference
Tavassoli, M. and Crosby, W. H. (1970) *Science NY* **169**, 291

Myeloid/erythroid (M/E) ratio

Mean normal values

Birth	1.85 : 1.0
2 weeks	11 : 1.0
1–20 years	2.95 : 1.0
Adult	3–4 : 1.0

M/E ratio increased

- Myeloid leukaemia.
- Most infections.
- Leukaemoid reactions.
- Red cell formation depressed.

M/E ratio normal

- Normal cases.
- Myelosclerosis.
- Myeloma.
- Aplastic anaemia.

M/E ratio decreased

- Myeloid cell formation depressed, e.g. agranulocytosis.
- Increased red cell activity.

Normoblastic hyperplasia

- Posthaemorrhage.
- Posthaemolysis.
- Iron-deficiency anaemia.
- Polycythaemia vera.

Megaloblastic hyperplasia

Quantitative marrow cell counts

The range of figures regarded as normal by various authorities is very wide. This variation is due to the uncontrollable dilution of aspirated marrow with peripheral blood, and the total nucleated cell count must be regarded as unreliable.

The degree of cellularity can be assessed in most cases from either stained films of marrow aspirate or histological sections made from marrow aspirate fragments blocked in paraffin.

Qualitative marrow cell counts

Much useful information can be obtained from a differential count of the nucleated cells obtained by bone marrow aspiration:

Normal differential

Haemocytoblast	0.1–1%
Myeloblast	0.1–3.5%
Promyelocyte	0.5–5%
Myelocyte	5–20%
Metamyelocyte } young forms	10–30%
Polystab forms }	
Polysegmented (adult polymorph)	7–25%
Eosinophilic myelocyte	0.1–3%
Adult eosinophil	0.2–3%
Basophilic myelocyte	0–0.5%
Adult basophil	0–0.5%
Lymphocyte	5–20%
Lymphoblast	Nil
Plasma cell	0.1–3.5%
Myeloma cell	Nil
Monocyte	0–0.2%
Megakaryocyte	0.1–0.5%
Reticulum cell	0.1–2%
Proerythroblast	0.5–5%
Basophilic normoblast }	2–20%
Polychromatic normoblast }	
Orthochromic (pyknotic) normoblast	2–10%
Megaloblast	Nil

A high proportion of the non-nucleated red cells in normal marrow are reticulocytes (approximately equal in number to the number of nucleated red cells present).

Note: The haematologist's opinion will always be included with a marrow cell count. 'Smear' cells and 'basket' cells, sometimes included in the count, are merely damaged and distorted cells produced during aspiration, or more probably during spreading of films, and are of no significance except that excessive numbers of these damaged cells are seen with a lymphocytosis.

Bone marrow biopsy

'Dry tap' or 'bloody tap'

On occasion no marrow sample is obtained following marrow aspiration or a small sample is obtained which is grossly diluted with peripheral blood. A useful marrow sample may be found in the tip of the needle.

Reference

Engeset, A., Foss, A. A. and Nesheim, A. (1971) *Nord. Med.* **85**,663

After errors in technique have been excluded, the following conditions may be underlying.

Marrow fibrosis

- Myelosclerosis.
- Leukaemia.
- Secondary carcinomatosis, involving bone marrow.
- Lymphoma.
- Tuberculosis (rare).
- Histoplasmosis.

Infiltration of marrow with tumour

- Secondary carcinoma.
- Lymphoma and lymphosarcoma.
- Hodgkin's disease.
- Sarcoidosis.

Hypoplasia of marrow

Aplastic anaemia.

Hyperplastic marrow

In both acute leukaemia and megaloblastic anaemia, the marrow may be extremely cellular, but because the majority of the cells are primitive, aspiration may be unsuccessful.

Note: In all cases where apparently no marrow specimen is obtained, it is well worth while attempting to expel any fragments from the needle, after its removal from the marrow, on to a slide for spreading. Also, where a large volume of peripheral blood is obviously present, it is worth adding the sample to 5% albumin solution containing EDTA. After mixing, the sample is centrifuged, and films are made from the 'buffy' layer which will contain any nucleated cells. Trephine biopsy avoids dilution of the sample by peripheral blood, and retains the original narrow architecture.

Bone marrow cells

Bone marrow eosinophils

Normal range

- Eosinophilic myelocytes: 0.1–3.0% of total.
- Adult eosinophils: 0.2–3.0% of total nucleated cell count.

The marrow content = 300 × number of circulating eosinophils in the blood. Increase in bone marrow eosinophils precedes peripheral blood eosinophilia by 1 day.

Pathological

Increased

- Carcinomatous invasion of bone marrow.
- Lymphadenoma.
- Hypersensitivity reactions.
- Some cases of myeloid leukaemias.
- Eosinophilic leukaemia: uncoordinated maturation of nucleus and cytoplasm. The cells give a strongly positive PAS (periodic acid–Schiff) reaction due to high glycogen content, and a relatively strong and acid phosphatase reaction (? a discrete disease, ? subdivision of chronic myeloid leukaemia).
- Some cases of pernicious anaemia in relapse.

References
Gross, R. (1957) *Dtsch. Med. Wochenschr.* **82**, 507
Kingsley, P. E. M., Marks, J. and Mitchell, J. S. (1956) *Br. J. Cancer* **10**, 458

Bone marrow basophils and mast cells

Normal range

This is 0–0.5%. Mast cells occur in bone marrow and most other tissues. Their large granules are not water soluble and do not overlie the cell nucleus. Basophils are present in small numbers. Their granules are water soluble and overlie the cell nucleus. They appear to be related to lymphoid follicles in the marrow.

Increased

1. Chronic myeloproliferative diseases:
    (a) polycythaemia vera;
    (b) chronic myeloid leukaemia.
2. Urticaria pigmentosa of childhood.
3. Systemic mastocytosis (? a reticuloendotheliosis).
4. May also be found in:
    (a) pancytopenia;
    (b) acute lymphoblastic leukaemia;
    (c) chronic lymphatic leukaemia;
    (d) secondary carcinomatosis infiltrating bone marrow.

The finding of increased basophils and/or mast cells is clinically useful in (2) and (3), otherwise it is incidental.

Bone marrow lymphocytes

Normally not more than 20% of the total nucleated cells are lymphocytes. Lymph follicles are normally present in the bone marrow, and may be seen in paraffin sections of marrow.

Physiological

In the newborn during the first few weeks, up to 40% of the marrow nucleated cells may be lymphocytes.

The normal adult level of less than 20% is reached by 1–2 years. Even so, up to 5 years of age the high lymphocyte count often present may at first sight suggest a diagnosis of lymphatic leukaemia.

Pathological

Increase

1. Lymphatic leukaemia:
    (a) acute lymphatic leukaemia;
    (b) chronic lymphatic leukaemia. In most cases of acute lymphatic leukaemia, and in advanced cases of chronic lymphatic leukaemia, there is an increase in the bone marrow lymphocyte count. Lymphoblasts are also seen, although in the chronic variety the number of lymphoblasts cannot be used safely as a prognostic index.
2. Lymphocytic lymphoma ⎞ The lymphocytes may be imma
3. Follicular lymphoma ⎬ ture, irregularly shaped or indented. Also, the number of nucleoli may be increased above two per cell.
4. Lymphosarcoma: so-called lymphosarcoma cells may also be seen (*see* 'Cells not normally found in bone marrow aspirate').
5. Infectious mononucleosis.
6. Aplastic anaemia.
7. Myelofibrosis.
8. Macroglobulinaemia.

Bone marrow lymphocytosis is accompanied by a normal peripheral blood white cell count and differential.

Note: Contamination with peripheral blood during bone marrow aspiration will result in a high lymphocyte count. Monocytes, normally absent from the marrow, are also seen.

Lymphoid nodules in marrow

Trephine biopsy enables lesions to be classified.

Normal

- Lymphoid follicles.
- Lymphoid infiltrates.

Abnormal

Cytologically normal, but increase in size or number of nodules

1. Predominantly lymphoid follicles.
2. Predominantly lymphoid infiltration;
    (a) chronic lymphatic leukaemia;
    (b) lymphosarcoma.

Cytologically abnormal

1. Malignant lymphomas
   (a) Hodgkin's lymphadenoma;
   (b) prelymphocytic or lymphoblastic leukaemia;
   (c) histiocytic (reticulum cell) sarcoma;
   (d) lymphohistiocytic lymphoma.
2. Granulomata.

In older adults, the bone marrow appearance with focal collections of lymphocytes in infectious mononucleosis and similar infections may suggest lymphoma.

References
Krause, J. R. and Kaplan, S. S. (1982) *Scand. J. Haematol.* **28**, 15
Rywlin, A. M., Ortega, R. S. and Dominguez, C. J. (1974) *Blood* **43**, 389

Bone marrow megakaryocytes

Mean normal count

About 3000/mm^3 or not more than 300 per 1 000 000 nucleated red blood cells. Megakaryocytes survive about 10 days – 3 days nuclear division, 7 days cytoplasmic maturation of platelets.

Thrombocytopenia produced by platelet-specific antiserum in rats is associated with increased number of megakaryocytes. ? A regulatory agent may act on a diploid precursor cell in response to thrombocytopenia.

References
Odell, T. T. Jr., Jackson, C. W., Friday, T. J. *et al.* (1969) *Br. J. Haematol.* **17**, 91
Tavassoli M. (1980) *Blood* **55**, 537

Physiological

Moderate decrease normally in old age.

Pathological

The morphology of megakaryocytes in disease is described.

Reference
Albrecht, M., Fülle, H. H. and Klenk, U. (1974) *Blut* **28**, 109

There appears to be a high correlation between various malignancies and uptake of marrow cells by megakaryocytes – this is emperipolesis (temporary presence of one cell within another, rather than phagocytosis).

Reference
Sahebekhtiari, H. A. and Tavassoli, M. (1976) *Scand. J. Haematol.* **16**, 13

Increase

1. Chronic myeloid leukaemia.
2. Polycythaemia vera: increased bone marrow cellularity, increased number of large megakaryocytes, plus increased red cell mass strongly support the diagnosis.

Reference
Lundin, P., Ridell, B. and Weinfeld, A. (1972) *Scand. J. Haematol.* **9**, 271

3. Megakaryocytic myelosis.
4. Myelofibrosis.
5. Infection (especially pneumonia).
6. Idiopathic thrombocytopenic purpura (some cases).
7. Thrombocytopenia due to destruction of platelets in peripheral blood:
   (a) sedormid sensitivity;
   (b) thrombotic thrombocytopenic purpura.
8. After acute haemorrhage:
   (a) secondary hypersplenism;
   (b) Gaucher's disease;
   (c) Felty's syndrome;
   (d) lymphomas;
   (e) disseminated lupus erythematosus.

Decrease

- Untreated pernicious anaemia.

Note: The percentage of polykaryocytes, i.e. multinucleate megakaryocytes, is increased. This is reversed following specific treatment.

- Cirrhosis of the liver (some cases).
- Acute infections (if very severe), especially in infants: congenital rubella infection; congenital toxoplasma infection; congenital cytomegalic inclusion disease; congenital syphilis.
- Toxic substances: benzene; cytotoxic drugs, etc.; drug sensitivity; long-term chlorothiazide therapy.
- Excessive X-ray irradiation.
- Aplastic anaemia.
- Bone marrow overgrowth with acute leukaemic deposits.
- Bone marrow overgrowth with carcinomatous deposits.
- Myelosclerosis (some cases).
- Congenital amegakaryocytic thrombocytopenia.
- Tidal platelet dysgenesis (compare normal female menstrual cycle in which bone marrow megakaryocytes do not vary in number).
- Congenital hypoplastic anaemias.
- Wiskott–Aldrich syndrome: megakaryocytes may be present in normal number or reduced.
- Pancreatic insufficiency and chronic neutropenia syndrome (Schwachman–Diamond–Oskil–Khaw syndrome).

References
Emery, J., Gordon, R. R., Rendle-Short, J. *et al.* (1957) *Blood,* **12**, 567 (two cases described and five other cases reviewed)
Engström, K., Lundquist, A. and Söderström, N. (1966) *Scand. J. Haematol.* **3**, 290

Bone marrow plasma cells

Normal range

This is 1–3.5%.

Reference
Dacie, J. V. (1956) *Practical Haematology*, 2nd ed., London: Churchill

Pathological

Increase

MYELOMA

Very high plasma cell counts may occur, e.g. 50% of the total nucleated cells in a marrow aspirate may be plasma cells. The atypical plasma cells, or myeloma cells, may occur as discrete clusters or may be disseminated evenly throughout the marrow. The fact that the cells may often be present in clusters explains why apparently normal marrow can be aspirated on occasions from cases of myeloma with bone marrow infiltration.

COLLAGEN DISEASES

- *Acute rheumatic fever:* there may be ten-fold increase in marrow plasma cells.

Reference
Good, R. A. and Campbell, B. (1950) *Am. J. Med.* **9**, 330

- *Rheumatoid arthritis:* the plasma cell count may rise to more than 6% of the total nucleated cell count.

Reference
Hayhoe, F. G. J. and Robertson-Smith, D. (1951) *J. Clin. Pathol.* **4**, 47

- *Ankylosing spondylitis:* the marrow was found to be hyperactive, with increased plasma cell counts in 10 out of 17 cases, and with increased marrow eosinophil counts in 4 out of 17 cases.

Reference
Kingsley Pillers, E. M. and Marks, J. (1956) *Lancet* **i**, 722

- *Ulcerative colitis:* bone marrow plasmacytosis has been mistaken for myeloma.

Reference
Bernstein, J. S. and Nixon, D. D. (1964) *Am. J. Dig. Dis.* **9**, 625

INFECTIONS (ESPECIALLY CHRONIC)

Increased plasma cell counts have been described in:
- Granulomata and chronic infections.
- Measles.
- Roseola infantum.
- Infectious mononucleosis.
- Boeck's sarcoid.
- Lymphogranuloma inguinale.
- Kala-azar.

SENSITIVITY TO ANTIGENS

- Serum sickness.
- In rabbits after hyperimmunization.

Reference
Bjoerneboe, M. and Gormsen, H. (1947) *Acta Pathol. Microbiol. Scand.* **20**, 649

- Hypersensitivity to *Trichinella*.

Reference
Carter, J. R. (1949) *Am. J. Pathol.* **25**, 309

HYPERSENSITIVITY TO DRUGS

Hypersensitivity to sulphonamides has been described in which there was serum hyperglobulinaemia, and the marrow plasma cell count was 50% of the total nucleated cell count.

Reference
Wolf, J. and Worken, B. (1954) *Am. J. Med.* **16**, 746

MALIGNANT CONDITIONS

Increased plasma cell counts have been found in:
- Carcinomatosis.
- Monocytic leukaemia.
- Hodgkin's disease.
- Giant follicular lymphoma.

OTHER CONDITIONS IN WHICH MARROW PLASMACYTOSIS MAY OCCUR

- Aplastic anaemia.
- Agranulocytosis.
- Cirrhosis of the liver.
- Primary amyloid disease.
- Post-irradiation.
- Macroglobulinaemia; plasma cell counts range from 2% to 6%.
- Collagen disorders.

Note: In all conditions except myeloma above, the marrow plasma cell count is usually not more than 10% of the total nucleated cell count.

References
Klien, H. and Block, M. (1953) *Blood* **8**, 1034 (a description of 60 cases with bone marrow plasmacytosis)
Liu, C. T. and Dahlke, M. B. (1967) *Am. J. Clin. Pathol.* **48**, 546

Bone marrow reticulum cells

Normal range

This is 0–1% of the total nucleated cell count.

Pathological

Increase

- Reticulum cell sarcoma.
- Myelofibrosis.

In both the above there may be an exaggerated normal pattern, or the pattern may be abnormal, with an increased number of fibroblasts.

Reference
Burston, J. and Pinniger, J. L. (1963) *Br. J. Haematol.* **9**, 172

- Pernicious anaemia (untreated).
- Polycythaemia vera.
- Megakaryocytic myelosis.
- Myeloma (some cases).
- Macroglobulinaemia.

Decrease

Aplastic anaemia.

Reference
Fadem, R. S. and McBirnie, J. E. (1950) *Blood* **5**, 191

Bone marrow fibroblasts

The bone marrow fibroblasts are mesenchymal in origin, unrelated to stem cells, and are relatively radio-resistant. In myelofibrosis the marrow fibroblasts are not different from normal fibroblasts.

Reference
Castro-Malaspina, H., Gay, R. E., Jhanwar, S. C. *et al.* (1982) *Blood* **59**, 1046

Bone marrow lymphoblasts

Normally present only in very small numbers.

Bone marrow myeloblasts

Normal range

This is 0.1–3.5%.

Pathological

Increase

ACUTE MYELOBLASTIC LEUKAEMIA

The majority of the nucleated cells in the marrow may be myeloblasts.

CHRONIC MYELOID LEUKAEMIA

Up to 50% of the nucleated cells may be myeloblasts. It is thought that the higher the proportion of myeloblasts the worse the prognosis.

ACUTE LEUCOCYTOSIS IN INFECTION

The myeloblast count may increase towards the upper limit of the normal range, and uncommonly may exceed it moderately (i.e. not more than 5%).

CHRONIC REFRACTORY ANAEMIA

This occurs when there is anaemia with granulocytopenia, thrombocytopenia and excessive numbers of myeloblasts.

Reference
Najean, Y. and Pecking, A. (1977) *Br. J. Haematol.* **37**, 25

Decrease

- Lymphoblastic and lymphatic leukaemia, when the marrow is infiltrated with the lymphoid cells.
- Monocytic leukaemia.
- Aplastic anaemia.
- Agranulocytosis with marrow failure.

Normal number

Chronic idiopathic neutropenia: a normal cellular marrow, except no cells more mature than myelocytes.

Reference
Lipton, A. (1969) *Arch. Intern. Med.* **123**, 694

Bone marrow myelocytes

Myeloid cells mature:

- Myeloblast 1 day.
- Premyelocyte 2 days.
- Myelocyte 2.9–3.4 days.
- Maturation pool 6.3–8.5 days.
- Myelocyte to entry in peripheral blood 11.4 hours.

This is 11 days' supply of myelocytes, metamyelocytes and neutrophils ($= 2000 \times 10^7$ per kg bodyweight). Neutrophil in peripheral blood 10.4 h (average). (Total blood granulocytes $= 70 \times 10^7$ per kg bodyweight.) Daily turnover 163×10^7 cells per kg bodyweight.

Pathological

Giant metamyelocytes in marrow in pernicious anaemia represent slow DNA synthesis with a 'pile up' in the G_2 compartment of interphase, eventually dying in the marrow, where they are phagocytosed.

The circulating hypersegmented neutrophils have diploid DNA and have not matured from giant metamyelocytes.

Reference
Wickramasinghe, S. N. and Bush, V. (1977) *Br. J. Haematol.* **35**, 659

Bone marrow-stainable iron (haemosiderin)

The bone marrow-stainable iron is a very good index of the presence or absence of iron deficiency. It disappears before changes appear in the peripheral blood, and is especially useful where the red blood cells do not appear hypochromic. The iron in this form is readily available, and rapidly disappears after haemorrhage. Storage iron consists of inorganic ferric iron surrounded by a protein shell, the complex being ferritin. Ferritin aggregates to form insoluble complexes – haemosiderin. Normal tissue iron stores consist mainly of ferritin. Haemosiderin is formed when there are excess tissue iron stores.

Iron therapy is only likely to benefit patients with reduced or no marrow-stainable iron.

Bone marrow iron deposits increase with age irrespective of disease.

Marrow-stainable iron increased

No increase in total body iron, merely redistribution

- Haemolytic anaemia.
- Infections.
- Uraemia.
- Refractory anaemia.

- Megaloblastic anaemias.
- Myelophthisic anaemia.
- Some cases of carcinomatosis.
- Haemolytic disease of the newborn.

Increased iron intake

ORAL IRON

- Excessive iron absorption in haemochromatosis.
- High iron content in diet with low phosphate content as in Bantus, with poor diet and iron cooking pots.
- Vitamin A deficiency may lead to duodenal damage and excessive iron absorption from normal diet.

INTRAVENOUS OR INTRAMUSCULAR INJECTIONS OF IRON PREPARATIONS

After iron–dextran injections, only 65% of the administered dose is available, even though the remainder is stainable. After iron–sorbital injections, 90% of the administered iron is available.

Reference
Olsson, S., Lundvall, O. and Weinfeld, A. (1971) *Acta Med. Scand.* **191**, 49

REPEATED BLOOD TRANSFUSIONS IN CASES WITHOUT BLOOD LOSS (E.G. APLASTIC ANAEMIA)

CHRONIC PANCREATIC INSUFFICIENCY

Marrow-stainable iron decreased

Iron deficiency

- Prelatent: reduced marrow-stainable iron, with normal blood count and normal serum iron. Marrow iron stores lower in adult male blood donors than in adult male controls.
- Latent deficiency: reduced marrow-stainable iron, with low serum iron and normal blood count.
- Manifest: reduced marrow-stainable iron, low serum iron and hypochromic anaemia.

References
Benzie, R. McD. (1963) *Lancet* **i**, 1074
Finch, C. A., Hegsted, M., Kinney, T. D. *et al.* (1950) **5**, 983
Hansman, K., Kuse, R., Meinecke, K. H. *et al.* (1971) *Klin. Wochenschr.* **49**, 1164

Bone marrow sideroblasts

The bone marrow sideroblasts form a small rapidly available pool. During acute haemorrhage, or in the initial phase of treatment of megaloblastic anaemia, bone marrow sideroblasts disappear completely. Following treatment of iron-deficiency anaemia with oral iron for a few days, bone marrow sideroblasts reappear.

When the whole blood haemoglobin level is normal, if no haemosiderin is seen in the marrow, the presence of sideroblasts indicates that some iron is still available. Absence of both marrow haemosiderin and sideroblasts is evidence of complete iron store depletion.

In infections, the bone marrow contains haemosiderin, and the marrow sideroblast count is normal (although in 10% of cases, no sideroblasts were found).

Reference
Weinfeld, A. and Hansen, H. A. (1962) *Acta Med. Scand.* **171** 23

Marrow reticulin and collagen fibres

Pathological

Increase

1. Myelosclerosis:
   (a) myeloid proliferation with cells giving positive alkaline phosphatase reaction;
   (b) excess bone reticulin and marrow fibrosis.
2. Some cases of polycythaemia vera.
3. Lymphoid myelosclerosis (rare): pancytopenia with peripheral blood lymphocytosis, hypoplastic marrow, proliferation of reticulin and collagen fibres without osteosclerosis.

References
Duhamel, G. (1971) *Acta Haematol.* **45**, 112
Pegrum, C. D. and Risdon, R. A. (1970) *Br. J. Haematol.* **18**, 475

Bone marrow necrosis and degeneration

Reported in one-third of 368 specimens from patients suffering from:

- Neoplastic disease.
- Disseminated intravascular coagulopathy (DIC).
- Various acute and chronic non-malignant disorders.

References
Hansen, P. V., Andersen, J. and Mygind, H. (1983) *Acta Med. Scand.* **214**, 331 (Report of a case and review)
Norgard, M. J., Carpenter, J. T. and Conrad, M. E. (1979) *Arch. Intern. Med.* **139**, 905

Vacuolated erythroblasts

- Acute alcohol poisoning.
- Severe malnutrition (marasmus, kwashiorkor).
- Aplastic anaemia.
- Erythroleukaemia
  Acute leukaemia } during therapy.
  Lymphoma
- Chloramphenicol toxicity.

- Rarely other conditions, including hyperosmolar non-ketotic coma.
- During treatment of phenylketonuria and also in experimental phenylalanine deficiency.
- Experimental riboflavin deficiency.

Reference
Lehane, D. E. (1974) *Arch. Intern. Med.* **134**, 763

PAS staining of erythroblasts

The periodic-acid–Schiff reaction (PAS) is used to stain glycogen and related polysaccharides. The following grades of reaction have been described.

Negative staining of erythroblasts

- Normal.
- Pernicious anaemia.
- Polycythaemia vera.
- Nutritional macrocytic anaemia.
- Aplastic anaemia.

Slight positive staining of erythroblasts

- Newborn infants (erythroblasts in cord blood).
- Fetal haemolytic anaemia.
- Acute and chronic leukaemia.
- Haemolytic anaemia.
- Reticulosis.
- Refractory anaemia.
- Myelosclerosis.

Strongly positive staining of erythroblasts

- Iron-deficiency anaemia.
- Thalassaemia major.
- Di Guglielmo's disease (erythraemic myelosis): strongly PAS-positive stain for glycogen useful in diagnosis, but negative results do not exclude this diagnosis. The abnormal erythroblasts show distinctive cytoplasmic budding and marked vacuolation.

Reference
Sondergaard-Petersen, H. (1975) *Acta Med. Scand.* **198**, 165, 175

(Up to 15% of peripheral blood lymphocytes may give positive results with PAS stains in macroglobulinaemia.)

PAS staining of other cells

- Myeloblasts – diffuse thin stain.
- Lymphoblasts – clear sharp granules. Negative in 20–30% of cases of ALL (particularly T-ALL and B-ALL).
- Monoblasts – fine granules.
- Haemocytoblasts – negative.
- Leukaemic lymphosarcoma.

Reference
Kass, L. and Hadi, M. Z. (1975) *Am. J. Clin. Pathol.* **64**, 503

Granulomatous disorders affecting the bone marrow

- Tuberculosis.
- Histoplasmosis.
- Infectious mononucleosis.
- Sarcoidosis.
- Brucellosis.

Reference
Ellman, L. (1976) *Am. J. Med.* **60**, 1

Cells not normally found in bone marrow

Normal cells which may be aspirated

- Blood vessel cells.
- Osteoblasts and osteoclasts.
- Cutaneous epithelial cells, glandular cells, hair follicles etc.

Abnormal cells which may be aspirated

1. Secondary deposits of carcinoma. Carcinoma cells may be seen in bone marrow aspirates in approximately 8% of advanced malignant disease.
   They are rarely found in:
   (a) extensive gastrointestinal malignancy;
   (b) extensive genitourinary malignancy;
   (c) extensive head and neck malignancy;

Reference
Mendoza, C. B., Moure, G. E. Jr. and Crosswhite, L. H. (1969) *Surg. Gynecol. Obstet.* **129**, 483

   (d) mammary carcinoma cells infiltrating bone marrow can be identified by immunocytochemical stain specific for epithelial membrane antigen. Micrometastases occur in 24% of cases with no histological lymph node involvement.

References
Dearnaley, D. P., Ormerod, M. G., Sloane, J. P. *et al.* (1983) *J. R. Soc. Med.* **76**, 359
Redding, W. H., Coombes, R. C., Monaghan, P. *et al.* (1983) *Lancet* **ii**, 1271

2. Secondary deposits of melanoma.
3. Secondary deposits of sarcoma, e.g.
   (a) fibrosarcoma;
   (b) round-cell sarcoma;
   (c) spindle-cell sarcoma;
   (d) lymphosarcoma;
   (e) osteoclast sarcoma.
4. Sternberg giant cells in Hodgkin's disease.
5. Neuroblastoma tumour cells (in young children).
6. Tuberculoma ⎫ Langhan's giant cells.
7. Boeck's sarcoid ⎭

8. Storage monocytes filled with cerebroside, in Gaucher's disease. Also in some cases of chronic myeloid leukaemia, glucocerebrosides derived from granulocytes accumulate in monocytes. Similar cells have been described in thalassaemia (+ HEMPAS CDA type II anaemia).

Reference
Albrecht, M. (1969) *Klin. Wochenschr.* **47**, 778

9. Giant monocytoid cells may be seen during fluoride treatment of osteoporosis.

Reference
Duffey, P. H., Tretbar, H. C. and Jarkowski, T. L. (1971) *Ann. Intern. Med.* **75**, 745

10. Excessive numbers of tissue basophils, occurring in any condition in which there is gross inhibition of haemopoiesis in bone marrow, e.g. pancytopenia, lymphatic leukaemia (both acute and chronic) or generalized bone marrow carcinomatosis.

11. Whipple's disease: typical large PAS-positive histiocytes are found, which contain rod-like inclusion bodies in their cytoplasm. On electron microscopy these inclusion bodies resemble bacteria.

Reference
Ransing, A. (1973) *Acta Med. Scand.* **193**, 5

12. Hermansky–Pudlak syndrome: albinism, haemorrhagic diathesis with increased bleeding time, plus pigmented macrophages in the marrow.

Reference
White, J. G., Edson, J. R., Desmick, S. J. *et al.* (1971) *Am. J. Clin. Pathol.* **63**, 319

13. 'Sea-blue histiocytes' in bone marrow. Recently cells resembling histiocytes and containing material which stained sea-blue with Giemsa stain have been described, associated with:
   (a) syndrome with a relatively benign course, mild purpura secondary to thrombocytopenia, with splenomegaly;
   (b) syndrome with progressive liver cirrhosis and poor prognosis;
   (c) syndrome associated with neurological disease;
   (d) occurring in patients suffering from: rheumatoid arthritis; sickle-cell anaemia; myeloproliferative disorder; thalassaemia; idiopathic thrombocytopenic purpura.

The status of the 'sea-blue histiocyte' has still not been finally settled.

References
Baumann, M. A. and Libnoch, J. A. (1983) *JAMA* **250**, 1459
Ozsoylu, S., Kocak, N. and Berkel, A. I. (1974) *Acta Paediatr. Scand.* **63**, 147
Rywlin, A. M. (1972) *Blood* **39**, 149
Rywlin, A. M., Hernandez, J. A., Chastain, D. E. *et al.*, (1971) *Blood* **37**, 587

Sawitsky, A., Rosner, F. and Chodsky, S. (1972) *Blood* **39**, 148
Silverstein, M. N., Ellefson, R. D. and Ahern, E. J. (1970) *N. Engl. J. Med.* **282**, 1

Note; Myeloma cells are discussed with plasma cells.

Foam cells in bone marrow

Lipid storage diseases

Sphingolipids

- Niemann–Pick disease.
- Gaucher's disease.
- GM$_1$ gangliosidosis.
- Lactosyl ceramidosis.
- Fabry's disease.

Non-polar lipids

- Wolman's disease.
- Cholesteryl ester storage disease.
- Cerebrotendinous xanthomatosis.

Hyperlipoproteinaemia

- Type I.
- Type II.
- Type III.
- Type IV.
- Type V.
- Secondary hyperlipoproteinaemia.

Miscellaneous

- Tangier disease.
- Lecithin cholesterol acetyl transferase deficiency.
- Chronic myeloid leukaemia.
- Von Gierke's glycogen storage disease.

The bone marrow malignancies

Malignant proliferation can develop in any of the many cell lines found in bone marrow and at several stages of development, e.g. pluripotential stem to mature lymphocyte.

Malignant proliferation may be rapid with poor differentiation and be associated with an acute clinical course, e.g. acute leukaemia, or it may be much slower with normal differentiation and a chronic clinical course as in chronic myeloid leukaemia or primary polycythaemia.

Aetiology

There is a clear association between retroviruses and bone marrow malignancies in some animals. Perhaps the best example would be leukaemias and lymphosarcomas in cats caused by feline leukaemia virus. In

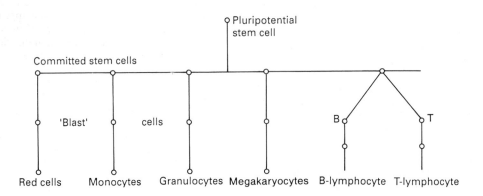

humans there is a strong association between the retrovirus HTLV-1 (human T-cell leukaemia virus) and a specific malignancy, adult T-cell leukaemia/lymphoma. However, to date no other clear viral associations have been found in bone marrow malignancy.

People accidentally or deliberately exposed to radiation have an increased risk of acute leukaemia, chronic myeloid leukaemia, lymphoma and perhaps myeloma. However, most patients diagnosed with bone marrow malignancy have no history of such exposure.

Several studies have shown an increased risk of acute leukaemia (mainly AML) and non-Hodgkin's lymphoma after chronic benzene exposure. These cases would only account for a small percentage of the total, however.

Bone marrow has the most active cell division of any organ and a predictable number of mutations will occur. Some of these are of no significance, some are lethal to the cell and a few may form abnormal clones. Whether these clones ultimately develop into a malignancy will certainly depend upon other factors; viral, chemical, radiation, or further mutation within the clone. We can find specific chromosomal abnormalities in some bone marrow malignancies, e.g. t(9, 22) in chronic myeloid leukaemia, t(15, 17) in acute promyelocytic leukaemia, t(8, 14) in Burkitt's lymphoma. It is of interest that some of these chromosomal changes are associated with activation of cellular oncogenes, i.e. *c-abl* in t(9, 22) CML, *c-myc* in t(8, 14) lymphoma. Activation of oncogenes may impart growth advantages to the abnormal clone.

The acute leukaemias

The rapid proliferation of an abnormal clone of cells arising from within the bone marrow and eventually spreading to the peripheral blood gives rise to acute leukaemia. Morphology, cytochemical staining, cytogenetics and antigen assessment using mono-

clonal antibodies can, in most cases, place the clone within one of the bone marrow cells lines.

Acute leukaemia affects all age groups and all races. The incidence varies geographically, but is usually 20–30/ million per year.

The presentation of acute leukaemia is that of bone marrow failure due to the very heavy marrow infiltration by abnormal 'blast' cells. At diagnosis, residual normal marrow is hard to find! In the past, the prognosis was universally bad, with death in a few weeks for most untreated cases. However, well-organized intensive chemotherapy has brought significant remission and cure rates.

Acute lymphoblastic leukaemia (ALL)

Although occurring in all age groups, ALL is most common in children, particularly in the range 3–6 years. Presentation is with anaemia, thrombocytopenia and neutropenia in most cases. Bleeding and potentially life-threatening infection are major problems. Bone pain and CNS disease (particularly in children) may be the presenting features in some patients. In addition to pancytopenia the peripheral blood will usually show a variable number of 'lymphoblasts' with high nuclear/cytoplasmic ratio and single nucleolus. The bone marrow is very heavily infiltrated (90% +) and provides plenty of material for diagnosis.

Morphology

ALL cells can be variable but are mainly monomorphic for each patient, falling into one of the following groups:

- L1: small monomorphic cells with little cytoplasm.
- L2: the cells are small and medium in size with rather more cytoplasm and more variable nucleus.
- L3: large blast cells with variable nucleus and blue vacuolated cytoplasm.

Patients who present with L1 morphology have a better prognosis.

Cytochemical stains

The periodic acid–Schiff (PAS) reaction will show 'block' positivity in about 75% of cases. It is important to identify magenta blocks of positive material in the cytoplasm, because monoblasts and myeloblasts may show a fine diffuse staining in their cytoplasm. The acid phosphatase reaction is said to show 'polar cap' positivity in cases of T-cell ALL (T-ALL).

Monoclonal antibodies

Monoclonal antibody techniques have largely replaced the use of cytochemistry in the diagnosis of ALL. Surface and cellular antigens can be identified using: immunofluorescence by microscopy or flow cytometry; immunocytology with immunoperoxidase or immunoalkaline phosphatase–antialkaline phosphatase (APAAP) and light microscopy.

References
Janossy, G. (1987) Immunofluorescence. In: Klaus G. G. B. Ed. *Lymphocytes–A Practical Approach,* pp. 67–108. Oxford: IRL Press
Mason, D. Y. (1986) Immunoenzymic labelling of haem samples with monoclonal antibodies. In: Beverley, P. C. L. Ed. *Methods in Haematology–Monoclonal Antibodies,* pp. 145–181. Edinburgh: Churchill-Livingstone

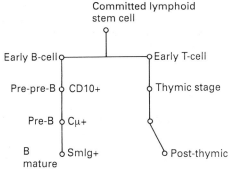

As antigens appear and disappear during maturation, cell types can be identified using a panel of monoclonal antibodies. Each antibody is coded CD (cluster designation) and then a number, e.g. CD19 and CD20 are B-cell markers, and CD2 and CD7 are T-cell markers.

Monoclonal antibody studies show that most cases of ALL are pre-pre-B-cell in type or so-called 'common-ALL'. Clinically this group also has the best prognosis. The groups are:

51%	common-ALL	pre-pre-B
25%	pre-B-ALL	
8%	null-ALL	
2%	B-ALL	
14%	T-ALL	

Null-ALL is in the B-cell series

CD10 is the common-ALL antigen, pre-B-ALL is distinguished from common-ALL by the appearance of cytoplasmic immunoglobulin (CyIg). More mature B-cells have surface membrane immunoglobulin (SmIg). Terminal deoxynucleotidyl transferase (TdT) is found in early B- and T-cells. HLA-DR is a marker for all B-cells (except plasma cells). It will also mark very early T-cells and mature but reactive T-cells.

It is important to identify which ALL group the patient falls into because of the difference in treatment and prognosis. Most studies show that common-ALL has the best prognosis and B-ALL the worst, the order being common-ALL > pre-B-ALL > null-ALL > T-ALL > B-ALL.

B-ALL is more difficult to get into remission and, together with T-ALL, needs more aggressive treatment programmes to achieve good results.

Cytogenetics in ALL

At least 70% of cases have a karyotype abnormality and, with improving techniques, this will increase further. Some of the changes are associated with specific clinical or immunophenotypic disease. Chromosomal breakpoints have been found associated with genes for growth factors and cell proliferation.

Cytogenetic changes are important in the diagnosis and prognosis of ALL. Patients with hyperdiploid states, particulary more than 50 chromosomes per cell, have a good prognosis. Translocation on the other hand appears to be associated with a worse prognosis, e.g. t(9, 22) Philadelphia chromosome positive ALL, which is seen in 2–3% of children with ALL and 20% of adults, is known to have a poorer prognosis.

Translocation at t(4, 11) is found in older children with a high presenting white cell count, organomegaly, undifferentiated blast cell phenotype and a poor prognosis. Abnormality t(1, 19) is present in one-third of pre-B-ALL.

There are many other abnormalities described including t(11, 14) in T-ALL and t(8, 14) in B-ALL.

Reference
Ahuja, H. G. and Cline, M. J. (1988) *Med. Oncol. Tumor Pharmacother.* **5** (4), 211–222 (Review on Genetic and cytogenetic changes in acute lymphoblastic leukaemia)

CD10+, CD19+, HLA-DR+, TdT+
CD10+, CD19, HLA-DR+, Tdt+,
    CyIg+(CM+)
CD19+, HLA-DR+, TdT+
    CD19+, HLA-DR+, CyIg+, SmIg+
CD2+, CD7+, Tdt+

Prognostic factors in ALL

Presenting features, such as age, sex, immunopheno-type and cytogenetics, will help the clinician to decide whether the patient should have a more or less intensive chemotherapy regimen. Interestingly, despite all the more sophisticated investigations, the single most important and accurate prognostic indicator is still the presenting white cell count.

Table 5.1   Prognostic factors in ALL

Good prognosis	Bad prognosis
Initial WBC < 20 × 10^9/l	WBC > 20 × 10^9/l
Age 2–10 years	Age < 2 or > 10 years
Female	Male
Common-ALL	B-ALL and T-ALL
(pre-pre-B immunophenotype)	t(9,22); t(4, 11)
Hyperdiploidy	CNS disease at presentation
L1 morphology	Mediastinal mass (lymph nodes)

Management

Improved therapy over the last 10 years means that a majority of children and a significant number of adults may be cured of acute lymphoblastic leukaemia. In the good prognostic group as many as 80% may be cured. With the improving chances for these patients, it is important they are treated in centres that have ALL expertise both on the ward and in the laboratory.

After initial assessment bone marrow is aspirated for morphology, cytochemical staining, im-munophenotyping, cytogenetics and possibly DNA analysis and in vitro cell culture. The patient may require red cell and platelet transfusions to stabilize their condition prior to chemotherapy. Aggressive treatment with appropriate antibiotic(s) may also be required.

The use of daily, high-dose prednisolone with weekly vincristine for 3–6 weeks brings about a smooth remission in 70–80% of cases with little in the way of side effects. Adding L-asparaginase to the induction regimen improves the remission rate to nearly 100% in the good prognostic group. For those patients in the bad prognostic group the further addition of daunorubicin will improve remission rates and probable long-term survival (UK ALL trials VIII–X). The use of more drugs, however, does bring increased morbidity, mainly from infections due to extended marrow suppression with neutropenia. It is important to remember that a neutropenic patient may not react with the normal symptoms and signs when infected. Fever, lethargy and loss of appetite may be all that is seen. Although blood cultures and swabs must be taken, it is important not to wait for results; broad-spectrum intravenous antibiotics (e.g. gentamicin, azlocillin) must be started immediately for any neutropenic pyrexia of undetermined origin. Some centres use prophylactic antibiotics in neutropenia; certainly the use of prophylactic co-trimoxazole (Sep-trin) reduces the incidence of opportunistic lung infection with Pneumocystis carinii. Viral and fungal infections are an increasing problem.

Whether the patient has had a three-drug regimen (vincrinstine, prednisolone, L-asparaginase – good prognosis disease) or a four-drug regimen (vincristine, prednisolone, L-asparaginase, daunorubicin – poor prognosis disease), once in remission they will require CNS prophylaxis. In the early 1970s, it became apparent that many patients, having achieved a good haematological remission, were relapsing initially in the CNS. It was found that these relapses could be prevented using intrathecal methotrexate and cranial irradiation. Most centres would currently use in-trathecal methotrexate injections and 18 Gy (1800 rad) to the cranium. However, with the reported side effects, such as poor learning, associated with this treatment, some are looking to drop the cranial irradiation in favour of systemic, high-dose methotrexate.

Following remission induction and CNS prophy-laxis there is debate about the need for early and/or late intensive consolidation therapy. Certainly, in the bad prognostic groups further intensive treatment seems to offer a better chance of long-term survival. Finally, patients are placed on maintenance chemo-therapy for up to 2 years using oral methotrexate and 6-mercaptopurine. Maintenance therapy reduces re-lapse rates, particularly if dosages are kept at optimal levels.

Relapse of ALL

About 50% of adults and 30% of children will ultimately relapse. For those that relapse whilst still on treatment the prognosis is very poor. A second remission can be achieved with chemotherapy in the majority of patients who relapse off treatment. Until the introduction of bone marrow transplantation, however, these second remissions did not lead to long-term survival.

With bone marrow transplantation, it may be possible to cure 60% of ALL in second remission and some centres are now advocating this treatment in first remission for bad prognosis ALL.

Acute myeloid leukaemia (AML)

This term covers all acute leukaemias other than lymphoblastic and the following 'FAB' classification is now widely used:

- M1: acute granulocytic leukaemia without maturation.
- M2: acute granulocytic leukaemia with some maturation.
- M3: acute promyelocytic leukaemia.
- M4: acute myelomonocytic leukaemia.
- M5: acute monocytic leukaemia.
- M6: erythroleukaemia.
- M7: acute megakaryoblastic leukaemia.

Acute myeloid leukaemia can occur at any age but has a much higher incidence in adults. It is clear that AML is a heterogeneous group of diseases, previously lumped together because there was no difference in management or prognosis.

Morphology and cytochemistry

M1 The dominant cell is the undifferentiated myeloblast with one or more nucleoli. Little maturation to promyelocytes or myelocytes is seen and there are very few Auer rods. Peroxidase and Sudan black stain will be positive in a small percentage of blast cells.

M2 The myeloblast makes up the majority of cells in the marrow, but now there is maturation to the promyelocyte stage and even beyond. Large numbers of Auer rods should be found. Peroxidase and Sudan black will be positive in a much higher percentage of cells.

M3 The marrow is heavily infiltrated by abnormal promyelocytes. Their cytoplasm is packed with granules and thin Auer rods. Cytochemistry will be as for M1 and M2. There is also a hypogranular M3 which has to be identified by electron microscopy and cytogenetics.

M4 Both granulocytic and monocytic differentiation of blast cells can be seen. The two cell population can be identified using peroxidase to stain myeloblasts and butyric esterase (brown) stains monocytoblasts.

M5 There are two subtypes:

- M5A: poorly differentiated monocytic leukaemia.
- M5B: differentiated monocytic leukaemia.

In M5A mainly monocytoblasts are found in the marrow and peripheral blood, whereas in M5B fewer blast cells are found in the marrow and large numbers of monocytes and promonocytes are seen in the peripheral blood. Esterase stains will identify the blasts.

M6 The predominant cells in marrow are the proerythroblast and large numbers of dysplastic nucleated red cells. Dysplasia may also be seen in remaining granulocytes and megakaryocytes. Iron stain may show ring sideroblasts; PAS staining may show diffuse or block positivity in the abnormal erythroid series.

M7 There may be marked fibrosis in the marrow making aspiration difficult. The blast cells are PAS positive, acid phosphatase positive and α-naphthyl acetate esterase positive. Electron microscopy detects platelet peroxidase activity.

Monoclonal antibodies

To date, monoclonal antibodies have not reached the same level of importance in AML as they have in ALL. Nevertheless, very useful information can be obtained, particularly in cases where cytochemistry is negative or equivocal. The following helps to pick out AML from ALL:

- CD11(a, b and c): positive on granulocytes and macrophages.
- CD13: positive on monocytes and granulocytes.
- CD14: positive mainly on monocytes.
- CD33: positive on early myeloid cells.
- CD34: immature myeloid cells, even stem cells.
- CDw41 ⎫ positive on platelets and mega-
- CDw42 ⎭ karyocytes.

Reference
Geller, R. B., Zahurak, Marianna, Hurwitz, C. A. *et al.* (1990) *Br. J. Haematol.* **76**, 340

Cytogenetics

Cytogenetics has become extremely useful in the investigation of AML. Over 60% of cases have a cytogenetic defect and some of these are very specific for M type. For example, t(8, 21) is found in M2 AML, mainly in younger patients, it is rare over the age of 50; t(15, 17) is found in more than 90% of cases of M3 AML and one-third have an associated trisomy

8. This karyotype has long duration of remission and a good prognosis. t(9, 11) and deletions at 11q23 are predominantly monocytic with 50% having M5A morphology. They are mostly seen in children.

Inversion/deletion structural changes of chromosome 16 with an associated trisomy 8 are seen in a variant of M4 (M4 EO). The morphology of M4 EO shows many abnormal eosinophils having aberrant positivity for chloroacetate esterase and often PAS-positive granules. Patients with M4 EO/inv 16 have a high complete remission rate and a better prognosis than other AMLs.

Trisomy 8 (888) is the most common change in AML, seen in 19% of all cases, particularly alone in M1, M4, M5 and as an additional change in M3.

Monosomy 7 (-7) is the second most common change in AML; however, as a sole anomaly it is seen only in 4% of M2 and M4. It is associated with previous chemotherapy and toxic agents, and is also seen in myelodysplastic syndrome.

Management of AML

The majority of cases are seen in adults and present with symptoms and signs of marrow failure. Originally, patients died almost equally of bleeding and infection: now with the great improvement in the availability and quality of platelet transfusions, most patients die of infection. As with ALL, intensive chemotherapy is used in an attempt to destroy leukaemic cells and allow normal marrow to regrow. However, there are no specific drugs, such as vincristine in ALL. As support care has improved in properly organized haematology units, chemotherapy has become more and more ablative so that now the aim is to create a temporary aplastic state from which it is hoped only the normal stem cells will recover to repopulate the marrow. This approach at present gives rise to higher remission rates and more long-term survivors – there are, however, more deaths in induction. Increasingly, allogeneic bone marrow transplantation in first remission of AML is seen as the best chance of long-term survival for those lucky enough to find a donor. Bone marrow rescue, using the patient's own stored first remission marrow, following highly ablative late intensification treatment, is also proving to be an effective therapy.

Following blood and bone marrow sampling and diagnosis using the investigations listed above, the patient must be properly prepared for intensive chemotherapy. A tunnelled central venous line is inserted as soon as possible, which will be used over the next few weeks for RBCs, platelets, chemotherapy, antibiotics, blood sampling, intravenous feeding and possible antifungal and antiviral treatment.

Blood and platelets are given prior to chemotherapy if required. Nose and throat swabs, baseline viral and fungal titres are also taken. Some centres believe in prophylactic systemic antibiotics and gut sterilization to reduce infection rates.

The most effective regimens are based on combinations of cytosine arabinoside with daunorubicin, but not forgetting highly trained medical and nursing staff caring for the patient on a unit, preferably with single rooms having filtered air to exclude fungal spores. Cytosine arabinoside $200 \, mg/m^2$ daily for 7 days with daunorubicin $50 \, mg/m^2$ on days 1, 2, and 3 is now a commonly used regimen.

A bone marrow sample at days 10–14 should be 'aplastic' with no leukaemic blasts; if blast cells persist a further course of chemotherapy is given immediately. The patient is then nursed until marrow recovery takes place, which may be from 15 to 30 days. The main danger during this period is from bacterial and fungal infection. In the 1970s, Gram-negative infections were the major problem, but the early use of broad-spectrum antibiotics has largely defeated these. Now more Gram-positive bacterial infections are seen – perhaps because of the use of Hickman lines? A bigger percentage of infections is also now caused by fungae, mostly *Candida* and *Aspergillus*, which are particularly difficult to treat during neutropenia. The early use of intravenous amphotericin B and the introduction of newer drugs such as fluconazole and itraconazole is helping to beat the fungal menace. The support of a good quality microbiology department is essential. During the neutropenic period, nursing staff must pay careful attention to the following: temperature, oral hygiene, skin care, Hickman line, fluid balance, nutrition, patient morale.

Complete remission rates of between 60% and 70% are achieved on well-organized units, much of the improvement in the last few years being due to better support care. Response rates are lower in M5, M6 and M7 types of AML. The M3 type has a better response rate, despite a high incidence of DIC (diffuse intravascular coagulation).

Consolidation therapy

Once remission has been achieved, various methods of consolidation have been attempted:

- Two or three further courses of the same chemotherapy or 'intensive consolidation' using high-dose cytosine arabinoside at 2 or $3 \, g/m^2$.
- Intensive consolidation with autologous marrow rescue.
- Bone marrow transplantation.

Wolff *et al.* (1985) have reported 51% 5-year survival using intensive consolidation chemotherapy, but it seems likely that bone marrow manipulation of some sort, if it can be made available to more patients, offers the best future hope for AML.

References

Ahuja, H. G. and Cline, M. J. (1988) *Med. Oncol. Tumor pharmacother.* **5**, 211–222

Drexler, H. G., Gignac, S. M., Minowada, J. *et al.* (1988) *Blut* **57**, 327–339

Griffin, J. D. (1987) *Haematol. Pathol.* **1**(2), 81–91

Lilleyman, J. S., Hinchcliffe, R. F. *et al.* (1989) *Br. J. Haematol.* **71**, 227–231

MIC Workshop Report (1988) *Br. J. Haematol.* **68**, 481

Priesler, H. D., Anderson, K., Rai, K. *et al.* (1989) *Br. J. Haematol.* **71**, 189–194

Stein, R. S. (1989) *Review Am. J. Med. Sci.* **297**, 26–34

Chronic myeloid leukaemia (CML)

This clonal abnormality at the level of the pluripotential stem cell initially produces a massive overproduction in the granulocyte series, the so-called *chronic phase* of the disease. Further changes within the clone may bring about less stable disease – the accelerated phase – or suddenly produce undifferentiated disease, as an acute leukaemia – the *blastic phase*.

Most patients present with anaemia, splenomegaly and a high WBC (mainly neutrophils and myelocytes). Bone marrow is packed with granulopoiesis, basophils are increased as may be vitamin B_{12}, uric acid and LDH. The neutrophil alkaline phosphatase score is always low and may be zero. This is a good, quick, test for the diagnosis of CML and immediately distinguishes from a high WBC due to infection, where the neutrophil alkaline phosphatase score would be raised.

The definitive test for CML is the clonal marker, first described by Hungerford and Nowell in 1954, the Philadelphia chromosome – Ph' – originally described as a deletion abnormality of chromosome 22. It is now known to be a translocation between 9 and 22, as t(9, 22)(q34: q11).

The Ph' chromosome is found in more than 95% of cases of CML and the figure increases with better cytogenetic techniques.

Recently the breakpoint on chromosome 22 has been shown to be restricted to a small area of 5.8 kilobases (kb) called the 'breakpoint cluster region' or bcr. The balanced translocation with chromosome 9 brings together the cellular proto-oncogene Abelson (*c-abl*) and the bcr gene on chromosome 22. The newly formed bcr/abl gene produces a 8.5 kb mRNA and a protein of molecular weight 210 000 (P210). This protein has tyrosine kinase activity, which has been shown in culture studies to increase granulopoiesis.

Interestingly, in Ph' ALL (as distinct from ALL arising in the blastic phase of CML), a 7.0 kb mRNA is produced giving a protein of molecular weight 195 000 (P190).

Management

CML can occur at any age, though it is rare in children and has a peak incidence in the third and fourth decades. Prognosis is variable but can be anything between 1 and 10 years. Survival for most patients depends on the length of the chronic phase, because once the accelerated or blastic phase is entered life is short.

Chronic phase

The initial high WBC and enlarged spleen can be reduced using oral busulphan or hydroxyurea, when the anaemia will correct without the need for blood transfusion. Intermittent courses of these drugs will keep the disease controlled for an average of 3–4 weeks, the natural history without drug intervention being 18–20 months. During the chronic phase the patient enjoys a good quality of life.

Accelerated phase

The accelerated phase is not well defined, but can be recognized by rising cell counts, enlarging spleen, poor response to busulphan etc., increased blast cells and basophils in the peripheral blood, weight loss, bone pain and further chromosomal changes.

If looked for carefully, this phase will be found in most patients and lasts for only 6–18 months.

Blast phase

The blast phase develops in 70–80% of patients, is usually resistant to treatment and is followed by death in 2–3 months. It is accompanied in most cases by chromosomal changes in the abnormal clone, e.g. (1) a second Ph' chromosome; (2) trisomy 8; (3) *isochromosome 17*.

Transformation can be due to acute myeloid leukaemia (70%), acute lymphoblastic leukaemia (20%, usually $CD10^+$) or 'undifferentiated leukaemia' (10%).

The ALL will respond to vincristine, prednisolone and daunorubicin, but remissions are usually short-lived.

Recent progress

Because of the poor results of therapy in the accelerated and blastic phase, new regimens either to extend the chronic phase or to eliminate the Ph' clone are being pursued, e.g. intensive combination chemotherapy, interferon therapy, bone marrow transplantation.

According to some centres it is possible to achieve complete, though temporary, suppression of the Ph' clone using intensive chemotherapy. Such treatment should be started early in the course of the disease, while normal stem cells still exist. Evidence suggests that significant reduction of the Ph' clone is associated with longer survival.

An alternative approach is to use subcutaneous interferon following initial control of the disease with busulphan. The interferon is given at a dose of 3 MU three to five times weekly. Side effects include depression and thrombocytopenia but it is possible to reduce the Ph' clone and perhaps prolong the chronic phase.

The most exciting advance in the treatment of CML is bone marrow transplantation. Allogeneic BMT in good centres gives a 3-year survival of 60% with a real chance of cure. Unfortunately the best results are only obtained when BMT is carried out in the chronic phase. Most of the deaths from BMT occur in the first year, so inevitably some patients will be forfeiting many years of survival in the chronic phase. The balance of risks must be clearly explained to patients. Some help may be obtained from 'scoring systems', which attempt to predict length of chronic phase, e.g. age, spleen size, platelet count, percentage of circulating blasts, where increase in any of these is related to worse prognosis. The formula may be quite accurate for outcome at 2 years (Sokal *et al.*), and hence relevant to the timing of BMT.

References
Kantarjian, H. M., Talpaz, M. and Gutterman, J. H. (1988) *Haematol. Pathol* **2**(2), 91–120
Talpaz, M. (1988) *Am. J. Med. Sci.* **296**(2), 95–97
Italian study group in CML (1988) *Br. J. Haematol.* **69**, 463
Sokal, J. E., Cox, E. B., Baccaranu, M. *et al.* (1984) *Blood* **63**, 789

Myelofibrosis

With anaemia, splenomegaly and sometimes a high WBC, there are similarities to CML, however the peripheral blood is leucoerythroblastic, with marked tear drop poikilocytosis, and the bone marrow is fibrotic to a much greater extent than seen in CML. Further the neutrophil alkaline phosphatase score is normal or high in myelofibrosis and the Ph' chromosome is not found! Indeed no consistent chromosomal abnormalities are found, although −7 (bad prognosis), trisomy 8 and 5q- (better prognosis) are seen.

The clinical course in myelofibrosis is very variable, survival being anything from 1 to 30 years. The diagnosis is often coincidental. A significant number of patients have a preceding primary polycythaemia. Attempts have been made to establish prognostic criteria along the lines shown in Table 5.2.

In the low-risk group median survival is 15 years whereas in the high-risk group it may be as low as 2 years.

Management

Most patients are over 50 years of age at the time of diagnosis, but about 30% are asymptomatic and require no immediate intervention. As there is presently no cure, management revolves around controlling the anaemia, WBC and problems with massive splenomegaly.

ANABOLIC STEROIDS

- Anaemia responds in 50% of cases (92% of patients with normal karyotype respond; 78% with abnormal karyotype do not).
- Oxymethalone has hepatic side effects.
- Danazol may be better.

Table 5.2   Prognostic factors in primary polycythaemia

Low-risk (long-lived) group		High-risk (short-lived) group
<50	age (years)	>50
>12	Hb (g/dl)	<12
<24	Plasma/blood immature cells	>24
No	Red cell aplasia	Yes
Normal/increased	Marrow cellularity	Reduced
Minimal	Marrow fibrosis	Massive
No	Bruising (platelet abnormality)	Yes
No	Fever, night sweats, weight loss	Yes

SPLENIC IRRADIATION

For symptomatic splenomegaly, temporary result.

SPLENECTOMY

Can improve quality of life in patients with symptoms such as massive splenomegaly and pancytopenia. However, it is not without danger, particularly in patients with platelet defects who may have profound bleeding during and after surgery. Good quality platelet support is thus essential.

CHEMOTHERAPY

Busulphan has been used to control WBC, although it tends to be less effective on spleen size. Hydroxyurea has been found to be more useful, with considerable reduction in fibrosis in some patients.

α-INTERFERON

Limited experience so far suggests that it may be possible to reduce WBC, platelets and spleen size.

Outcome

Death is due to:

- Infection (40%).
- Cardiovascular haemorrhage (40%).
- Acute leukaemia (20%).

Bone marrow transplantation has recently been shown to be an effective treatment in younger patients (<50 years).

References
Barosi et al. (1988) Br. J. Haematol. **70**, 397–401
Manoharan, A. (1988) Br. J. Haematol. **69**, 295
Pagliuca, A., Layton, D. M., Manoharan, A. et al. (1989) Br. J. Haematol. **71**, 493

Primary polycythaemia

Polycythaemia is a term used to describe high haemoglobin and packed cell volume levels, usually more than 18 g/dl and 0.54 for men and more than 16 g/dl and 0.48 for women. It does not necessarily mean an increase in red cell mass, as a decrease in plasma volume will have the same effect.

Polycythaemias are divided into:

- Primary polycythaemia which is a bone marrow disorder.
- Secondary polycythaemia, where the bone marrow functions normally.
- Apparent polycythaemia, in which the red cell mass is in the normal range.

Secondary causes and apparent polycythaemia must be excluded before a diagnosis of primary polycythaemia is made.

Measurement of the red cell mass will exclude apparent polycythaemia where a lowered plasma volume is found. Causes of apparent polycythaemia include stress, heavy cigarette smoking, alcohol, diuretic therapy and hypertension.

In secondary polycythaemia, an increased red cell mass is found, but there is a physiological or pathological reason not directly concerning the bone marrow. Causes include high altitude, cyanotic heart disease, hypoxic lung disease (e.g. chronic bronchitis), renal (renal carcinoma, benign renal tumour, hydronephrosis, polycystic kidneys), Cushing's syndrome, cerebellar haemangioblastoma and hepatoma.

Most patients with primary polycythaemia do not present a difficult diagnosis. They show high haemoglobin, PVC and red cell mass, high WBC and/or platelet count, splenomegaly, high neutrophil alkaline phosphatase score and pruritus (especially after a hot bath).

The plasma/blood is unremarkable, but the bone marrow shows expansion of all cell lines and fibrosis: indeed many of these patients will ultimately develop myelofibrosis. However, some patients present with only an increased red cell mass, when a confident diagnosis of primary polycythaemia is difficult. Erythropoietin levels and erythroid colony growth in culture may help to overcome this problem. Patients with a certain diagnosis of primary polycythaemia have endogenous erythroid colony growth, i.e. colony growth in culture without the addition of erythropoietin. They also have normal or low circulating erythropoietin levels.

When patients present with only high red cell mass and no other criteria for primary polycythaemia, they have no endogenous erythroid colony growth and normal or raised erythropoietin levels. Further, none of the patients in this latter group, in a recent study (Reid et al., 1988), developed primary polycythaemia during a 3-year follow-up period.

Management

Attention to the underlying cause and venesection are used to manage cases of secondary and apparent polycythaemia.

Primary polycythaemia is treated with:

- Venesection to bring the PCV into the normal range, when high haemoglobin is the main problem. Careful management of the PCV will help prevent thromboembolic complications.
- Chemotherapy with busulphan or hydroxyurea when high WBC, high platelets or very large spleen become a problem. [32]P can also be used to control the disease.

In well-controlled disease, the prognosis is good with median survival reported between 10 and 15 years. Most patients die from thromboembolic disease, haemorrhage, transition to acute leukaemia, progression to myelofibrosis or related disorders.

Reference
Reid, C. D., Fidler, J., Kirk, A. *et al.* (1988) *Br. J. Haematol.* **68**, 395–400

Myeloma

Myeloma is the proliferation of B-lymphocytes, the end result of which is the accumulation of large numbers of monoclonal plasma cells. These abnormal plasma cells give rise to the following pathological and clinical findings:

- Infiltration of the bone marrow with plasma cells, leading to marrow failure, i.e. anaemia, thrombocytopenia, neutropenia.
- Lytic lesions in bone, causing pain and pathological fractures due to secretion of osteoclast activiting factor by the plasma cells.
- Production of complete or incomplete immunoglobulin by the abnormal plasma cell pool, which can be detected as a monoclonal protein on electrophoresis of the serum or urine.

The excess protein can lead to problems:

- Increase in the viscosity of blood, with adverse effects on the cardiovascular system.
- Excretion of immunoglobulins (particularly light chains) in the urine can lead to renal failure.
- Interference with normal haemostasis (inhibition of platelets and fibrin polymerization).

Prognostic factors

Myeloma is a disease of the elderly and associated with a median survival of 3–4 years. A worse prognosis is found when:

- The haemoglobin is less than 8.5 g/dl at presentation.
- There is significant reduction in creatinine clearance.
- There is light chain disease (only light chains secreted by the tumour, which then appear in the urine).
- The β_2-microglobulin level is greater than 4 mg/l.

Management

Until recently no attempt has been made to 'cure' myeloma – merely to control it, with chemotherapy for systemic disease and radiotherapy for specific painful bony lesions.

Melphalan with prednisolone has been the standard chemotherapy, given in courses of 5–7 days, 4–6 weeks apart. Treatment is continued until the monoclonal protein level falls to a plateau. There is no evidence that continuing melphalan and prednisolone on the plateau improves survival: 60–70% of patients respond to melphalan and prednisolone. These patients inevitably relapse, but 80% will achieve a second remission (i.e. having once responded most remain sensitive).

Recent studies have shown ABCM (Adriamycin (doxorubicin) 30 mg/m^2 BCNU (carmustine) 30 mg/m^2 on day 1; cyclophosphamide 100 mg/m^2, melphalan 6 mg/m^2 (on days 21–24)) to be better than melphalan and prednisolone, particularly in younger patients (less than 65 years).

Even more aggressive regimens, such as high-dose melphalan (140 mg/m^2) and bone marrow transplantation (for younger patients) are being used in an attempt to bring longer survival or even 'cures'. It is too early to comment on the effectiveness of such treatments.

For patients who do not respond to initial chemotherapy, or who relapse very early (less than 6 months), palliative treatment is probably the best choice:

- High-dose dexamethasone 40 mg daily for 4 days, repeated as required.
- Hemi-body radiotherapy, top half followed by bottom half 4–6 weeks later which gives very good relief of pain and is an excellent treatment in carefully selected patients.

References
Barlogie, B., Alexanian, R., Dickie, K. A. *et al.* (1987) *Blood* **70**, 869–872
Buzaid, A. C. and Durie, B. G. (1988) *J. Clin. Oncol.* **6**, 889–905
Durie, B. G. (1988) *Hematol. Oncol.* **6**, 77–81
Rostom, A. Y. (1988) *Hematol. Oncol.* **6**, 193–198

Chronic lymphocytic proliferations

These are mainly seen in the elderly and comprise the following group of disorders:

- Chronic lymphatic leukaemia.
- Prolymphocytic leukaemia.
- Diffuse lymphocytic lymphoma.
- Hairy cell leukaemia.
- Waldenström's macroglobulinaemia.

Chronic lymphatic leukaemia (CLL)

CLL is a chronic, usually benign, proliferation of small mature lymphocytes. The peripheral blood lymphocyte count is more than 10×10^9/l and the bone marrow will be variably infiltrated. The vast majority (more than 90%) will mark as monoclonal B-cells. A smaller number have T-cell markers; these patients also have a lower median age.

A large number of CLL patients are diagnosed purely coincidentally, with no symptoms or signs relevant to the underlying disease, the only finding being a raised lymphocyte count on routine haematology. Others may present with anaemia, lymphadenophy or splenomegaly.

Because of the variable prognosis in CLL many attempts have been made to predict outcome using:

- Marrow function, organomegaly, lymphadenopathy, as in the Rai and Binet classifications.
- Multivariate regression analysis of prognostic factors, showing that uric acid, alkaline phosphatase, lactate dehydrogenase, lymphadenopathy and age had the strongest predictive relation to survival time. This method is able to divide patients into low, intermediate and high risk, having 5-year survival of 75%, 59% and 14% respectively.
- Bone marrow histology, which can divide CLL into diffuse and non-diffuse histological types: diffuse shows 30–40% 5-year survival; non-diffuse shows 70–80% 5-year survival.

Management

For patients who have early stage disease and good prognostic indicators, no treatment is given. Patients are observed at regular follow-up in outpatients and treatment started only when there is a rising lymphocyte count (more than $50 \times 10^9/l$), marrow failure, gross lymphadenopathy or organomegaly intervene.

For those patients requiring treatment, chlorambucil and prednisolone are used, e.g. chlorambucil 10 mg daily for 14 days; prednisolone 40 mg daily for 14 days.

This course of treatment can be repeated monthly for 6–8 months or until the CLL is well controlled. Splenic irradiation has also been used to control CLL in patients who cannot tolerate chemotherapy.

A significant number (10%) develop autoimmune haemolytic anaemia and/or autoimmune thrombocytopenia during the course of their CLL. Infections, particularly lung infections, due to immunosuppression can be a repeated problem and may be helped by immunoglobulin infusions. The disease may progress to a more aggressive form, but even without morphological progression may ultimately become resistant to treatment. Many patients, however, will die of unrelated disease.

Prolymphocytic leukaemia (PLL)

The lymphocytes are larger with prominent central nucleolus, the peripheral lymphocyte count is high (more than $100 \times 10^9/l$), and there is splenomegaly in most cases.

PLL is always progressive and requires combination chemotherapy with regimens, such as 'CHOP' (C = cyclophosphamide; H = hydroxydaunorubicin (Adriamycin); O = Oncovin (vincristine) and P = prednisolone).

Diffuse lymphocytic lymphoma (DLL)

This is predominantly a B-cell disease, which is morphologically identical to CLL. At diagnosis patients with CLL have blood and bone marrow infiltration, whereas those with DLL have lymphadenopathy and hepatosplenomegaly and often normal peripheral blood. The 'two' diseases merge one with the other, however, and the differences are really only clinical. Treatment of DLL is along the same lines as CLL.

Hairy cell leukaemia (HCL)

This uncommon disease was first described in 1958 as a variant of CLL. Patients have progressive pancytopenia and massive splenomegaly. The cells have abundant cytoplasm with characteristic projections. The marrow trephine biopsy is very helpful, showing diffuse infiltration; the cell nuclei appear well spaced due to the clear cytoplasm surrounding them. The cells are strongly acid phosphatase positive, the reaction being unaffected by tartrate. Electron microscopy is virtually diagnostic.

Management

Splenectomy is an excellent treatment and can give long-lasting remissions. It is particularly recommended for patients with very large spleens.

α-Interferon is of proven benefit and will bring about normal blood counts in 90% of cases. At least 1 year's treatment is recommended and relapses will occur, but resistance is rare and patients can be retreated.

2'-Deoxycoformycin, which is an adenosine deaminase inhibitor, is very effective in the treatment of HCL. Ninty per cent of patients will respond and complete remission has been reported in 60%.

Reference
Dearden. C. and Catovsky, D. (1988) *Eur. J. Haematol.* **41**, 193–196

Waldenström's macroglobulinaemia

This is a B-cell malignancy which in some ways is a cross between a low grade lymphoma and myeloma. The marrow is infiltrated by 'small plasmacytoid lymphocytes', which secrete monoclonal IgM. Marrow failure and very high viscosity levels may be achieved. It is best treated with chlorambucil and prednisolone to control the tumour, but also plasma exchange if the high viscosity causes clinical symptoms.

Myelodysplastic syndromes (MDSs)

The myelodysplastic syndromes are a set of previously apparently heterogeneous disorders characterized by:

- Hypercellular marrow.
- Trilineage dysplasia.
- Peripheral pancytopenia.

These have been brought together into a new classification by Bennett *et al.* (1982):

RA   refractory anaemia
RAS   refractory anaemia with ring sidero-blasts
RAEB   refractory anaemia with excess blasts
RAEB-T   refractory anaemia with excess blasts in transformation
CMML   chronic myelomonocytic leukaemia

RA

Patients present with a macrocytic anaemia (but normal vitamin B_{12} and folate) and the features of MDS. The trilineage dysplasia is described as the following:

ERYTHROPOIESIS

- Vacuolated normoblasts.
- Normoblasts with non-pigmented areas in the cytoplasm.
- Megaloblastic features.

GRANULOPOIESIS

- Pelger–Hüet cells.
- Neutrophils with agranular cytoplasm.

MEGAKARYOCYTES

Three abnormal types are described:

- Micromegakaryocytes with a solitary nucleus.
- Polynuclear megakaryocyte with several small round separate nuclei.
- Large megakaryocytes with single nuclei.

RAS

The same as RA, but often with a dimorphic peripheral blood film and diagnostically 15% or more 'ring sideroblasts' in the bone marrow.

RAEB

The marrow blast cell count is increased at 5–20%.

RAEB-T

The blast cell count is between 20% and 29%. At above 30% the condition is considered to have transformed into an acute leukaemia.

CMML

Here there is trilineage dysplasia but the peripheral blood monocyte count is more than 1×10^9/l. There may also be splenomegaly.

Management of MDSs

RA and RAS have a good prognosis with fairly long survival times. There may be no need for immediate treatment. When symptomatic, anaemia can be corrected by blood transfusion.

RAEB and RAEB-T have a poor prognosis with, not surprisingly, a high incidence of transformation to acute leukaemia. Treatment at this stage is not very rewarding: neither intensive chemotherapy nor low dose cytosine arabinoside, for instance, being helpful in most cases.

There is evidence that RA and RAS can progress to RAEB, RAEB-T and hence acute leukaemia. There is also good evidence that some apparent de novo acute leukaemias are in fact previously undiagnosed, and now transformed, myelodysplastic syndromes.

There have been successful reports of bone marrow transplanation in younger patients with MDSs.

References
Bagby, G. C. (1980) *Ann. Intern. Med.* **92**, 55
Bennett, J. M. *et al.* (1982) *Br. J. Haematol.* **51**, 189–199
Brito-Babapulle, V., Catovsky, D. and Galton, D. A. G. (1987) *Br. J. Haematol* **66**, 445–450
Elias, J. A. (1985) *Blood* **66**, 298–301
Mufti, G., Stevens, J. R., Oscier, D. G. *et al.* (1985) *Br. J. Haematol.* **59**, 425–433
Spriggs, D. R., Stone, R. M. and Kufe, D. W. (1986) *Clin. Haematol.* **15**, 1081–1107

Aplastic anaemia

The anaemia is usually normocytic or moderately macrocytic with associated leucopenia, thrombocytopenia and low reticulocyte count. No immature red cells or white cells are seen in the peripheral blood. The erythrocyte sedimentation rate is increased as the PCV falls. These findings are due to the failure of the bone marrow to produce the normal cells circulating in the peripheral blood. Prognosis is worse in cases with persistent thrombocytopenia. In some cases aplastic anaemia is primarily due to a sinusoidal microcirculation defect in the bone marrow. Once the supporting tissue in the marrow is damaged, e.g. by irradiation, erythropoiesis cannot restart and bone marrow grafts do not take.

Reference
Crosby, W. H. and Knospe, W. H. (1971) *Lancet* **i**, 20

In the human developing red cell the nuclear membrane is closely related to the endoplasmic reticulum (ER). The ER is the primary site for cell detoxication and metabolism. Since the red cell ER is relatively small, it is possible that the nuclear membrane has similar functions. Each individual chromosome is probably anchored at many points to the nuclear membrane, and chromatin fibres converge and attach to annuli of pores in the nuclear membrane. The nuclear membrane is associated with the activation of DNA synthesis and the nuclear pores regulate RNA efflux, only opening when adequate concentration is reached in the cell. Thus change in the endoplasmic reticulum, nuclear membrane, or nuclear membrane pores may glossly interfere with red cell production.

Reference
Frisch, B., Lewis, S. M. and Sherman, D. (1975) *Br. J. Haematol.* **29**, 545

Patients with a total granulocyte count of less than $0.5 \times 10^9/l$, platelets less than $20 \times 10^9/l$, reticulocytes less than $15 \times 10^9/l$ and non-myeloid marrow cellularity more than 75%, have 100% mortality in 3 months. Twenty per cent of patients with three or less of these findings survive 3 months at least.

Primary idiopathic aplastic anaemia

Due to unknown causes

Familial hypoplastic anaemia, without developmental anomalies

Familial hypoplastic anaemia, with developmental anomalies (Fanconi's syndrome)

- Pigmentation of the skin.
- Hypoplasia of the testes.
- Skeletal deformities.

Pure red cell aplasia

Erythropoietin acts at the level of erythroid colony-forming unit (CFU-E). Erythoid burst-forming unit (BFU-E) is regulated by cell-to-cell interactions.

Diamond–Blackfan anaemia [R]

Congenital hypoplastic anaemia has an insidious onset at birth or in early infancy. The white cell count and platelet counts are normal, but the red cells show fetal characteristics, including macrocytosis, increased i-antigen content, raised haemoglobin F concentration and fetal enzyme pattern.

Corticosteroid therapy with maintenance on low doses of prednisolone results in correction of the anaemia in 70–80% of cases. It has been suggested that some patients have defective erythropoietin-insensitive progenitors, partially corrected by corticosteroids. In others, it is possible that pregenitors are absent with failure of commitment of stem cells to erythroid differentiation.

Acquired red cell aplasia in children [R] (transient erythroblastopenia of childhood)

This condition, in which red cells with fetal characteristics are absent, often follows acute virus infection. It has been found that serum from patients suppress both BFU-E and CFU-E (IgG antibody found in 8 of 12 cases, with no evidence of anti-erythropoietin activity).

Pure red cell aplasia of adults [R]

This heterogeneous condition includes

1. Self-limiting disease associated with infections, drugs etc.
2. Chronic disease:
   (a) associated with thymoma, lymphoproliferative disease, connective tissue disease;
   (b) idiopathic.

An IgG antibody has been demonstrated which interferes with erythroblast activity.

References
Krantz, S. B. (1974) *N. Engl. J. Med.* **291**, 345
Peschle, C., Marmont, A. M., Marone, G. *et al.* (1975) *Br. J. Haematol.* **30**, 411
Sief, C. (1983) *Br. J. Haematol.* **54**, 331

Secondary aplastic anaemia

Known bone-marrow depressants (dose-related)

- Aminopterin, α-methopterin.
- Benzene.
- Busulphan.
- γ-Benzene hexachloride.
- 6-Mercaptopurine.
- Nitrogen mustards.
- *p*-phenylenediamine.
- Triethylene melamine.
- Trinitrotoluene.
- Urethane.

Drugs which may cause bone-marrow depression

(i.e. drugs to which a personal idiosyncrasy may develop):

Antiepileptics

- Aloxidone.
- Methyl hydantoin.
- Paramethadione.
- Phenylacetylurea.
- Trimethyladione.

Antibiotics

- Chloramphenicol.
- Streptomycin.
- Sulphonamides.

Antirheumatics

- Gold salts.
- Phenylbutazone.

Other drugs

- Acetazolamide.
- Hydralazine.
- Mepacrine.
- Organic arsenicals.

Irradiation injury

Local irradiation exposure to 40–50 Gy (4000–5000 rad) results in marrow aplasia which resolves slowly, often incompletely, over several years. There was no increase in aplastic anaemia in the atomic bomb exposure survivors in Japan, whereas the incidence of aplastic anaemia is higher than in the general population in ankylosing spondylitis patients treated with courses of irradiation and in radiologists.

Infections

Virus

- Hepatitis (usually non-A, non-B) 0.3–0.5% of cases, with a poor prognosis; 25% of patients with aplastic anaemia have abnormal liver function test results at diagnosis, suggesting subclinical infection or exposure to hepatotoxic agents.

Reference
Zeldis, J. B., Dienstag, J. C. and Gale, R. P. (1983) *Am. J. Med.* **74**, 64

- Infectious mononucleosis.
- Dengue ⎫
- Influenza ⎭ not common.

Bacteria

- Tuberculosis and atypical mycobacterial infections.
- Brucellosis.

Parasitic diseases

Associated with peripheral cell destruction or hypersplenism.

Other conditions

- Paroxysmal nocturnal haemoglobinuria: aplastic anaemia develops in up to 25% of cases; 5–10% of aplastic anaemia cases progress to paroxysmal nocturnal haemoglobinuria.
- Leukaemia: 1–5% of patients with aplastic anaemia have leukaemia. Rapid normalization of blood count following steroid therapy suggests underlying ALL rather than aplastic anaemia.
- Graft-versus-host disease: some cases progress to aplastic anaemia.
- Patients with primary or secondary cellular immune deficiency.
- Thymoma.
- X-linked lymphoproliferative system.
- Pre-ALL in childhood.
- Aplastic crises during sickle-cell disease, hereditary spherocytic anaemia, pyruvate kinase deficiency, and thalassaemia intermedia, are often associated with parvovirus infection.

Reference
Davis, L. R. (1983) *B. J. Haematol.* **55**, 391

Treatment of aplastic anaemia

As has been seen, the causes of aplastic anaemia are many and varied. Some cases will recover after a period of support with red cell and platelet transfusions. However, severe aplastic anaemia, with platelets less than $20 \times 10^9/l$ and neutrophil count less than $0.5 \times 10^9/l$, has an appalling prognosis and requires more than blood transfusion support.

Anabolic steroids

Oxymethalone has been used extensively to treat aplastic anaemia. Whilst it will often increase the red cell count and haemoglobin, they have no consistent effect upon platelets or neutrophils. Steroids are not the treatment of choice in severe aplastic anaemia.

Antilymphocyte globulin (ALG)

ALG prepared in the horse or the rabbit has been shown to be of value in severe aplastic anaemia. Most centres use horse ALG first, the injection being covered with steroids to prevent 'serum sickness' which would otherwise occur during the first week in most cases.

Response may take up to 3 months, but is seen in 40–50% of cases. If no response is seen at 4 months, an injection of rabbit ALG may be given, as some patients will respond to the second ALG. Responses may not be complete, but provided blood transfusion support can be avoided they are worthwhile.

Bone marrow transplantation (BMT)

The treatment of choice in severe aplastic anaemia is BMT. There is no doubt that early transplantation with a matched related donor gives the patient the best chance of long-term survival. Results from most centres show a 60–80% success rate.

A recent report on the follow-up of 137 survivors of severe aplastic anaemia showed that the 34 treated with BMT had no haematological disease 8 years later. However, of the 103 patients treated with ALG, 20 (19%) developed complications of MDS, acute leukaemia, paroxysmal nocturnal haemoglobinuria. The risk of developing a late complication increases with time, being 58% at 8 years.

Reference
Tichell, A., Gratwahl, A., Würsch, A. *et al.* (1988) *Br. J. Haematol.* **69**, 413–418

There have been tremendous advances in the clinical application of BMT and there is much more knowledge now about the mechanisms involved.

BMT can be divided into:

1. Allogeneic BMT.
   (a) matched related (sibling) donors;
   (b) matched unrelated donors (MUD).
   The best matched related donors are of course identical twins!

2. Autologous BMT: this procedure involves using the patient's own stored (usually frozen) marrow, taken at the time of 'remission' which is reinfused after intensive ablative therapy. It is not a 'transplant' in the strict sense of the word and perhaps should be called autologous marrow rescue.

Bone marrow transplantation is now used in the following conditions:

- Aplastic anaemia – allogeneic BMT is the treatment of choice in severe cases.
- Severe combined immune deficiency syndrome – allo-BMT.
- Chronic myeloid leukaemia – allo-BMT gives the only chance of cure at the present time; 50–60% disease free survival at 4 years, starting from chronic phase.
- Acute myeloid leukaemia – allo-BMT: in first remission offers a higher chance of cure than present chemotherapy (more than 50% survival at 3 years). Auto-BMT as an intensive consolidation therapy may improve long-term survival.
- Acute lymphoblastic leukaemia – allo-BMT: in second remission ALL can achieve 30–40% 3-year disease-free survival. Some are advocating its use to obtain better cure rates in first remission bad prognosis ALL.
- High grade lymphomas – allo and auto-BMT have been used both in first remission and after relapse.
- 'Solid tumours' such a breast and lung – so far results are not good but they will certainly get better.
- Myeloma.
- Myelodysplastic syndrome – allo-BMT has been successful in younger patients (less than 50 years). This of course only applies to a minority of these groups.
- Thalassaemia, sickle-cell disease – very good results have been obtained in well-selected cases.

Advantages of BMT

1. The chance of higher cure rates than conventional treatment in:
   (a) aplastic anaemia;
   (b) acute myeloid leukaemia;
   (c) relapsed acute lymphoblastic leukaemia;
   (d) bad prognosis acute lymphoblastic leukaemia;
   (e) high grade lymphoma.
2. The chance of cure where none previously existed in:
   (a) chronic myeloid leukaemia;
   (b) myeloma;
   (c) myelodysplastic syndrome;
   (d) thalassaemia;
   (e) sickle-cell disease.

Disadvantages of BMT

There is a risk of early death from the procedure, which in chronic disease such as CML or sickle-cell disease has to be weighed against possible length and quality of survival.

Autologous BMT can only be used when 'normal' marrow is available, i.e. it cannot be used in aplastic anaemia or thalassaemia.

In leukaemia and lymphoma there is the danger of 'transplanting' (even in remission) malignant cells – hence relapse!

Allogeneic BMT is restricted by availability of donors, only 1 : 4 siblings will be matched, matched unrelated donors are difficult to find and in any case at the moment carry a high incidence of graft versus host disease (GVHD).

Conditioning therapy

In order to prepare someone for a bone marrow transplant they need to be pre-treated to destroy any existing marrow and (in the case of malignancy) any remaining disease.

Most early conditioning regimens have contained total body irradiation (TBI) with, for example, high-dose cyclophosphamide. TBI, however, has a number of early and late side effects:

- Early: nausea, vomiting, fever, mucositis, diarrhoea, erythema, alopecia, parotitis, idiopathic interstitial pneumonia, hepatic veno-occlusive disease.
- Late: cataract formation, reduced growth in children, reduced endocrine function, carcinogenesis.

In order to avoid these, trials with intensive chemotherapy only have been carried out, i.e. busulphan + cyclophosphamide, high-dose melphalan.

The results have been at least as good as regimens that include TBI!

Graft versus host disease (GVHD)

One of the biggest problems with allo-BMT is GVHD. Several attempts have been made to overcome this.

- Post-transplant immunosuppression using methotrexate and/or cyclosporin A: these will reduce the incidence and severity of GVHD; cyclosporin A is usually given at controlled levels for 100 days post-transplant.
- T-cell depletion of the donor marrow will significantly reduce the incidence of GVHD. However, there will be a higher graft failure rate and, in the case of leukaemia and lymphoma, a higher relapse rate.

Infection

This is a major cause of death in BMT, both early and late. Common infections are bacterial, fungal, viral (*note:* CMV) and *Pneumocystis carinii.*

There is no doubt that results from BMT will continue to improve and that it has an important role in the management of aplastic anaemia and haematological malignancies.

References

Apperly, J. F., Goldman, J. *et al.* (1988) *Br. J. Haematol.* **69**, 239–245
Conde, R., Iriondo, A., Rayon, C. *et al.* (1988) *Br. J. Haematol.* **68**, 219–226
Kanfe, E. J., McCarthy, D. M. (1989) *Br. J. Haematol.* **71**, 447–450
Storb, R. (1988) *Am. J. Med. Sci.* **296**, 87–94
Weisdorf, D. J., McGlave, R. B., Ramsay, N. K. *et al.* (1988) *Br. J. Haematol.* **69**, 351–381

Chapter 6

Bleeding, clotting and transfusion

Plasma Coagulation Factors

Nomenclature of blood-clotting factors

Accepted International Symbol	Synonym
Factor I	Fibrinogen
Factor II	Prothrombin
Factor III	Tissue factor
Factor IV	Calcium
Factor V	Factor V
	Labile factor
	Plasma ac-globulin
	Proaccelerin
	Plasma prothrombin conversion factor
Factor VII	Factor VII
	Stable factor
	Cofactor V
	Proconvertin
	Serum prothrombin conversion accelerator
Factor VIII	Factor VIII
	Antihaemophiliac globulin A
	Thromboplastinogen
	Thromboplastin plasma component
	Prothrombokinase
	Thrombocytolysin
Factor IX	Factor IX
	Christmas factor
	Plasma thromboplastin component
	Antihaemophiliac globulin B
	Plasma thromboplastin component B
	Antihaemophiliac globulin B
	Plasma thromboplastin component B
Factor X	Factor X
	Prower factor
	Stuart factor
	Stuart–Prower factor
Factor XI	Factor XI
	Plasma thromboplastin antecedent
Factor XII	Factor XII
	Hageman factor
Factor XIII	Factor XIII
	Fibrin-stabilizing factor
	Fibrinase

Blood coagulation

A quarter of a century ago, the first comprehensive 'cascade' or 'waterfall' of sequential activation of plasma zymogens resulting in the formation of fibrin clot was published. Since then, the knowledge of platelet function has advanced, a number of natural anticoagulants as well as more coagulant factors have been discovered and the fibrinolytic system and its antagonists have been studied, with dramatic effects on treatment of bleeding and clotting disorders.

Our clotting system has evolved so that locally adhering and aggregating platelets can repair a minute tear in the endothelium of a large artery, or a lacuna in a minute capillary, whilst fibrin clot can plug a complete tear through a blood vessel, with subsequent repair back to normal or, at least, survival. At the same time, whilst this repair system is locally effective, the coagulation system (activated platelets and fibrin clotting) is confined strictly to the local damaged site.

Inappropriate clotting or the formation of platelet aggregates in the wrong place at the wrong time, with progressive extension throughout the circulation, is prevented by a system of anticoagulants and fibrinolytics, which, in turn, are prevented from damaging the local repair.

Ineffective clotting will result in bleeding, while excessive clotting will result in thromboses and emboli.

References
Davie, E. W. and Ratnoff, O. D. (1964) *Science* **145**, 1310
Macfarlane, R. G. (1964) *Nature* **202**, 498

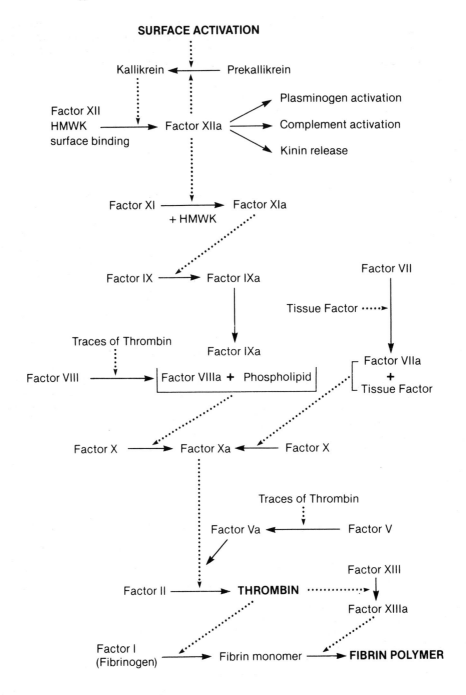

'Cascade' mechanism of blood coagulation. HMWK – high molecular weight kinninogen. Circulating plasma clotting factors (zymogens) are converted to activated forms (solid arrows). Activated clotting factors accelerate the conversion of zymogens to activated factors (dotted lines).

Fibrinogen (factor I)

Normal plasma concentration

Newborn infant

The value is 1.81 ± 0.61 g/l, lower in pre-term infants. Synthesis of fetal fibrinogen persists for up to 7–8 days after birth. Adult levels of fibrinogen are reached by 2 months.

Adult

The value is 2–4 g/l, increasing with age and increasing in women after the menopause. Plasma fibrinogen is a positive risk factor for ischaemic heart disease, myocardial infarction and stroke.

Late pregnancy

The value is 4–6.5 g/l, associated with increased ESR and plasma viscosity. It is also increased by oral contraceptives.

References
Desvignes, P. and Bonnet, P. (1981) *Clin. Chim. Acta* **110**, 9
Foley, M. E., Isherwood, D. M. and McNicol, G. P. (1978) *Br. J. Obstet. Gynaecol.* **85**, 500
Wilhelmsen, L., Svärdsudd, K., Korsan-Bengsten, K. *et al.* (1984) *N. Engl. J. Med.* **311**, 501

Fibrinogen synthesis

This occurs in the hepatocytes under genetic control, with possible genetic control of fibrinolysis also affecting the plasma fibrinogen concentration. Circulating fibrin degradation products, fragments D and E, stimulate its production. It is an acute phase protein and increases in response to inflammatory stimuli.

References
Bell, W. R., Kessler, C. M. and Townsend, R. R. (1983) *Br. J. Haematol.* **53**, 599
Humphries, S. E., Cook, M., Dubowitz, M. *et al.* (1987) *Lancet* i, 1452

Platelet fibrinogen is synthesized in the megakaryocytes and carried in the α-granules.

Structure of fibrinogen

The molecule has a molecular weight of 340 000, and consists of a dimer with A-, B- and γ-polypeptide chains connected by disulphide bridges, and the two halves in turn joined by disulphide bridges (Aα, Bβ, γ)$_2$. The predominant γ-chain species in normal human fibrinogen has a molecular weight of 50 000, with higher-molecular-weight variants which have a low affinity for platelet binding. The fibrinopeptide B is negatively charged and keeps fibrinogen molecules apart in the plasma.

References
Peerschke, E. I. B., Francis, C. W. and Marder, V. J. (1986) *Blood* **67**, 385
Weisel, J. W., Stauffacher, C. V., Bullitt, E. *et al.* (1986) *Science* **230**, 1388

The molecule has the electrophoretic mobility of a γ-globulin, and has a half-life in the circulation of about 4–5 days, the molecule decreasing in size the longer it is in the circulation.

Increase

Physiological

During the last trimester of pregnancy, and with increasing age (after the menopause in women); oral contraceptives.

Pathological

- Inflammatory disorders, including bacterial infections, tissue damage due to trauma or surgery with peak values at 5–10 days, burns, post-X-ray therapy, pulmonary embolism, venous thrombosis. In acute pancreatitis and following myocardial infarction, the level of increase and its persistence is related to the severity of the attack.
- Liver disease, including cirrhosis, chronic hepatitis, hepatoma and obstructive jaundice, in which the fibrinogen may be abnormal in structure and fail to polymerize.
- Rheumatoid arthritis and other so-called 'collagen diseases'.
- Nephrosis: fibrinogen antagonistic to PGI$_2$-mediated inhibition of platelet aggregation in vitro. This effect is abolished by albumin, but plasma albumin is very low in nephrosis, encouraging thrombosis.
- Diabetes mellitus.
- Tobacco smoking: both tobacco smoking and plasma fibrinogen are risk factors for ischaemic heart disease.
- Hypertriglyceridaemia.

References
Ernst, E. (1991) *Brit. Med. J.* **303**, 596
Markowe, H. L. J., Marmot, M. G., Shipley, M. J. *et al.* (1985) *B. Med. J.* **291**, 1312
Mikhailidis, D. P., Barradas, M. A., Maris, A. *et al.* (1985) *J. Clin. Pathol.* **38**, 1166
Simpson, H. C. R., Mann, J. I., Meade, T. W. *et al.* (1983) *Lancet* i, 786

Decrease

Physiological

Newborn and pre-term babies.

Pathological

Acquired

- Depressed synthesis – liver damage, severe cachexia.
- Disseminated intravascular coagulopathy, with consumption of fibrinogen.
- Therapeutic defibrination with ancrod (Arvin).

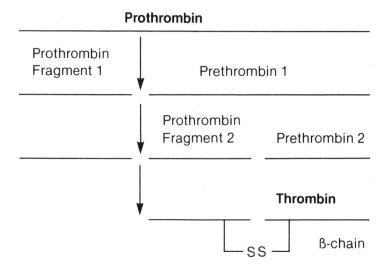

Prothrombin

Prothrombin Fragment 1	Prethrombin 1
	Prothrombin Fragment 2	Prethrombin 2
		Thrombin

—S S—   ß-chain

Activation and conversion of prothrombin to thrombin.

- Clofibrate therapy reduces increased plasma fibrinogen.
- Moderate alcohol, ticlopidine, propanolol, stanozolol.
- Subjects treated with unsaturated fish oils show a significant fall in plasma fibrinogen and triglycerides with increased fibrinolytic activity, without any bleeding tendency developing.

References
Celerblad, G. and Korsan-Bengsten, K. (1976) *Clin. Chim. Acta* **66**, 9
Saynor, G. and Gillott, T. (1988) *Br. Med. J.* **297**, 1196

Congenital

AFIBRINOGENAEMIA [R] [AR]

Heterozygotes are symptomless. Homozygotes (over 25 cases reported) suffer from haemarthroses after injury, and abnormal bleeding after injury or surgery. Plasma fibrinogen levels are less than 100 mg/l. Clotting tests are normal after addition of fibrinogen to the patient's plasma.

FIBRINOGENOPENIA [R]

Symptomless, possibly heterozygotes of congenital afibrinogenaemia. Plasma fibrinogen 100–1000 mg/l.

DYSFIBRINOGENAEMIA [AR] [R]

Fourteen families have been studied. Signs and symptoms range from abnormal bleeding to thrombophilia. There may be persistence of fetal fibrinogen, an unstable fibrinogen molecule with excessive catabolism, or poor delayed polymerization of fibrin.

ANTIBODIES AGAINST FIBRINOGEN

These very rarely develop in afibrinogenaemia following transfusion.

Reference
Bithell, T. C. (1985) *Clin. Chem.* **31**, 509 (review of dysfibrinogenaemia)

Factor II (prothrombin)

Prothrombin is a glycoprotein containing 6% of carbohydrate, with a molecular weight of 72 000, an isoelectric point of pH 4.2, an electrophoretic mobility of an α_2-globulin and consists of a single polypeptide chain. It is moderately stable in stored blood, stable in deep-frozen plasma, relatively heat stable and withstands 56°C for 7 h.

Normal plasma level

About 100 μg/ml (60–155 μg/ml varying with method used). Prothrombin is synthesized in hepatic ribosomes and acquires up to 10 γ-carboxyl groups on glutamyl residues near the amino-terminal of the molecule by means of a post-translational vitamin K-dependent microsomal carboxylase reaction. These groups allow normal prothrombin to bind calcium ions during clotting, to associate with phospholipid during clotting, and to adsorb onto barium sulphate in vitro. Levels of 40% of normal prothrombin concentration are required for satisfactory haemostasis. Factor Xa and factor II are adsorbed and concentrated on phospholipid-rich surfaces via calcium ion bridges on (Gla)residues. Wounds and accompanying cell damage provide adequate phospholipid-rich sites, and factor II is activated by the protease Xa. (Gla)residues are necessary for VII, IX and X, and all the vitamin-K-dependent factors (other than factor II) contain (Gla)residues in their final activated form. When factor II is activated, 'fragment 1' is released (residues 1–156) contains all 10 (Gla)residues in the original prothrombin molecule, and these can competitively inhibit further activation of II by Xa. Prothrombin half-life following transfusion is about 50 h. During clotting, factor Xa (protease) in the presence of factor Va, calcium ions and phospholipid, cleaves prothrombin into two polypeptide chains, fragment 1–2 with a molecular weight of 35 500, and prethrombin 2 with a molecular weight of 37 500. Prethrombin 2 then undergoes a second proteolytic cleavage, converting it to thrombin, and thrombin converts plasma fibrinogen to fibrin. Fragment 2 protects thrombin from the action of antithrombin III in the immediate vicinity of a clot. Increased amounts of fragments F_{1+2} are found in the plasma of most patients with repeated episodes of venous thrombosis or pulmonary embolism, while symptom free, suggesting a prethrombotic state.

Stypven generates thrombin from prothrombin by activating factors X and V in the presence of phospholipid and calcium. Taipan venom generates thrombin and prothrombin fragments by direct action. *Echis carinatus* venom activates prothrombin directly to thrombin.

References
Bauer, K. A. and Rosenberg, R. D. (1987) *Blood* **70**, 343 (review of prethrombotic state)
Blanchard, R. A., Furie, B. C., Jorgensen, M. *et al.* (1981) *N. Engl. J. Med.* **305**, 242
Swars, H., Hafner, G., Erbel, R. and Ehrenthal, W. (1991) *Lancet* **337**, 59

Pathological decrease

Infants

In pre-term infants factor II levels are approximately 30% of normal. Full-term infant factor II levels are approximately 50% of normal, reaching full adult levels by 60–120 days.

Vitamin K deficiency

- Absence of vitamin K from the diet.
- Malabsorption of vitamin K, in association with a malabsorption syndrome.
- Liver disease: there is an abnormal depression of both active prothrombin and inert prothrombin precursor. A disproportion of IIAg and IIC indicates vitamin K deficiency, which should respond at least partially to vitamin K supplements.
- Vitamin K antagonists, such as the anti-vitamin K anticoagulant, warfarin. Active prothrombin levels fall, with increase in the des-γ-carboxy form, which

is inactive. Normally factor II precursor is carboxylated and glycosylated before secretion by the hepatocytes.
- Malnourished patients with low serum vitamin K_1 levels are at risk of developing hypoprothrombinaemia when they are treated with some cephalosporins or other antibiotics. The prothrombin clotting time is relatively insensitive to depletion of body vitamin K_1 stores.

Reference
Cohen, H., Scott, S. D., Mackie, I.J. *et al.* (1988) *Br. J. Haematol.* **68**, 63

Congenital [R]

- Hypoprothrombinaemia.
- Abnormal molecular variant of prothrombin (dysprothrombin).

These rare conditions are associated with excessive bleeding, mucous membrane haemorrhage, menorrhagia in females and postoperative haemorrhage.

The one-stage prothrombin time is abnormally prolonged, and is not corrected by adsorbed normal plasma, aged serum or Russell's viper venom. The activated partial thromboplastin time (APTT) may be increased.

Immunological factor II is reduced in hypoprothrombinaemia, and is normal in dysprothrombinaemia.

References
Montgomery, R. R., Otsuka, A. and Hathaway, W. E. (1978) *Blood* **51**, 299
Owen, C. A. Jr., Henriksen, R. A., McDuffie, F. C. *et al.* (1978) *Mayo Clin. Proc.* **53**, 29

- Structurally abnormal variants with normal coagulant activity occur.

Reference
Board, P. G. (1982) *Ann. Hum. Genet.* **46**, 293

Factor III (tissue factor)

This glycoprotein is produced in the cell surface in response to injury, and vascular endothelial cells produce the procoagulant when stimulated. Membrane-bound tissue factor complexes with factor VII and activates it to factor VIIa. It also augments the proteolytic attack of factor VIIa on factors IX and X. It is not released by normal undamaged vascular endothelial cells.

Human leucocytes develop procoagulant activity (tissue factor) in response to bacterial endotoxin, antigen–antibody complex, some plasma lipoproteins, lytic products of the fifth component of complement and phytohaemagglutinins. These responses are inhibited by corticosteroids.

Tissue factor activity in the subendothelium of blood vessel walls possibly plays a part in both the arrest of bleeding and the promotion of thrombin formation at the site of vascular injury. Its highest specific activity occurs in the brain, lung and placenta, and it is released into the circulation following severe shock, trauma, intravascular haemolysis and amniotic embolism.

Tissue thromboplastin is species specific and its mode of preparation affects its potency. This is important in the laboratory in the standardization of the prothrombin time.

Reference
Weiss, H. J., Turitta, V. T., Baumgartner, H. R. *et al.* (1989) *Blood* **73**, 968

Thrombin

Thrombin has a specificity for arginine–lysine bonds, and also cleaves an arginine–threonine bond in prothrombin to release prethrombin, followed by an arginine–lysine cleavage to release active thrombin. Free thrombin is only found in the circulation when the rate of formation exceeds its elimination. Release of thrombin into the circulation can be demonstrated by:

- A rise of fibrinopeptide A levels above baseline values (biological half-life of 3 min).
- Positive fibrin gel tests.
- Detection of thrombin–antithrombin III complexes.
- Fragments F_{1+2} from prothrombin cleavage in the circulation.

Thrombin actions

Once thrombin has been formed, it releases more thrombin from prothrombin. Thrombin cleaves fibrinopeptide A from the Aα chains, then it cleaves fibrinopeptide B from Bβ chains of fibrinogen. In the coagulation cascade, thrombin activates factors IX to IXa, V to Va, VIII to VIIIa and XIII to XIIIa.

In the localization of a clot, thrombin combines with thrombomodulin to activate protein C, and hence to inactivate factors Va and VIIIa, interfering with the action of factor Xa in the immediate vicinity of the clot.

Thrombin neutralization

Although fragment 2, released during conversion of prothrombin to thrombin, inhibits the inactivation of active thrombin by antithrombin III (AT-III) plus heparin at the local clot site, thrombin is rapidly neutralized as it enters the general circulation, and has a biological half-life of only 37 seconds. When thrombin combines with thrombomodulin before its activation of protein C, it loses its thrombotic activities. Thrombin is also adsorbed onto fibrin as it is formed, to be released and neutralized later during clot retraction. Combining irreversibly with AT-III and heparin, the thrombin complex is then removed from the circulation, thrombin being eliminated and heparin being released back into the circulation.

Traces of thrombin take part in thrombin-mediated feedback reactions with the generation of more thrombin. Traces of tissue factor in the presence of platelets produce explosive thrombin generation, and small amounts of thrombin induce procoagulant activity in platelets. Heparin inhibits this at concentrations of as little as 0.1–0.15 IU/ml, a major activity of heparin being the scavenging of minute amounts of thrombin before they induce feedback reactions.

Reference
Béguin, S. L., Lindhout, T. and Hemker, H. C. (1989) *Thrombos. Haemostas.* **60**, 457; **61**, 25

Factor IV (calcium)

In vitro it is possible to interfere with the one-stage prothrombin estimation (for example) by adding too much or too little calcium chloride to the system.

However, in vivo, the serum calcium variation in disease is not sufficient to interfere with the coagulation mechanisms. Hypocalcaemia sufficient to interfere with coagulation would be incompatible with life.

Factor V

Plasma factor V is a single-molecule glycoprotein (20% carbohydrate content), with a molecular weight of 350 000. It is synthesized in hepatocytes and reticuloendothelial cells in the liver, and has a biological half-life of 15–24 h. Each molecule carries one high affinity binding site for calcium.

Factor V in the platelet (platelet factor I) is stored in the α-granules, and is not present on the surface of the intact platelet. Coagulant activity indistinguishable from plasma factor V is released following platelet aggregation and release by collagen.

Factor V is heat labile, storage labile (although it keeps well in fresh-frozen plasma) and is not adsorbed on gels. It circulates in an inactive form and is activated by thrombin to factor Va, which is capable of accelerating conversion of factor II to thrombin by factor Xa. Activation of factor Va consists of proteolysis of the molecule in at least two places, releasing three to five polypeptides, with molecular weights of 70 000 and 100 000 from each end of the molecule, and one of 150 000. The active part has a molecular weight of

94 000. Thus factor V is consumed during coagulation.

Factor Va binds to factors Xa and II, whilst factor V does not. Platelets bind factor Va to their surface. After activation, platelets bind both factors V and Va avidly to receptor sites in the platelet membrane. When bound, both factors Va and Xa are protected from the action of inhibitors (e.g. protein-C and AT-III).

Physiological

Both the full-term and pre-term newborn infant have plasma factor V levels similar to those of older children and adults. Cord blood plasma factor V activity is 54–155%. During normal pregnancy there is a moderate increase in maternal plasma factor V.

Pathological

Deficiency

Congenital deficiency [R]

About 150 cases of this rare autosomal bleeding diathesis have been reported. It exists in two molecular forms: one with low coagulant and antigenic activities, and one with low coagulant but with antigenic activity present (i.e. an abnormal molecular form). The condition is associated with bruising, epistaxis, oral bleeding, bleeding following minor lacerations and following tooth extraction. Muscle haematomas, haemarthroses and intracranial haemorrhages are rare.

Reference
Chiu, H. C., Whitaker, E. and Colman, R. W. (1983) *J. Clin. Invest.* **72**, 493

LABORATORY TESTS

Prolonged bleeding times are found in a third of cases (?abnormal platelet factor V).

Both the prothrombin clotting time and the APTT are abnormally prolonged, and corrected by the addition of adsorbed normal plasma, but not by aged serum or Russell viper venom.

The thromboplastin generation test shows abnormal results with the patient's absorbed plasma. (*Note:* normal platelets cannot be used, as they contain factor V.) The inability of plasma from the patient to correct the thromboplastin generation time (TGT) of stored human oxalated plasma indicates probable factor V deficiency. Specific estimation of the factor in the patient's plasma is then helpful.

Bleeding can be corrected using fresh frozen plasma 10 ml/kg body weight. A minimum of 20% factor V activity is required for haemostasis.

Acquired deficiency

1. In severe liver disease, reduced plasma factor V levels are a better index of liver damage than either estimation of factor XIII or plasminogen.

Reference
Biland, L., Duckert, F., Prisender, S. *et al.* (1978) *Thromb. Haemost.* **39**, 646

2. Rarely;
   (a) melaena neonatorum;
   (b) promyelocytic leukaemia;
   (c) associated with depression of other clotting factors: radio-phosphorus therapy [R]; and following severe haemorrhage with rapid replacement with stored blood.

Factor V inhibitors

Low potency antibodies of short duration may develop in apparently normal patients following surgery, or treatment with antibiotics (e.g. cephaloridine and especially the aminoglycosides) neutralizing both plasma and platelet factor V.

Factor VII

Factor VII is a single-chain glycoprotein with a molecular weight of 48 000, and with initial amino acid sequence homology with other vitamin K-dependent proteins. It is synthesized in the liver, has an electrophoretic mobility of a β-globulin, and circulates in the plasma in a semi-active form in the plasma, even in the absence of tissue factor. Vitamin K is essential for the carboxylation of glutamyl residues to form γ-glutamic acid residues on the molecule, necessary for calcium binding, and hence ability to take part in clotting.

Factor VII is a serine protease with obligate dependence on a lipid cofactor. Activation of factor VII to factor VIIa follows hydrolysis to a double chain form with disulphide linkage, without release of a peptide fragment during activation. Factors XIIa, Xa, and IXa can all activate factor VII and, since both factors XII and IX can be activated by kallikrein, the so-called 'intrinsic' and 'extrinsic' clotting systems are linked (probably explaining why the prothrombin time and thrombotest are both shortened when plasma is shaken with glass beads).

Factor VIIa complexes with tissue factor, and its ability, in the presence of calcium ions, to activate factor X to factor Xa is markedly increased. Cells from non-vascular tissues initiate clotting by increasing the activity of factor VIIa, directly related to the number of factor VIIa receptors on the cell surface – important in enhancing clotting after tissue damage. Factor VII is not consumed during clotting, and is therefore present in both plasma and serum.

References
Masys, D. R., Bajaj, S. P. and Rapaport, S. I. (1982) *Blood* **60**, 1143
Rodgers, G. M., Broze, G. J. Jr. and Shumax, M. A. (1984) *Blood* **63**, 434

The normal plasma factor VII range is 70–125%, about 50% in the full-term normal newborn infant, and about 36% in the pre-term infant. It has a biological half-life of 70–375 min.

Increase

Physiological

- Increases three- to four-fold during late pregnancy.
- Oestrogen-containing contraceptive pill.

Pathological

Factor VII is a risk factor for myocardial infarction, and factors VIIC and VIIAg are correlated directly with the plasma triglyceride concentration. Also, patients, immediately following an acute myocardial infarction, have increased plasma factor VIIC levels, especially when there are complications.

Reference
Sousa, J. C., Azevedo, J., Soria, C. et al. (1988) Rev. Iberoam. Thromb. Hemost. **S1**, 52

Decrease

Physiological

In the newborn and pre-term newborn infant.

Pathological

Acquired

- Haemorrhagic disease of the newborn, occurring in infants born to mothers who are severely vitamin K deficient, on treatment with warfarin, anticonvulsants or antituberculous drugs. During the first 24 hours, intracranial, intrathoracic or intra-abdominal bleeding may develop. Typically, bleeding develops between 1 and 7 days after birth, from the gastrointestinal tract, from the nose, into the skin, from the vagina or from postcircumcision wounds in male infants. It may also develop later, after 1–3 months in infants with diarrhoea and malabsorption.

The bleeding tendency persists until vitamin K is given (and large doses are unnecessary, and may be toxic), or until normal bacterial flora have colonized the infant gut and begun synthesis of vitamin K, which is then absorbed.

Reference
Hathaway, W. F. (1987) In: Oski, F. A., Ed. *Haematology/Oncology Clinics of North America*, Vol. 3, p. 367. London: W. B. Saunders

- Kwashiorkor.
- Liver disease: synthesis of both factors VIIC and VIIAg falls. When the raised prothrombin ratio fails to respond to vitamin K within 24 h, this indicates severe liver damage.

- Treatment with anti-vitamin K anticoagulant drugs (e.g. warfarin, coumarins), factor VII is formed without γ-glutamyl calcium-binding residues and factor VIIAg is not reduced (compare liver damage).

Congenital

INHERITED FACTOR VII DEFICIENCY [R] [AR]

About 120 cases have been described, and three main classes exist:

1. VII$^-$: the majority of cases have very low factor VIIC with unmeasurable factor VIIAg, because of genetic suppression of synthesis of factor VII.
2. VII$^+$: plasma contains very low levels of factor VIIC with normal factor VIIAg, because of synthesis of normal levels of markedly defective factor VII molecules. There is variable response to the action of different animal thromboplastins (helpful in detection).
3. VII^R: plasma contains low factor VIIC with low factor VIIAg, the result of decreased capacity to synthesize a defective factor VII molecule. Homozygotes have a life-long bleeding tendency, with ecchymoses, epistaxis and bleeding from the gums. Haematuria and intrauterine bleeding are common. Gastrointestinal bleeding and haemathrosis may occur. The prothrombin ratio is greater than 3.5 in homozygotes, and this can be corrected by the addition of Russell's viper venom in the presence of cephalin and calcium ions. The bleeding time, clotting time, thrombin time and APTT are all normal. Heterozygote carrier detection is now possible.

References
Briet, E., Loeliger, E. A., van Tilburg, N. H. et al. (1976) Thrombos. Haemost. **35**, 289
Girolami, A., Fabris, F., Zanon, R. D. D. et al. (1978) J. Lab. Clin. Med. **91**, 387
Mariani, G., Mazzucconi, M. G., Hermani, J. et al. (1981) Br. J. Haematol. **48**, 7
Mariani, G., Hermans, J., Orlando, M. et al. (1985) Br. J. Haematol. **60**, 687
Triplett, D. A., Brandt, J. T., Batard, M. A. et al. (1985) Blood **66**, 1284

Plasma levels of 10–15% factor VIIC make surgery safe, and replacement therapy in the form of prothrombin complex or factor VII concentrate can be given at the time of operation. There is a lack of correlation between reduced factor VII levels and surgical bleeding.

Reference
Yorke, A. J. and Mant, M. J. (1977) *JAMA* **238**, 424

Factor VII inhibitors

Tissue factor VII inhibitors also inhibit factor Xa, and inhibition of factor VIIa/tissue factor activity is triggered by the factor Xa it generates. This could explain the need for factor IXa/VIIIa/ phospholipid activation to continue generation of factor Xa during haemostasis, another localizing control system in clotting.

References
Broze, G. J. Jr., Warren, L. A., Novotny, W. F. et al. (1987) *Blood* **71**, 335
Rao, L. V. M. and Rapoport, S. (1987) *Blood* **69**, 645

Factor VIII

Definitions

VIII/vWF	factor VIII/von Willebrand factor
VIIIC	factor VIII procoagulant activity as measured by clotting assay techniques
VIIICAg	factor VIII procoagulant activity as measured by immunological techniques using homologous antibodies to VIIIC
VIIIRAg	factor VIII-related antigen as measured by immunological techniques using heterologous antibodies to VIII/vWF. High-molecular-weight multimers are necessary for the sticking of platelets to the blood vessel wall, and to support ristocetin-induced aggregation of platelets
VIIIRRCo	ristocetin cofactor activity, the factor VIII-related activity required for the aggregation of human platelets by the antibiotic ristocetin
VIIIRWF	von Willebrand factor activity, bleeding time factor
vWF	von Willebrand factor: that part of the VIII/vWF protein which has VIIIRRCo, VIIIRWF, and VIIIRAg, but is devoid of VIIIC and VIIICAg

Factor VIII coagulant activity (VIIIC)

Neither the molecular weight nor the site of synthesis is known, although it is probably formed in the liver. The normal plasma activity is 100 u/dl (50–200), and 1 u is defined as that activity present in 1 ml of fresh normal plasma as standardized internationally. VIIIC is unstable on storage, and is rapidly lost from bank blood. It can be stored for long periods as fresh frozen plasma, or concentrated as (*a*) cryoprecipitate, or (*b*) factor VIII concentrate.

Following transfusion it has a biological half-life of 4–11 h. Factor VIIIC is activated by traces of thrombin and is consumed during clotting. It interacts with IXa and phospholipid during the activation of factor X to Xa.

Newborn infants have levels of factor VIIIC activity similar to those of adults.

Hereditary decrease of VIIIC

Haemophilia A [XR]

This sex-linked recessive bleeding diathesis is characterized by abnormal prolonged or repeated bleeding, with haemarthrosis, deep tissue bleeding and, less commonly, external blood loss. The severity of bleeding varies from affected family to family.

Using factor VIIIC assays, clinical grading includes:

- 'Symptomless haemophilia' – factor VIIIC 30–50% normal – 0.3–0.5 U/ml.
- Mild haemophilia – factor VIIIC 5–30% normal – 0.05–0.3 U/ml.
- Moderate haemophilia – factor VIIIC 2–5% normal – 0.02–0.05 U/ml.
- Severe haemophilia – factor VIIIC less than 1%–less than 0.01 U/ml.

Moderate and mild haemophilias (A) include:

- Cases with no factor VIIICAg.
- Cases with factor VIIICAg in amounts less than or equal to the corresponding plasma factor VIIIC levels.
- Cases with factor VIIICAg in amounts greater than the corresponding plasma factor VIIIC levels.

Plasma factor VIIIC activity probably forms a dissociable complex with macro-molecular factor VIIIRAg (which is normal in haemophilia A but abnormal in von Willebrand's disease).

Reference
Ljung, R., Holmberg, L. and Nilsson, I. M. (1981) *Acta Med. Scand.* **209**, 11

LABORATORY TESTS

The plasma APTT is abnormally prolonged and the prothrombin time (single stage) is normal. Factor VIIIC is abnormally reduced, and factor VIIICAg is variable. It is important to check that the APTT reagents are sensitive to factor VIII coagulant activity deficiency.

Reference
Barrowcliff, T. W. and Gray, E. (1981) *Thromb. Haemost.* **46**, 629

TREATMENT

Plasma factor VIIIC levels should be maintained above: 15–20% for minor spontaneous bleeding, 20–40% for severe haemarthroses, and for haemostasis in minor surgery, 80–100% for major surgery or trauma, using cryoprecipitate or factor VIII concentrate. Prothrombin concentrate (factors II, VII, IX and X) can be used for resistant haemophiliacs who have developed antibodies, but there is then a risk of thrombosis.

To reduce the requirement for cryoprecipitate or factor VIII concentrate in mild and moderate haemophiliacs due to undergo minor surgery or tooth extraction, tranexamic acid 1 g stat and 500 mg three times daily postoperatively plus DDAVP 32 g intravenously 12-hourly should be given in the absence of urinary tract haemorrhage or intracranial bleeding. The synthetic androgenic hormone danazol increases plasma factor VIII levels in classic haemophilia.

Reference
Boulton, F. E. and Smith, A. (1979) *Lancet* **ii**, 535

ARGININE VASOPRESSIN (DDAVP) IN FACTOR VIII DEFICIENCY

DDAVP stimulates release of factor VIIIAg into the circulation in normal subjects, but not in nephrogenic diabetes insipidus (?detecting X-linked carriers). It has been found useful in raising factor VIII levels in both mild haemophilia due to factor VIII deficiency, and in von Willebrand's disease. In von Willebrand's disease it may be useful in type I and some type IIa cases, is ineffective in type III disease, and is contra-indicated in type IIb disease as it causes thrombocytopenia. The bleeding time and APTT are reduced towards normal in von Willebrand's disease, with increases in plasma factors VIIIc, VIIIAg, vWF and platelet adhesion in types I and IIa.

References
Gralnick, H. R., Williams, S. B., McKeown, L. P. *et al.* (1986) *Blood* **67**, 465
Kobrinsky, N. L., Israels, E. D., Gerrard, J. M. *et al.* (1984) *Lancet* **i**, 1145
Kobrinsky, N. L., Doyle, J. J., Israels, E. D. *et al.* (1985) *Lancet* **i**, 1293
Mannucci, P. M. (1988) *Blood* **72**, 1449 (review)

COMPLICATIONS OF PROLONGED REPLACEMENT THERAPY IN HAEMOPHILIA

1. Antibodies against factor VIIIC (predominantly IgG): Antibodies develop in up to 10% of severely affected haemophiliacs, and treatment can then be modified:
   (a) overload infusion of factor VIII (short term);
   (b) plasmapheresis to remove antibody (short term);
   (c) ?immunosuppressive therapy;
   (d) (II, VII, IX, X) prothrombin concentrate, bypassing the deficiency of factor VIIIC. Some preparations are thrombotic.

References
Lederman, M. M., Ratnoff, O. D., Scithea, J. J. *et al.* (1983) *N. Engl. J. Med.* **308**, 79
Menilove, J. E., Aster, R. H., Casper, J. T. *et al.* (1983) *N. Engl. J. Med.* **308**, 83

2. Chronic active hepatitis.
3. Acquired immune deficiency disease (AIDS).

DETECTION OF CARRIERS

The only female carriers who can be reliably detected as symptomless carriers are (using comparison of VIIC/VIIIRAg):

- Daughter of a proven haemophiliac father.
- Mother with a haemophiliac son plus a previous family history of the disease.
- Mother with more than one haemophiliac son.

Reference
Peake, I. R., Newcombe, R. G., Davies, B. C. *et al.* (1981) *Br. J. Haematol.* **48**, 651

PRENATAL DIAGNOSIS

With amniocentesis at 14–15 weeks it is possible to detect a haemophiliac male fetus. Using DNA and conventional methods, the mothers must be heterozygous both for a disease gene and a marker gene. The final results are 'probabilistic', and multiple marker genes are often in linkage disequilibrium.

References
Graham, J. B., Green, P. P., McGraw, R. A. *et al.* (1985) *Blood* **66**, 759
Mibashan, R. S., Peake, I. R. Rodeck, C. H. *et al.* (1980) *Lancet* **ii**, 994

Acquired decrease of factor VIIIC

Disseminated intravascular coagulopathy. Factor VIIIC is consumed during clotting.

Antibodies against factor VIIIC rarely develop after childbirth temporarily, and also rarely in the course of some autoimmune diseases, but do not cause serious bleeding.

Factor VIIIC activity falls temporarily after dextran infusion, especially in von Willebrand's disease.

Increase in factor VIIIC

- Late pregnancy (200–500%) and also during treatment with contraceptive pill.
- Post-exertion.
- DDAVP (also catecholamines, insulin and hypoglycaemia).
- Postmenopausal women (?associated with increased risk of ischaemic heart disease).

Reference
Meade, T. W., Haines, A. P., Imeson, J. D. *et al.* (1982) *Lancet* **i**, 22

- Cushing's syndrome.
- Postoperation (in the absence of excessive bleeding).
- After acute myocardial infarction.

Reference
Cuciana, M. P., Missits, I., Olinic, N. *et al.* (1980) *Thromb. Haemost.* **43**, 41

- Atherosclerosis without occlusive accidents.
- Cirrhosis.

Reference
Baele, G., Matthius, E. and Barber, F. (1977) *Acta Haematol.* **57**, 290

- Postheparin therapy, and sudden cessation of warfarin therapy.

Reference
Denson, K. W. E. and Redman, C. W. G. (1977) *Lancet* ii, 1028

- Hyperthyroidism.
- Renal damage.
- Carcinomatosis.

Increase in factor VIIIRAg

- Nephritis.
- Myocardial infarction.
- Diabetic angiopathy.
- Primary necrotizing arteritis (Wegener's syndrome).
- Chronic relapsing polyarteritis nodosa.
- Some cases of scleroderma.

Reference
Editorial (1988) *Lancet* i, 1203

Von Willebrand factor

Megakaryocytes and the vascular endothelial cells synthesize von Willebrand factor (vWF). The endothelium also synthesizes tissue plasminogen activator (t-PA) and both are released following physical exercise, stress, venous occlusion, adrenaline and DDAVP injection. vWF is present in the α-granules and membranes of platelets, and is released in response to ADP, thrombin, collagen and ristocetin, to bind to specific sites on the activated platelet. It is responsible for platelet adhesion that is high shear rate dependent to the vascular subendothelium at sites of damage to the endothelium, with platelet adhesion to types I and III collagen fibrils. vWF also acts as a carrier protein for factor VIII procoagulant. The factor VIII/ vWF has a subunit molecular weight of 230 000, and exists as a series of disulphide-linked multimers of molecular weight $0.4–20 \times 10^6$.

Normal platelets are agglutinated by ristocetin in the presence of vWF. Bernard–Soulier platelets do not agglutinate, as they lack the glycoprotein with vWF binding sites.

References
Jeanneau, Ch., Bachouchi, N. O., Gorin, I. *et al.* (1987) *Br. J. Haematol.* **67**, 79
Ruggeri, Z. and Zimmerman, T. S. (1987) *Blood* **70**, 895

Deficiency

Acquired von Willebrand's disease

Twenty cases are described, including autoimmune disease, systemic lupus erythematosus, Felty's syndrome, lymphoreticulopathy, 'benign' monoclonal gammopathy, and Waldenström's macroglobulinaemia. Acquired type II deficiency, with lack of large factor vWF multimers, and discrepancy between factor vWF antigen measurement and functional assays, has been found in episodic haemolytic uraemic syndrome, disseminated intravascular coagulopathy and non-cyanotic heart disease.

References
Gill, C., Wilson A. D., Endres-Brook, J. *et al.* (1986) *Blood* **67**, 758
Mazurier, C., Parquet-Gernier, A., Descamps, J. *et al.* (1980) *Thrombos. Haemostas.* **44**, 115

Congenital von Willebrand's disease

Clinical manifestations

The condition affects both sexes. Minor injuries lead to abnormal bleeding. Spontaneous bleeding occurs from the gums, nose and gastrointestinal tract. Deep tissue haematomas are rare, and haemarthroses do not occur. Menorrhagia and postpartum haemorrhage occurs in affected females.

Laboratory findings

The bleeding time is frequently increased above normal, but plasma factor vWFAg and its activity do not correlate with the bleeding time in mild von Willebrand's disease, although there is excellent correlation between the bleeding time, and platelet factor vWF activity and factor vWFAg. Obviously, platelet factor vWF plays a very important part in the early stages of haemostasis. The capillary fragility test is often abnormal. Platelet adhesiveness, measured by a Salzman glass bead column, is abnormal in most cases. Ristocetin-induced aggregation of platelets is reduced or absent (compare haemophilia A). Transfusion with fresh frozen plasma or cryoprecipitate is followed by high levels of factor VIIIC in the plasma, rising to a peak at 24 h and falling by 36 h. This pattern of temporary induction of factor VIIIC synthesis and release characterizes von Willebrand's disease from haemophilia A. Various types and subtypes of von Willebrand's disease have been defined.

TYPE I [AD] Quantitative deficiency of all factor vWF multimers, with reduction in factors VIIIC, VIIIvWF and VIIIRCo (ristocetin cofactor activity).

TYPE II Types IIA [AD], IIB [AD], IIC [AR], IID, IIE, IIF and 'platelet type' von Willebrand disease, are characterized by distinct structural and functional abnormalities of factor vWF in the plasma and platelets, properties of factor vWF in functional tests and in the mode of inheritance.

Types IIA, IIC and IID lack high- and medium-molecular-weight multimers, with altered 'triplet' structure to the multimer bands. Type IIA – large vWF multimers are absent from the plasma, and also from the platelets in some cases. Ristocetin-induced platelet aggregation is markedly decreased or absent (compare type IIB).

Type IIB – high-molecular-weight multimers lacking with normal banding. The platelets show a heightened response to ristocetin, and there is age-dependent thrombocytopenia.

TYPE III [AR] [R] A rare and most severe form, with marked reduction of synthesis and/or rapid catabolism of vWF.

'PLATELET TYPE' OF VON WILLEBRAND'S DISEASE There is mild to moderate thrombocytopenia with enhanced ristocetin-induced platelet aggregation. Washed platelets show increased binding of normal factor vWF in the presence of ristocetin. Cryoprecipitate enhances the patient's platelet aggregation.

References

Gralnick, H. R., Rick, M. E., McKeown, L. P. *et al.* (1986) *Blood* **68**, 58
Holmberg, L., Nilsson, I. M., Borge, L. *et al.* (1983) *N. Engl. J. Med.* **309**, 816
Mazurier, C., Parquet-Gernez, A., Goudemand, J. *et al.* (1988) *Br. J. Haematol.* **69**, 499
Ruggeri, Z. and Zimmerman, T. S. (1987) *Blood* **70**, 895
Weiss, H. J., Meyer, D., Rabinowitz, R. *et al.* (1982) *N. Engl. J. Med.* **306**, 326
Zimmerman, T. S. and Ruggeri, Z. M. (1983) *Clin. Haematol.* **12**, 175

Treatment

Cryoprecipitate or factor VIII concentrate is given 12–24 h before a planned operation. Factor VIII concentrate or cryoprecipitate is given immediately to cover emergency surgery, recent trauma or spontaneous bleeding. In mild cases, tranexamic acid plus DDAVP may also be given to reduce the volume of concentrate needed to control haematemesis.

Reference

Aledort, L. M. (1991) *Mayo Clin. Proc.* **66**, 841

Inhibitors

Precipitating antibodies may develop against factors VIIIvW and VIIIRAg. Inhibitors against factors VIIIRCo and VIIIRAg may develop in:

- Von Willebrand's disease in severely affected cases after repeated transfusions.
- Systemic lupus erythematosus.
- Paraproteinaemia.
- Lymphadenoma.
- Diabetes mellitus.
- Occasionally in some otherwise normal individuals.

Reference

Mannucci, P. M., Meyer, D., Ruggeri, Z. M. *et al.* (1976) *Nature* **262**, 141

Factor IX

Factor IX, the zymogen of a serine protease, is a single-chain glycoprotein with a molecular weight of 54 000, which is synthesized in the liver. Vitamin K-dependent γ-carboxyglutamyl residues are essential for its activity. Adsorbable on gels, it is stable for 30 min at 56°C, and is stable for a few days in fresh bank blood, for many months in fresh frozen plasma and can be prepared as a stable concentrate. Its biological half-life is 20 h. Factor IX is activated by factor XIa in two stages to activated factor IX, two polypeptide chains linked by disulphide bonds. It can also be activated by factor VII–tissue factor complex, and to a moderately active form by Russell viper venom. After activation, in the presence of calcium ions, phospholipid and factor VIII/VIIIa, it cleaves factor X to activate it.

Decrease

Physiological

Newborn full-term infants – 28%. Lower levels in pre-term babies.

Pathological

Acquired

- Severe vitamin K deficiency, or blocking of vitamin K action by oral anticoagulants (warfarin, coumarins).
- Liver disease.
- Very rarely reported in nephrosis, congestive cardiac disease, untreated hypothyroidism. In vitro activity is reduced in Gaucher's disease without a bleeding diathesis.

Reference

Boklan, B. F. and Sawitsky, A. (1976) *Arch. Intern. Med.* **136**, 489

Congenital

This takes the form of inherited factor IX deficiency (haemophilia B, Christmas disease) [XR]. It affects 1 in every 20 000 male births in the USA and is about 10 times less frequent than haemophilia A (factor VIII deficiency) in the UK, with variations in severity from family to family. Cases present as clinical haemophilia, although some cases are only mildly affected and remain symptom free until subjected to trauma. Four different types have been described.

1. B⁻ with absence of measurable IX antigen: 70% of cases.
2. B⁺ with reduced IX coagulant activity and normal IX antigen – the third most common.

3. B^R with reduced IXC and reduced IXAg – the second most common.
4. B^M and intermediate subtype B^+ with normal factor IXAg but prolonged prothrombin time using ox thromboplastin – the rarest type, discovered in Norway.

The abnormalities found in the factor IX molecule include defective proteolytic activation, defective calcium binding and defective serine protease activity.

References
Bloom, A. L. (Ed.) (1981) *Haemostasis and Thrombosis*, pp 335–338. London: Churchill-Livingstone
Thompson, A. R. (1986) *Blood* **67**, 565 (review of structure, function and molecular defects)

The plasma activated partial thromboplastin time is abnormally prolonged, and is corrected by alumina eluate and not by alumina-absorbed plasma (compare factor VIII). Factor IX levels are low. The platelet count and function, and prothrombin time are normal. Heterozygote carriers can be detected.

References
Gianelli, F., Anson, D. S., Choo, K. H. *et al.* (1984) *Lancet* **i**, 239
Peake, I. R., Furlong, B. L. and Bloom, A. L. (1984) *Lancet* **i**, 242

Treatment of haemorrhages or preparation for surgery requires fresh frozen plasma transfusion or factor IX concentrate.

Reference
Bloom, A. L. (Ed.) (1981) *Haemostasis and Thrombosis*, p. 372. London: Churchill-Livingstone

Antibodies against factor IX

One per cent of factor IX deficiency patients in the UK (up to 3% elsewhere) develop antibodies following transfusion. Similar antibodies may rarely develop during a normal pregnancy, or in some connective tissue diseases.

Reference
Reece, E. A., Clyne, L. P., Romero, R. *et al.* (1984) *Arch. Intern. Med.* **144**, 525

Factor X

Plasma factor X has a molecular weight of 56 000, and consists of a light chain (mol. wt = 16 500) joined to a heavy chain (mol. wt + 39 000), the heavy chain being homologous to prethrombin 2, the light chain being very similar to the Gla domain of prothrombin fragment 1.

Factor X has the electrophoretic mobility of an α_1-globulin, is adsorbed by gels and is heat labile (destroyed in 30 min at 56°C – compare factor VII).

Biological half-life = 1–3 days. It is not destroyed during clotting. During activation of factor X to factor Xa, cleavage occurs in the heavy chain, releasing a 51-residue peptide from the active enzyme. The amino acid sequence in factor Xa is similar to that of trypsin and pepsin.

Factor X is activated by factor VIIa plus tissue factor in the presence of calcium ions. Minimal generation of factor Xa activates more factor VII to factor VIIa, so that the rate of activation of factors IX and X increases dramaticallly. It is probably at this stage that low-dose heparin is most effective. Activation of factor X also occurs by the action of platelet phospholipid, factors IXa, VIII/VIIIa and calcium ions, or by direct platelet action. Both trypsin and Russell viper venom can activate factor X to factor Xa.

References
de Gaetano, G. (1981) *Clin. Haematol.* **10**, 297
Semeraro, N. and Vermylen, J. (1977) *Br. J. Haematol.* **36**, 107

Factor Xa activity

- 'Prothrombinase' complex of factors Xa, V/Va, calcium ions and phospholipid residues on platelet membrane cleaves two peptide bonds in the prothrombin molecule to generate thrombin. This activity develops rapidly to 100% activity in 30 s, being rapidly destroyed (15% activity after 10 min). Factor Xa binds to platelet membrane binding sites via factor Va attached to the platelet membrane surface. When bound, both factor Xa is protected from the inhibitory action of AT-III (with heparin as cofactor), and factor Va is protected from the inhibitory action of protein C. Using specific inhibitor of thrombin (dansyl-arginine-methyl-piperidine amide) it has been shown that factor Va at the platelet surface binding factor Xa ensures massive localization of thrombin generation and subsequent fibrin formation at the site of vascular injury.

References
Giles, A. R., Nesheim, M. E., Hoogendoorn, H. *et al.* (1982) *Br. J. Haematol.* **51**, 457
Walsh, P. N. (1978) *Br. J. Haematol.* **40**, 311

- Factors Xa, Va, calcium ions and platelet factor 3 activate prothrombin to thrombin much more slowly.
- In the presence of phospholipid and calcium ions factor Xa rapidly activates VII to VIIa. This may partly explain the very short biological half-life of factor VII in the circulation, if traces of factor Xa are repeatedly generated.

Reference
Masys, D. R., Bajaj, S. P. and Rapaport, S. I. (1982) *Blood* **60**, 1143

- Factor Xa plus phospholipid and calcium ions convert factor IX to inactive IX_α in humans (i.e. it does not activate factor IX).

Inactivation of factor Xa

Factor Xa combines irreversibly with AT-III and is inactivated, with heparin acting as cofactor. Low-dose heparin therapy during the peroperative period in surgery, results in significantly increased plasma anti-factor Xa activity.

Reference
Lowe, G., Belch, J. K. *et al.* (1982) *Thromb, Haemost.* **47**, 296

Congenital deficiency [R] [?AR]

The homozygote with this rare bleeding diathesis suffers from bleeding from the mucous membranes, bleeding after surgery, trauma and tooth extraction, and may develop haemarthroses. Heterozygotes are usually symptom free, but may have a mild bleeding tendency. Various varieties have been described.

Type Stuart

Severely decreased synthesis of a normal factor X molecule, with reduced factors XC and XAg.

Type Prower

Normal factor XAg levels with reduced coagulant activity, due to impaired ability of the abnormal molecule to be activated.

Variants

Selective defects in response to one or more activators (intrinsic, extrinsic, Russell viper venom and animal tissue thromboplastin). In factor X deficiency the APTT and prothrombin times are prolonged, and factor X assays reveal low levels. Treatment of the homozygote during a bleeding episode is with fresh frozen plasma or prothrombin concentrate.

References
de Stefano, V., Leone, G., Ferrelli, R. *et al.* (1988) *Br. J. Haematol.* **69**, 387
Girolami, A., Cosen, P., Brunetti, A. *et al.* (1975) *Acta Haematol.* **53**, 118

Acquired deficiency

Physiological

Pre-term and newborn infants – the plasma factor X concentration depends on the gestational age.

Pathological

- Warfarin therapy: depression of active factor II, VII, IX and X, with the formation of inert factors without calcium binding sites. Factor X activity falls after about 4 days of oral anticoagulant therapy.

- Vitamin K deficiency.
- Kwashiorkor.
- Liver disease (some cases).
- Amyloidosis: although 41% of 101 cases with amyloidosis bled, no isolated factor X deficiency was found. It was thought that bleeding was probably due to amyloid infiltration of blood vessels.

Reference
Yood, R. A., Skinner, M., Rubinow, A. *et al.* (1983) *JAMA* **249**, 1322

Further investigation has revealed that factor X deficiency does not occur in secondary amyloidosis, but may occur in primary amyloidosis (with AL amyloid).

Reference
Cohen, D., Pras, M., Franklin, E. C. *et al.* (1983) *Am. J. Med.* **74**, 513

Increased factor X

- During normal pregnancy.
- During treatment with oral contraceptives.

Factor XI

Factor XI is a glycoprotein with a molecular weight of 160 000. It consists of two identical disulphide-linked chains, each with a molecular weight of 80 000, and has an eletrophoretic mobility of a γ-globulin. Platelet factor XI has a molecular weight of 52 000, and occurs as a tetramer. It is stable on storage, not adsorbed by gels or removed by filtration, and is stable at 56°C for 30 min. Following transfusion, it has a circulation half-life of about 60 min. The normal plasma range = 65–140%. Factor XI is activated by limited proteolysis by factor XIIa. In turn, factor XIa activates factor IX to IXa, by cleaving two internal peptide bonds. Factor XIa can also activate factor XII and plasminogen. High-molecular-weight kininogen reversibly associates with prekallikrein and factor XI.

Factor XIa is inhibited by $C\bar{I}$ inhibitor, and also by antithrombin III (with heparin acting as cofactor).

Activation of factor XI by platelets requires the presence of collagen. Platelet membrane factor XI can substitute for plasma factor XI in coagulation. Damaged endothelial cells release an enzyme which cleaves and activates factor XII, which as factor XIIa, activates factor XI (to XIa) and prekallikrein (to kallikrein).

References
Mannhalter, C. and Schiffman, S. (1980) *Thromb. Haemost.* **43**, 124
Walsh, P. N., Sinha, D., Koshy, A. *et al.* (1986) *Blood* **68**, 225

Decrease

- Pre-term infants – plasma factor XI concentration about 20%.

- Normal term infants – plasma factor XI concentration about 30%.
- Adult levels of factor XI are not reached until about 6 months.
- Normal pregnancy – plasma factor XI levels fall to 60–70% at term.

Pathological decrease

Congenital deficiency

Inherited as an autosomal trait, there is poor correlation between plasma factor XI levels and a tendency to bleed, and the nature of the bleeding tendency is unpredictable. The most common manifestations include excessive bruising, menorrhagia, epistaxis and postoperative and postdental extraction bleeding. Haemarthoses and intramuscular bleeds are rare. In most cases there is depression both of factor XI antigen and clotting activity, rarely the factor XI antigen level is normal but clotting activity is severely reduced (a defective molecule).

The APTT is prolonged, whilst the bleeding time and prothrombin time are normal. Surgery is safe if plasma factor XI activity is 30–40% of normal or more. Homozygotes are severely affected, whilst many heterozygotes have levels of plasma factor XI activity high enough for safe surgery.

References
Bolton-Maggs, P. H. B., Wan-Yin, B. Y., McGraw, A. H. *et al.* (1988) *Br. J. Haematol.* **69**, 521
Mannhalter, C., Hellstern, R. and Deutsch, E. (1987) *Blood* **70**, 31

Acquired deficiency

- Liver disease.
- Disseminated intravascular coagulopathy.

Inhibitors of factor XI

- Congenital factor XI deficiency following multiple transfusions.
- Some patients not congenitally deficient in factor XI, including some patients with lupus erythematosus.
- One case of factor XI deficiency, never transfused, suffering from carcinoma.

Reference
Chediak, J., Madej-Zevin, P., Ratnoff, O. D. *et al.* (1986) *Br. J. Haematol.* **63**, 123

Factor XII

Factor XII, a single chain glycoprotein with a molecular weight of 80 000, is a serine protease zymogen, with a plasma concentration of 40 μg/ml. It has an electrophoretic mobility of a β-globulin, and is probably synthesized in the liver.

Activation

Activation occurs following damage to vascular endothelium (anoxia, acidosis, antigen/antibody deposition, heat damage), and activation in vitro is caused by glass, kaolin or ellagic acid. Surface binding enhances activation by kallikrein.

α-Factor XIIa has a molecular weight of 52 000, and β-factor XIIa has a molecular weight 28 000. The heavy and light chains are linked by disulphide bonds. α-Factor XIIa binds to negatively charged surfaces. β-Factor XIIa activates prekallikrein to kallikrein. α-Factor XIIa activates both prekallikrein and factor XI.

Actions of activated XIIa

- Converts prekallikrein to kallikrein, which in turn converts more factor XII to factor XIIa.
- Activates factor XI to factor XIa.
- Factor XIIa fragments activate factor VII to VIIa.
- Factor XIIa and fragments activate plasminogen to plasmin.
- Activates the complement system.
- Generation of permeability enhancing agents depend on factor XIIa.
- Induces chemotactic activity in neutrophils.
- Factor XIIa cross-links with fibrin, α_2-plasmin inhibitor, fibronectin and vWF, forming a link between fibrin clot and the subendothelium.

Reference
Hada, M., Kaminski, M. and Bockenstedt, P. *et al.* (1986) *Blood* **68**, 95

Physiological deficiency

- Newborn infants have moderately lower levels than in adults.
- Factor XII levels fall moderately in pregnancy.

Pathological deficiency

Congenital [AR] [R]

Homozygotes have a thrombotic tendency. Most cases have markedly reduced factor XII antigen and factor XII coagulant activity, rare cases have normal factor XII antigen levels. The activated partial thromboplastin time is abnormally prolonged and the prothrombin time is normal, with normal factor VIII and IX levels. Platelet counts and function tests are normal. Kaolin-induced euglobulin clot lysis is slower in Hageman trait plasma.

Reference
Saito, H., Scott, J. G., Movart, H. Z. *et al.* (1979) *J. Lab. Clin. Med.* **94**, 56 (49 cases reported)

Acquired

- Nephrosis.

- Disseminated intravascular coagulopathy, with conversion of factor XII to factor XIIa, and subsequent elimination.
- Factor XII is reduced in cirrhosis, but not in chronic active hepatitis.
- Following hypophysectomy.

Reference
Cordova, C., Violi, F., Alessandri, C. *et al.* (1986) *J. Clin. Pathol.* **39**, 1003

Inhibitors

Activation of factor XII occurs in angioneurotic oedema (inherited); inhibition of factor XIIa by AT-III is accelerated by heparin. α_2-Antiplasmin inhibits clot promotion and prekallikrein activating activity of factor XII fragments.

Increase

- After intravenous DDAVP factor XII is increased (also factors VIIIRAg and VIIIC).
- Marked increase in factor XII with oral contraception, due to oestrogen action.

References
Gordon, E. M., Douglas, J. G., Ratnoff, O. D. *et al.* (1985) *Blood* **66**, 602
Nenci, G. G., Berrettini, M., de Cunto, M. *et al.* (1983) *Br. J. Haematol.* **54**, 489

Antibodies against factor XII are rare, and are associated with a bleeding tendency.

Factor XIII

Plasma factor XIII is an inactive transglutaminase (fibrinoligase) until it is activated. It consists of two A subunits joined as a dimer, connected to two B subunits (A_2B_2). Each A subunit has a molecular weight of 75 000, and each B subunit has a molecular weight of 80 000, making an aggregate molecular weight of the whole molecule of 320 000.

The normal plasma concentration is about 20 μg/ml, and the inactive factor XIII has a biological half-life of 6–10 days (the activated form has a half-life in the circulation of about 1 h).

Platelet factor XIII consists of only A subunits, and is synthesized in the megakaryocytes. It accounts for about 50% of the total blood factor XIII activity, and there is a linear relationship between factor XIII level and platelet counts.

References
Adang, R., Kiss, A and Muszbek, L. (1987) *Br. J. Haematol.* **67**, 167
Rider, D M., McDonagh, R. P. and McDonagh, J. (1978) *Br. J. Haematol.* **39**, 579

When activated by thrombin to factor XIIIa in the presence of calcium ions, a two-stage reaction occurs

soon after thrombin has catalysed release of fibrinopeptide A from fibrinogen. Fibrin polymers accelerate thrombin-catalysed plasma factor XIIIa formation.

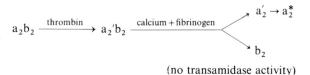

(no transamidase activity)

$a_2' =$ intermediate form, $a_2^* =$ active XIIIa.

Factor XIIIa cross-links fibrin to fibrin to form insoluble polymerized fibrin, fibronectin to fibrin, fibronectin to collagen, plasma factor vWF to fibrin during gel formation, and cross-links to α_2-plasmin inhibitor. The binding of factor XIII to fibrin and fibrinogen may serve to regulate factor XIIIa formation, and may prevent free factor XIIIa circulating in the plasma. Factor XIII is released 24 h later from formed clot. Clot deficient in factor XIII does not support growth of fibroblasts as well as normal fibrin clot does.

References
Board, P. G., Coggan, M. and Hamer, J. W. (1980) *Br. J. Haematol.* **45**, 633
Hada, M., Kaminski, M., Bockenstedt, P. and McDonagh, J. (1986) *Blood* **68**, 95
Lorand L., Losowsky, M. S. and Miloszewski, K. J. M. (1980) In: Spaet, T. K. (Ed.) *Progress in Haemostasis and Thrombosis*, Vol. 5. p. 245. New York, Grune & Stratton

Deficiency

Congenital deficiency [R] [?AR ?some XR]

Over 100 cases of this uncommon bleeding diathesis have been described. Prolonged bleeding, with onset a few hours after trauma, occurs after injury, and includes bleeding from the umbilical stump and perinatal intracranial haemorrhage. There is delayed wound healing with excessive keloid formation. Superficial bruising, haematomas and bleeding from the mucous membranes in the mouth and the gastrointestinal tract occur. Haemarthrosis has been described. Habitual abortion may occur in females.

LABORATORY TESTS The fibrin clot is abnormally soluble in 5 mol/l urea solution or in 1% monochloracetic acid. Tests for deficiency of other plasma clotting factors or platelet function abnormality, are normal.

Two forms are found: (1) the 'a' chain is absent from the molecule, and (2) the factor XIII is present as an abnormal ineffective variant.

TREATMENT Treatment is transfusion of stored blood, dried plasma, processed plasma or cryoprecipitate. Paradoxically the most severe cases are treated because severe bleeding develops soon after injury or surgery, whereas mild cases may develop severe post-surgery keloid formation, as they suffer from slow oozing of blood persisting over periods of possibly weeks, before the condition is considered.

Acquired deficiency

- Liver disease – acute hepatitis; cirrhosis; secondary liver malignancy ('a' chains are synthesized in the liver).
- Thrombocytopenia – factor XIII activity is below normal, because of loss of 'a' chains normally carried by platelets.
- Disseminated intravascular coagulopathy: factor XIII is consumed.
- Postmyocardial infarction.
- Glomerulitis.

Reference
Alkjaersig, N., Fletcher, A. P., Lewis, M. *et al.* (1977) *Thromb. Haemost.* **38**, 863

- Leukaemia, some cases, especially in promyelocytic leukaemia.
- Dermatological disease with vasculitis.
- Burns.
- Surgical procedures with extracorporeal circulation.
- Schönlein–Henoch purpura: levels of less than 50% associated with complications.

Reference
Dalens, B., Travade, P., Libbé, A. *et al.* (1983) *Arch. Dis. Child.* **58**, 12

- Inhibition by myeloma paraprotein of factor XIII activity may occur in some cases of myeloma.

Reference
Klingemann, H.-G., Egbring, R. and Havemann, K. (1981) *Scand. J. Haematol.* **27**, 253

- Sickle-cell disease crisis.
- Pre-term infant. (Severe bleeding due to acquired factor XIII deficiency must be very rare.)
- Inhibitors of factor XIII activity: (1) one case of factor XIII deficiency treated with repeated transfusions; (2) isoniazid therapy. Drug-induced SLE [R]. The inhibitor is an IgG acting against factors XIII and XIIIa.

Increase in factor XIII

Increase in plasma factor XIII has been described in both type IV hyperlipoproteinaemia and in combined hyperlipidaemia.

Reference
Cucianu, M. P., Miloszewski, K., Porotin, D. *et al.* (1976) *Thromb. Haemost.* **36**, 542

Prekallikrein

The single-chain glycoprotein, with a molecular weight of 88 000, exists in the inactive prekallikrein form in plasma, pancreas and intestine, and in the active, kallikrein, double-chain form in salivary glands and kidneys. Prekallikrein combined with factor XI and high-molecular-weight kininogen (HMWK) activates factor XII to XIIa, and factor XIIa in turn activates prekallikrein to kallikrein, and also activates factor XI to XIa, before factor XIa activates factor IX to IXa. It also liberates kinins from low-molecular-weight kininogen (LMWK) and HMWK. The heavy chain of kallikrein assists in the aggregation of neutrophils and the release of elastase.

Reference
Colman, R. W., Wachtfogel, Y. T., Kucich, U. *et al.* (1985) *Blood* **65**, 311

Decrease

Physiological

Low levels in newborn and pre-term infants.

Pathological

Acquired

Reduced in liver disease, nephrosis and dengue.

Reference
Fisher, C. A., Schmaier, A. H., Addonizo, V. P. *et al.* (1982) *Blood* **59**, 963

Congenital [AR] [R]

Fewer than 10 cases have been reported. The APTT is longer than normal, and is shortened by prolonged incubation with kaolin, or by ellagic acid which activates factor XII without requiring kallikrein. It is not associated with a bleeding tendency.

Passevoy factor deficiency [R] [AD]

Twelve members of five kindreds have been described, who suffered from easy bruising and excessive bleeding after minor trauma. The deficient factor is removed from plasma by aluminium hydroxide, and is neither Fletcher factor nor Fitzgerald, Flaujeac factor.

The patients' APTT is prolonged, which is corrected by plasma, or plasma absorbed with celite. The prothrombin time, thrombin time and platelet functions are all normal. Plasma levels of factor VIII, IX, XI, XII prekallikrein and HMWK are all normal

References
Hougie, C., McPherson, R. A. and Aronson, L. (1975) *Lancet* **ii**, 290
Hougie, C., McPherson, R. A., Brown, J. E. *et al.* (1978) *N. Engl. J. Med.* **298**, 1045

Kininogen (HMWK and LMWK)

Kininogen exists as a high-molecular-weight form (HMWK) with a molecular weight 110 000–120 000, and a low-molecular-weight form (LMWK) with a molecular weight of 50 000–60 000. HMWK transports and optimally positions prekallikrein and factor XI on a negatively charged surface (platelet membrane), allowing them to be activated by surface-bound factor XIIa. HMWK circulates in the plasma as a pro-cofactor, to be cleaved by kallikrein or factor XIIa. It has then developed the ability to bind to a negatively charged surface, and to activate factor XII, prekallikrein and factor XI. Activated platelets express HMWK on the external platelet membrane, and platelet enzymes cleave and increase the coagulant activity of exogenous HMWK.

Bradykinin is liberated from HMWK and LMWK by the action of kallikrein. It is a peptide concerned with vasodilatation, increased vascular permeability and pain generation.

Deficiency

Physiological

The low levels of HMWK and LMWK in the plasma of newborn and pre-term infants explain the prolonged APTT found in the newborn.

Pathological

In congenital kininogen deficiency, of the named affected families, Fitzgerald and Reid lack HMWK, whilst Williams and Flaujeac lack both HMWK and LMWK. The condition is asymptomatic, with both decreased fibrinolytic activity and kinin formation.

Reference
Schmaier, A. H., Smith, P. M., Purdon, A. D. *et al.* (1986) *Blood* **67**, 119

The coagulation–kinin pathway

Patients deficient in factor XII, prekallikrein or HMW kininogen, detected by prolonged APTT, do not bleed.

Reference
Kaplan, A. P. and Silverberg, M. (1987) *Blood* **70**, 1 (review).

Histidine-rich glycoprotein (HRGP)

HRGP is a procoagulant plasma protein, interacting with fibrinogen and fibrin, reducing the binding of plasminogen to fibrin, binding heparin and neutralizing its activities and inhibiting heparin cofactor II. It forms complexes with platelet thrombospondin, controlling the degree of fibrinolysis in the region of a platelet plug. Plasma levels of HRGP are increased following myocardial infarction and deep vein thrombosis. The normal plasma concentration is about 125 μg/ml, and 1% of the total circulating HGRP is platelet associated. When platelets are stimulated, HRGP is expressed on their surfaces.

Abnormally high plasma levels of HRGP, a condition of dominant inheritance, is associated with a thrombotic tendency, as there is inhibition of fibrinolysis as well as reduction in the inhibition of the spread of coagulation from a local microsite.

References
Engesser, L., Kluft, C., Briet, E. and Brommer, E. S. P. (1987) *Br. J. Haematol.* **67**, 355
Lerch, P. G., Nydegger, U. E., Kuyas, C. and Haeberli, A. (1988) *Br. J. Haematol.* **70**, 219

Clotting factors in the newborn

For normal values of coagulation factors in infants from birth to six months see Andrew *et al.* (1987).

Reference
Andrew, M., Paes, B., Milner, R. *et al.* (1987) *Blood* **70**, 165

Clotting factors in various species

- Clot retraction is poor in fowls.
- Low prothrombin and factor VII concentrations occur in opossum, chicken, duck, sheep and cow.
- The levels of factor V are greatly increased in other mammals when compared with humans. Lower levels of factor V are found in fowls.
- Higher levels of factor VIII (AHG) are present in cows and sheep than in humans, whilst in dogs the level is 300–400% of normal adult human levels.
- The adult guinea-pig has reduced levels of factor VII, II and X, when compared with adult humans.
- Factor IX (Christmas factor) is present in the same concentration in all mammals. No factor IX is present in fowls' blood.
- Factor X (Stuart–Prower factor) is present in very low levels (1–5% of adults human levels) in newborn and adult cats.
- Hageman factor is present in all mammals, but is absent from the blood of chickens and duck; the level is low in horses.
- Thromboplastin generation is negligible in the chicken and the duck (not unexpectedly, since factor XII is absent and factor XI is present in reduced amounts).
- Thromboplastin from the various species exhibits species specificity.

- The plasma clotting factors are present in amounts similar to the levels found in the newborn human and in the newborn dog.
- Interaction of the various coagulation factors present produces a normal haemostatic mechanism in each species.

References

Didisheim, P., Hatori, K. and Lewis, J. (1959) *J. Lab Clin. Med.* **53**, 866

Hathaway, W. E., Hathaway, H. S. and Belhasen, L. P. (1964) *J. Lab. Clin. Med.* **64**, 784

Kerr, C. B. (1965) *J. Med. Genet.* **2**, 254 (reviews clotting in invertebrates, fishes, birds, reptiles and mammals)

Kisker, C. T. (1987) *Thromb. Haemost.* **57**, 118 (compares humans, rabbit, dog and sheep coagulation factor activities)

Natural Anticoagulants

- Inactivation of the early stages of plasma clotting.
- α_1-Antitrypsin.
- CI inactivator.
- α_2-Macroglobulin.
- Protein C.
- Protein S.
- Thrombomodulin.
- Antithrombin III.
- Heparin cofactor II.
- β_2-Glycoprotein I.

Inactivation of the early stages of plasma clotting

β_2-Glycoprotein 1 in plasma inhibits contact activation of the intrinsic blood coagulation pathway. Plasma kallikrein is inhibited by CI inactivator, α_2-macroglobulin and AT-III. Factor XIIa is inhibited by CI inactivator (with minimum activity by AT-III and α_2-antiplasmin inhibitor). Plasma factor XIa is inhibited by CI inactivator (and to a much lesser extent by α_1-antitrypsin, AT-III and α_2-antiplasmin inhibitor).

Reference

Schousboe, I. (1985) *Blood* **66**, 1086

α_1-Antitrypsin

α_1-Antitrypsin has a molecular weight of 54 000. It is less effective than antithrombin III or α_2-macroglobulin, with no antithrombin activity under physiological conditions. Patients with deficiency state have no thrombotic tendency, but tend to suffer from pulmonary emphysema and liver damage.

Plasma concentration 290 ± 45 mg/100ml. Acts against plasmin and elastase and factor XIa.

An abnormal antitrypsin associated with a life-long bleeding diathesis has been described.

Reference

Owen, M. C., Brennan, S. O., Lewis, J. H. *et al.* (1983) *N. Engl. J. Med.* **309**, 694

CI inactivator

The molecular weight of this glycoprotein is 104 000. Inhibits factor XIIa and XIa and kallikrein. Deficiency state is associated with angioneurotic oedema, but no hypercoagulability.

α_2-Macroglobulin

α_2-Macroglobulin is synthesized by the liver and ? by lymphocytes. It is a glycoprotein with a molecular weight of 725 000, and 8% is carbohydrate. It consists of two half-molecules, each composed of two polypeptide chains with a molecular weight of 85 000.

α_2-Globulin complexes with trypsin, plasmin and thrombin, and 25% of the total thrombin inhibiting activity of the plasma is due to this substance. Heparin prevents binding between α_2-macroglobulin and thrombin. Plasma levels are maximal by 1–3 years, falling to adults levels (2g/l) by 25 years. It is thought that its main function is to protect against endopeptidases. It has limited action against thrombin (but not against factors Xa or XIIa), against kallikrein, and against plasmin and plasminogen activator. Familial α_2-macroglobulin deficiency is asymptomatic.

Increase

- Nephrosis.
- Cirrhosis.

Decrease

- Familial deficiency.
- During streptokinase therapy.

Reference

Berquist, D. and Nilsson, I. M. (1979) *Thromb. Haemost.* **42**, 219

Protein C

Protein C, a vitamin-K-dependent glycoprotein, consists of two disulphide-linked polypeptide chains, and has a molecular weight of 62 000. It is synthesized in the liver, and has 10 calcium-binding γ-carboxyglutamyl residues per molecule. The zymogen of this serine protease is activated by thrombin, traces of α-thrombin, trypsin and the factor X activator of Russell viper venom. Thromboglobulin from the vascular endothelial cells binds thrombin and, in addition to reducing its ability to catalyse clot formation, converts thrombin into a potent protein C activator, increasing protein C activity 1000-fold. Activated protein C (APC) inactivates the platelet-dependent activation of prothrombin by factor Xa, inactivating platelet-bound factor Va by destroying factor Xa binding sites. It also inactivates factor VIIIa, which is essential for factor IXa activity. Phospholipid membrane surface and free calcium ions are essential for APC activity. This high affinity membrane interaction also requires the presence of protein S. Thrombomodulin with calcium ions inhibits cleavage of protein S by thrombin. In addition, APC neutralizes plasminogen activator inhibitor (PAI) and therefore also enhances fibrinolysis. In vitro, APC accelerates whole blood clot lysis, and is probably one factor in the prolongation of the APTT of over-incubated activated plasma. APC is slowly inactivated by a plasma protease inhibitor.

References
de Fouw, N. J.,van Hinsbergh, V. M. W., de Jong, Y. F. *et al.* (1987) *Thromb. Haemost.* **57**, 176
Sakata, Y., Loskutoff, D. J. and Gladson, C. L. *et al.* (1986) *Blood* **68**, 1218
Suzuki, K. (1984) *Semin. Thromb. Hemost.* **10**, 154

Physiological decrease

● Third trimester of pregnancy.
● Newborn infant: levels correlate with gestational age, and are related to the rate of synthesis of protein C in the liver, and not to the rate of γ-carboxylation. There is a slow increase after birth.

Pathological deficiency

Congenital

Inherited protein C deficiency [AR]

Two types are found:

1. Defective production of normal protein C, with a normal ratio between biological activity and antigen estimation.
2. Normal antigen levels but reduced biological activity, i.e. abnormal molecular structure.

Clinical presentation

HOMOZYGOTE

Rare, with thromboembolism occurring soon after birth and death early in childhood.

Reference
Seligsohn, U., Berger, A., Abend, M. *et al.* (1984) *N. Engl. J. Med.* **310**, 559

HETEROZYGOTE

Increased incidence of venous thrombosis, including intracranial venous thrombosis, and thromboembolism, often beginning in early adult life and requiring lifetime treatment with warfarin. Only a few cases of arterial thrombosis due to protein C deficiency have been described. Whilst purpura fulminans associated with protein C deficiency in a newborn infant responded to coumarin therapy, coumarin skin necrosis associated with hereditary protein C deficiency has been successfully treated with vitamin K and heparin.

Reference
Horellou, M. H., Conard, J., Bertina, R. M. *et al.* (1984) *Br. Med. J.* **289**, 1285

Acquired

● Liver disease.
● Warfarin therapy: protein C falls in the first 12–24 hours, before falls in factors II, VII, IX and X. As this may be associated with an increased risk of thrombosis in the early stages of oral anticoagulant therapy, loading doses of warfarin are contraindicated. Similarly, warfarin should be withdrawn slowly.

Reference
Schofield. K. P., Thomson, J. M. and Poller, L. (1987) *Clin. Lab. Haematol.* **9**, 255

● Severe infections: protein C levels fall, and with increase in C4b protein, which carries protein S, free active protein S is decreased, reducing protein C activation.
● Depressed by the third day after surgery or injury.
● Acute phase of major venous thrombosis.
● Consumed in disseminated intravascular coagulation.
● Adult respiratory distress syndrome without consumption coagulopathy.
● L-asparaginase therapy.

Protein S

Protein S, a vitamin-K-dependent plasma protein with a molecular weight of 69 000, circulates in a free active form and in an inactive form bound to C4b binding protein. C4b binding protein is a regulatory protein in the complement system and is an acute phase reactant. Protein S is also released by thrombin stimulation from platelet α-granules.

Action

Protein S acts as a cofactor for activated protein C by increasing the affinity of protein C for the negatively charged phospholipid of platelets, increasing the destruction of factor Va. It also enhances fibrinolysis.

Thrombin-cleaved protein S is seven times less effective than native protein S. Thrombomodulin, in the presence of free calcium ions, inhibits cleavage of protein S.

Plasma concentration reduced below normal adult levels

- Various substances, including bacterial endotoxin, tumour necrosis factor, and immune mediator interleukin 1.
- Hereditary deficiency of protein S [AD inheritance]: Patients suffer from a combination of deep vein thrombosis, superficial thrombophlebitis and pulmonary embolism. The age at first thrombosis ranges from adolescence to old age and no obvious precipitating cause of thrombosis may be found in half the cases.
- There is a significant reduction in protein S in pregnancy, with lowest level in the second trimester, returning to normal after delivery. Oral contraceptives also depress protein S activity.

References
Comp, P.C. and Esmon, C. T. (1984) *N. Engl. J. Med.* **311**, 1525
Engesser, L., Broekmans, A. W., Briët, E. *et al.* (1987) *Ann. Intern. Med.* **106**, 677
Malm, J., Laurell, M. and Dahlbäck, B. (1988) *Br. J. Haematol.* **68**, 437
Schwartz, H. P., Heeb, M. J., Wencel-Drake, J. D. *et al.* (1985) *Blood* **66**, 1452

Thrombomodulin

Thrombomodulin is a glycoprotein, with a molecular weight of 74 000, produced by endothelial cells in the circulation, including lymphatic endothelium, which helps to maintain liquid lymph. It is an integral protein located in the surface of all endothelial cells, except those in the brain microcirculation. Highest concentrations occur in the lung and the placenta. It can be detected in other tissues, including the extracerebral intracranial blood vessels, including the basilar and internal carotid arteries, the choroid plexus, and the endothelium of the pia arachnoid.

Thrombin complexes with thrombomodulin, its ability to clot fibrinogen and to activate platelets and factor V is inhibited, but there is a 1000-fold increase in protein C activation.

Pathological decrease

Factors which decrease thrombomodulin, protein C and protein S, increase tissue factor, increasing the tendency to thrombosis in infections and in the presence of some tumours. Recent work with very effective low-dose warfarin therapy strongly suggests that protein C and protein S activities, with antithrombin III, are also very important in preventing thrombosis after surgery or injury.

Reference
Esmon, C. (1987) *Science* **235**, 1348
Ishii, H., Salem, H. H., Bell, C. E. *et al.* (1986) *Blood* **67**, 362

Antithrombin III (AT-III)

AT-III is a proteinase inhibitor which is synthesized both in the liver and in vascular endothelial cells. It consists of a single polypeptide chain, with a molecular weight of 58 000, has the electrophoretic mobility of an α_2-globulin and a high degree of homology with α_1-antitrypsin. AT-III combines stoichiometrically and irreversibly with thrombin, inhibiting its activities, including the aggregation of platelets, and accounts for 75% of the antithrombin activity in the blood. It also inhibits the activities of factors IXa, Xa, XIa, XIIa, plasmin, urokinase and kallikrein.

Heparin acts as cofactor and greatly accelerates its activities. The presence of 50% or more of normal AT-III activity in the plasma gives normal protection against venous thrombosis. Vessel wall-associated AT-III, combined with vessel wall heparin and heparin-like glycosaminoglycans, protect the vessel wall by complexing with any thrombin. Platelet factor 4 (PF4), released from activated platelets, inhibits the binding of AT-III to the vessel wall. When endothelial cells are damaged, the production of tissue factor (procoagulant) is induced, encouraging local thrombus for repair.

During the conversion of factor II (prothrombin) to thrombin, fragment 2 is released, which protects thrombin from local AT-III. Similarly, when factor Xa is bound to the phospholipid of platelet membrane by factor Va, it is also protected from AT-III activity. AT-III with heparin inactivates thrombin faster than factor Xa.

Biological half-life

This is 2.7 $\pm$ 0.3 days, and is reduced in the presence of thrombosis.

Normal plasma levels

These are 85–120% bioassay, and 75–128% by immunoassay – 150 μg/l.

Reference
Beeler, D. L., Marcum, J. A., Schiffman, S. and Rosenberg, R. D. (1986) *Blood* **67**, 1488

Deficiency of AT-III activity is associated with increased risk of venous thromboembolism, without increased risk of arterial thrombosis.

Deficiency

Physiological

- Normal full-term infant: 40–87% of adult activity, reaching adult levels by 6 weeks after birth.
- Pre-term infant at 28–32 weeks – 29%, at 37–40 weeks – 51%.
- Infants with respiratory distress syndrome, with increased thrombotic tendency.

Reference
McDonald, M. M., Hathaway, W. E., Reeve, E. B. *et al.* (1982) *Thromb. Haemost.* **47**, 56

Pathological

Acquired

- Following heparin infusion.
- Liver disease, including cirrhosis, hepatitis, hepatic coma.
- Nephrosis: AT-III lost in the urine ? related to tendency for renal vein thrombosis and other thromboses.
- Disseminated intravascular coagulopathy: early and significant decrease.
- Extensive thrombosis: a temporary fall in AT-III is of no diagnostic value for detecting venous thrombosis after myocardial infarction. Normal AT-III levels in patients with active thrombosis excludes inherited AT-III deficiency.
- Gram-negative septicaemia: low AT-III levels persist.
- Postoperation: fall by the third day is restored to preoperative value by the fifth day. The degree of depression of AT-III varies with the operation site.
- L-Asparaginase therapy.
- Levamisole therapy.

Congenital

Hereditary antithrombin III deficiency (AD) – perhaps 3.5% of patients with a hereditary increased tendency to thrombosis. The AT-III molecule has two distinct critical binding sites: (1) coagulation serine proteases, (2) heparin binding sites. Both are essential for normal AT-III activity.

TYPE I DEFICIENCY

The majority of patients suffer from this form, with a high incidence of recurrent or extensive venous thrombosis, affecting especially the deep leg veins and iliac veins, with also a high incidence of pulmonary embolism. It is thought that the homozygous state is incompatible with life. Heterozygotes have plasma AT-III levels of 25–50% of normal. Kindred with low platelet AT-III concentrations suffer more severely from multiple thromboses.

They have reduced AT-IIIag with reduced antithrombin, anti Xa and heparin cofactor activities. Oral anticoagulants are highly effective in preventing thrombosis, and warfarin induces AT-III production and release. Surgery can be covered by giving AT-III concentrates.

Reference
Hambley, H., Davidson, J. F., Walker, I. D. and Menzies, T. (1987) *Clin. Lab Haematol.* **9**, 27

TYPE IIa DEFICIENCY

Less tendency to thrombosis. Normal AT-IIIag, but reduced anti-IIa, anti-Xa and heparin affinity.

TYPE IIb DEFICIENCY

Less tendency to thrombosis. Normal AT-IIIag, normal heparin affinity, but reduced anti-IIa and anti-Xa.

TYPE OR DEFICIENCY

Less tendency to thrombosis. Normal AT-IIIag, normal anti-IIa activity and normal heparin affinity, but reduced anti-Xa activity.

TYPE III DEFICIENCY

Less tendency to thrombosis. Normal AT-IIIag, anti-IIa and anti-Xa. Reduced heparin affinity.

References
Fisher, A. M., Beguin, S., Sternberg, C. and Dautzenberg, M. D. (1987) *Br. J. Haematol.* **66**, 213
Vinazzer, H. A. (1988) *Rev. Iberoam. Tromb. Hemost.* **1**, 12

Heparin cofactor II (HC-II)

Heparin cofactor II is a glycoprotein synthesized in the liver, with a molecular weight of 65 000, which neutralizes thrombin (factor IIa), but not factor Xa, more slowly than AT-III. Its activity is greatly increased by dermatan sulphate, present in the intima and media of large arteries, skin, heart valves and tendons. Dermatan sulphate has no effect on AT-III. HC-II activity is enhanced to a lesser extent by heparin, and its activity enhanced by dermatan sulphate or heparin is prevented in the neighbourhood of a thrombus by released PF4. HC-II is involved in preserving the fluidity of blood in intact vessels; in addition, it inhibits chymotrypsin in the circulation very efficiently.

Pathological deficiency

- Type I inherited HC-II deficiency [AD]: there is reduced HC-II in the plasma, with a risk of thrombosis in the homozygote. Heterozygotes (?0.9% of the population) may have a slightly increased thrombotic tendency.
- Disseminated intravascular coagulopathy.
- Liver failure.

References

Bertina, R. M., van der Linden, I. K., Engesser, L. *et al.* (1987) *Thromb. Haemost.* **57**, 196
Sie, P., Dupouy, D., Pichon, J. *et al.* (1985) *Lancet* **ii**, 414
Tollefsen, D. M. and Pestka, C. A. (1985) *Blood* **66**, 769
Tran, T. H., Marbet, G. A. and Duckert, F. (1985) *Lancet* **ii**, 413
Vinazzer, H. A. (1988) *Rev. Iberoam. Tromb. Hemost.* **1**, 12

β_2-Glycoprotein I

This substance neutralizes negatively charged macromolecules that enter the blood stream, and diminishes unwanted activation of coagulation factors in the blood. It also inhibits the contact phase of activation of coagulation. Its concentration is reduced in disseminated intravascular coagulation.

Reference
Schousboe, I. (1985) *Blood* **66**, 1086

Abnormal menstrual bleeding (due to haematological abnormalities)

Inherited plasma clotting deficiencies
- von Willebrand's disease.
- Factor IX deficiency carriers.
- True haemophilia carriers.

Platelets

Platelet count

Normal peripheral blood count
- Newborn: $150–250 \times 10^9$/l.
- Children (1–15 years): $175–500 \times 10^9$/l.
- Adults (> 15 years): $150–400 \times 10^9$/l with slightly higher counts in women than men ($+ 40–70 \times 10^9$/l).

The platelet count rises during the first 3 months. Each individual has a fairly constant platelet count while healthy, within the normal range. The inheritance of the platelet count has not yet been determined – e.g. what are the platelet counts of the offspring of parents with platelet counts, say, of 150×10^9/l and 450×10^9/l respectively ? There is a non-linear inverse relation between the mean platelet volume (MPV) and the platelet count, and there do not appear to be any racial differences.

References
Graham, S. S., Traub, B. and Mink, I. B. (1987) *Am. J. Clin. Pathol.* **87**, 365
Lewis, S. M. (1982) In: Hardisty, R. M. and Weatherall, D. J. Eds *Blood and its Disorder*, 2nd Ed, p. 44. Oxford: Blackwell Scientific
Saxena, S., Cramer, A. D., Weiner, J. M. and Carmel, R. (1987) *Am. J. Clin. Pathol.* **88**, 106

Physiological changes

Increase

- Sudden exercise lasting for more than 40 min results in an increase of $+ 25\%$ in the platelet count, following release of platelets from the spleen, with increase in platelet sensitivity to ADP, adrenaline, 5-hydroxytryptamine (5-HT) and collagen.

Reference
Peatfield, R, C., Gawel, M. J., Clifford, F. *et al.* (1985) *Med. Lab. Sci.* **42**, 40

- At ovulation, by up to 140×10^9/l.
- Postpartum thrombocytosis, returning to normal after a few days.

Decrease

- Fall at menstruation, rising to normal again by the fourth day.
- Mild harmless thrombocytopenia in up to 8% of normal pregnancies, more marked during the third trimester, with an increase in the MPV during the last 4 weeks.

References
Burrows, R. F. and Kelton, J. G. (1988) *N. Engl. J. Med.* **319**, 142
Fay, R. A., Hughes, A. O. and Farron, N. T. (1983) *Obstet. Gynecol.* **61**, 238
Sejeny, S. A., Eastham, R. D. and Baker, S. R. (1975) *J. Clin. Pathol.* **28**, 812

Pathological changes

Increase

- Following trauma, fractures of bones or surgery. Platelet counts fall during the first 48 h, then rise to peak values by about the tenth day, with peak platelet adhesiveness at this time.
- Acute blood loss, with peak values at about 7–10 days.
- Some cases of cancer. ? The value of screening patients with persistent thrombocytosis for an underlying malignancy.
- Following asphyxia.
- Inflammatory conditions, infections, including inflammatory bowel disease, coeliac sprue, Crohn's regional ileitis, chronic tuberculosis.
- Iron deficiency, returning to normal following adequate treatment.
- Reticulocytosis: the platelet count increases immediately before an increase in reticulocytes.
- Post splenectomy increase is followed by high platelet counts with risk of thrombosis. This also follows splenic vein thrombosis. Platelets are normally stored in the spleen.
- Rheumatoid arthritis during disease activity, with reduced platelet survival.

Reference
Farr, M., Scott, D. L., Constable, T. J. *et al.* (1983) *Ann. Rheum. Dis.*
42, 545

- Myeloproliferative disorders, including chronic myeloid leukaemia with counts often exceeding 1000×10^9/l, polycythaemia vera, primary thrombocythaemia.

Reference
Jabaily, J., Iland, H. J., Laszlo, J. *et al.* (1983) *Ann. Intern. Rev.* **99**, 513

- Folinic acid, or citrovorum factor, produces thrombocytosis lasting some days.
- Vincristine therapy. The platelets become spherical, following loss of their microtubules.
- Lithium treatment after 4 weeks.

Reference
Joffe, R. T., Kellner, C. H., Post, R. M. *et al.* (1984) *N. Engl. J. Med.* **311**, 674

- Rarely in Boeck's sarcoid.
- Rarely in myelosclerosis. Thrombocytopenia is more common.
- Hypothyroidism: generally an increase in number of small platelets, with the count falling to normal following treatment with tri-iodothyronine (T_3).

Reference
van Doormaal, J. J., van der Meer, J., Oosten, H. R. *et al.* (1987) *Thromb. Haemost.* **58**, 964

Decrease

Primary

HEREDITARY THROMBOCYTOPENIA

1. Macrothrombocytes:
   (a) normal platelet lifespan;
   (b) shortened platelet lifespan – Bernard–Soulier syndrome;
   (c) Epstein's syndrome: giant platelets, congenital nephritis and nerve deafness [AD] [R];
   (d) grey platelet syndrome: large platelets with specific α-granule deficiency [R];
   (e) familial giant platelet syndrome: easy bruising, thrombocytopenia, defective platelet aggregation, with impaired arachidonic acid mobilization.

Reference
Greaves, M., Pickering, C., Martin, J. *et al.* (1987) *Br. J. Haematol.* **65**, 429

2. Microthrombocytes:
   (a) sex-linked recessive inheritance with shortened platelet lifespan – Wiskott-Aldrich syndrome;
   (b) dominant inheritance: functional platelet defects predominate with only minimal thrombocytopenia.

3. Normal platelet size:
   (a) dominant inheritance with either normal platelet lifespan, or shortened lifespan;
   (b) autosomal recessive inheritance;
   (c) May–Hegglin anomaly, with thrombocytopenia in one-third of patients [R];
   (d) Chédiak–Higashi syndrome [R].

CONGENITAL [R]

- Transient benign thrombocytopenia in the newborn, with transient marrow megakaryocyte aplasia.
- Congenital aplasia of bone marrow megakaryocytes, which may be associated with congenital deformities.
- Infant of mother suffering from idiopathic thrombocytopenic purpura, with transplacental transfer of maternal antiplatelet factor. Purpura persists for a few weeks, with subsequent complete recovery.
- Isoimmune neonatal purpura.

Reference
Chandler, D. and Daniel S. J. (1985) *Am. J. Clin. Pathol.* **83**, 766

- Haemolytic disease of the newborn.

Secondary

CHEMICAL

- Dose-related marrow depressants, e.g. nitrogen mustards and other cytotoxics.
- Drug antibody response, e.g. quinidine, quinine, sedormid, butobarbitone, salicylates etc. In purpura due to quinine and quinidine, the antibodies are directed against platelet membrane glycoproteins GPV, GPIb, and GPIIb/IIIa.

References
Christie, D. J., Mullen, P. C. and Aster, R. H. (1987) *Br. J. Haematol.* **67**, 213
Stricker, R. B. and Shuman, M. A. (1986) *Blood* **67**, 1377
Tomiyama, Y., Kurata, Y., Mizutani, H. *et al.* (1987) *Br. J. Haematol.* **66**, 535

- Vinyl chloride disease.
- Gold therapy: thrombocytopenia with reduced platelet survival. Increased phagocytosis of platelets by macrophages with increase in bone marrow megakaryocytes.
- Alcoholic thrombocytopenia due to suppression of megakaryocyte development.
- Erucic acid, $C_{22:1}$ (ω-9), a contaminant of edible oils reduces platelet numbers [R].

PHYSICAL AGENTS

- X-ray irradiation.
- Following severe burns: a similar pattern to other injuries; the platelet count falls to low levels by the fourth day, rising towards normal by the seventh

day, with a subsequent peak between the seventh and twentieth days, when there is a risk of thrombosis.

- Severe heat stroke, with reduced plasma factors I, II, V and VIII.
- Hypothermia, with sequestration of platelets in the spleen.

BIOLOGICAL AGENTS

- Snake bite.
- Insect or spider bite.
- Vaccine injections.

DISORDERED HAEMOPOIESIS

- Leukaemia, especially acute varieties.
- Aplastic anaemia: since cyclosporin increases the platelet count in some cases, there may be an autoimmune element.

Reference
Stryckmans, P. A., Dumont, J. P., Velu, Th. *et al.* (1984) *N. Engl. J. Med.* **310**, 655

- Hypersplenism.
- Thrombotic thrombocytopenic purpura: in this condition the platelet life is reduced to a few hours only.
- Megaloblastic anaemia: in pernicious anaemia, vitamin B_{12} induces the production of a thrombopoietic factor before the increase in reticulocytes occurs.
- Hodgkin's lymphadenoma, due to reduced platelet production and shortened platelet lifespan.
- Acquired amegakaryocytic thrombocytopenic purpura, with selective reduction or total absence of megakaryocytes in an otherwise normal bone marrow.
- Kwashiorkor.
- Nutritional iron deficiency in infants: up to 28% have thrombocytopenia.

HAEMOPOIESIS CAUSED BY INFECTIONS

- Viral, e.g. infectious mononucleosis (in 50% of cases during the first 4 weeks). The thrombocytopenia is thought to be due to circulating platelet antibodies, and there is usually a dramatic response to cortisone.
- Bacterial, e.g. meningococcal meningitis, tularaemia etc. Gram-negative bacteria have a substance in their endotoxic lipopolysaccharide which reacts with platelets, causing intravascular coagulation, septic shock and thrombocytopenia.
- Malaria (*Plasmodium vivax*) in the early stages of the disease. In most cases there is no evidence of intravascular coagulation, there is increased plasma IgM, and the lowest platelet counts are

found between diagnosis and the fourth day of treatment. There is invasion of platelets by the parasites, with subsequent removal of damaged platelets from the circulation.

BLOOD FACTORS

- Following incompatible blood transfusion: this can occur immediately after the transfusion, or days later when Pl^{A1} and anti-HLA antibodies may have developed.
- Following massive replacement with stored blood of severe blood loss.
- Disseminated intravascular coagulopathy, including Kasabach–Merritt syndrome with chronic DIC (thrombocytopenia associated with solitary or multiple haemangioma).

Reference
Warrell, R. P and Kempin, S. J. (1985) *N. Engl. J. Med.* **313**, 309

- Idiopathic thrombocytopenic purpura: antiplatelet antibodies develop and cause platelet destruction.
- Platelet count reduced in 55% of cases of uncompensated portal cirrhosis, with depression of factors V and IX.
- Cor pulmonale: thrombocytopenia due to excessive utilization of platelets in the circulation is present in up to 30% of cases. There is an inverse relationship between the pulmonary arterial pressure and the platelet count. Thrombocytopenia is more common in older patients with hypoxaemia and polycythaemia.

Reference
Terai, M., Nakazawa, M., Takao, A. and Imai, Y. (1987) *Br. Heart J.* **57**, 371

- Cyanotic heart disease, with reduced plasma factor V levels.
- Eclampsia and pre-eclampsia.

Drugs causing thrombocytopenia

The following drugs and chemicals are not listed in order of severity or frequency of incidence. It will be seen that many of them, in certain cases, may severely affect the bone marrow as a whole, causing aplastic anaemia and incidental secondary thrombocytopenia (with reduced numbers of megakaryocytes in the bone marrow). The incidence of drug-induced thrombocytopenia will obviously vary with local prescription habits.

Sensitized state (megakaryocytes present in the bone marrow)

Acetazolamide
Amidopyrine
p-Aminosalicylates

Antipyrine
Arsenicals, organic
Bismuth
Carbutamide
Chloramphenicol
Chlorophenothane (DDT)
Chlorothiazide (especially with long-term therapy)
Chlorpropamide
Dinitrophenol
Marfanil sulphathiourate
Meprobamate
Mercurial compounds
Organic hair dyes
Oxytetracycline
Phenobarbitone and other barbiturates
Phenylbutazone (butazolidine)
Quinidine
Quinine
Ristocetin
Sedormid
Sodium salicylate
Streptomycin
Sulphonamides
Thiourea and thiouracils
Tolbutamide
Troxidone

Amegakaryocytic thrombocytopenia

All drugs and chemicals listed as causes of aplastic anaemia.

Artefactual increase in blood platelet count

With the increasing use of machines for the counting of platelets in whole blood, it has been found that certain artefacts can be counted as though they were platelets especially when electro-optical automated platelet counters are used.

- Malarial parasites.
- Howell–Jolly bodies.
- Nucleated red cells.
- Fragments from leukaemic cells, in leukaemia with high white cell counts.
- Aggregating red cell stroma secondary to red cell antibody agglutination or agglutination by paraproteins.
- Heinz bodies.
- Pappenheimer bodies, especially in splenectomized patients with haemolysis. These artefacts only affect the whole blood platelet count if they are present in large numbers.

Reference
Morton, D., Orringer, E. P., Lahart, L. A. *et al.* (1980) *Am. J. Clin. Pathol.* **74**, 310

Pseudothrombocytopenia

Under certain conditions, platelets can be undercounted:

- Platelet satellitosis.
- Platelet cold agglutinins.
- Platelet giant forms 'mistaken' for red or white blood cells.
- Platelet clumping with EDTA. This is the most frequent cause (up to nearly 2%), associated with platelet glycoprotein IIb, IIIa or both.

References
Payne, B. A. and Pierre, R. V. (1984) *Mayo. Clin. Proc.* **59**, 123
Pegels, J. G., Bruynes, E. C. E., Engelfriet, C. P. *et al.* (1982) *Blood* **59**, 157

Platelet volume

Normal range

This is 7–10.5 fl.

Reference
Giles, C. (1981) *Br. J. Haematol.* **48**, 31

The platelet volume distribution is log-normal with a right skew, and there is an inverse relationship between the mean platelet volume (MPV) and the total platelet count. Northern Europeans tend to have higher platelet counts with smaller platelets, whilst Southern Europeans tend to have lower platelet counts with larger platelets. Megakaryocytes mature to cytoplasmic disintegration in three ploidy classes: $8n$, $16n$, and $32n$. Light (less dense) platelets are derived from $32n$ ploidy, and are more liberally endowed with surface canaliculi than those derived from $16n$ ploidy. Dense platelets, derived from $8n$ ploidy, have a greater content of granules and mitochondria than the average platelet. Large platelets, probably derived from $8n$ ploidy, selectively aggregate with a lower dose of ADP, have a greater ability for serotonin uptake, higher lactate dehydrogenase activity, and a greater 'release' potential. Light platelets are more active in the uptake of particles, and have a greater content of membrane lipid, as a source of arachidonic acid, a precursor of prostaglandins and thromboxanes.

The MPV of platelets in blood collected into EDTA increases over 2–3 h when standing at 23–25°C.

Reference
Lippi, U., Capelletti, P., Schinella, M. *et al.* (1985) *Am. J. Clin. Pathol.* **84**, 111

Increase

Physiological

Adhesive platelets are larger than non-adhesive platelets. During normal pregnancy the platelet count tends to fall with an increase in MPV.

Pathological

1. Activation of platelets in the circulation:
   (a) immediately after surgical operation;
   (b) after acute myocardial infarction;
   (c) rheumatic heart disease with valve impairment, and also after prosthetic heart valve replacement;
   (d) septicaemia without thrombocytopenia, with the MPV returning to normal following successful antibiotic therapy;

Reference
van der Lelie, J. and von dem Borne, A. K. (1983) *J. Clin. Pathol.* **36**, 693

   (e) diabetes mellitus with retinopathy;
   (f) disseminated intravascular coagulopathy.
2. Megaloblastic anaemia due to vitamin B_{12} deficiency.
3. Response to antibodies:
   (a) systemic lupus erythematosus;
   (b) idiopathic thrombocytopenic purpura.
4. Inherited platelet disorders:
   (a) Bernard–Soulier syndrome;
   (b) grey platelet syndrome;
   (c) May–Hegglin anomaly, with thrombocytopenia and normal platelet function;
   (d) Hereditary thrombocytopenia, deafness and renal disease, with giant platelets.
5. Others:
   (a) macroglobulinaemia;
   (b) myeloproliferative disorders with great variation in platelet volume distribution;
   (c) somes cases of hypersplenism.

Decrease

Pathological

- During haemostasis.

Reference
Thompson, C. B. (1985) *Br. Med. J.* **291**, 95

- Sepsis with thrombocytopenia and marrow suppression.

Reference
Bessman, J. D. and Gardner, F. H. (1983) *Surg. Gynecol. Obstet.* **156**, 177

- Wiskott–Aldrich syndrome.

Platelet structure and contents

1. Bone marrow megakaryocytes and platelet formation.
2. Platelet structure.
3. Specific binding sites on the platelet surface.
4. Platelet contents:
   (a) microtubules;
   (b) platelet granules;
   (c) enzymes.
5. Platelet coagulation factors:
   (a) fibrinogen;
   (b) factor V;
   (c) factor XIII;
   (d) high-molecular-weight kininogen;
   (e) α_2-antiplasmin;
   (f) factor XI;
   (g) von Willebrand factor.
6. Platelet anticoagulation factors: platelet antithrombin III.
7. Platelet surface glycoproteins:
   (a) glycoprotein I;
   (b) glycoproteins II and III;
   (c) actin and myosin;
   (d) thrombospondin.
8. Calcium and calmodulin.
9. Platelet factor 4.
10. β-Thromboglobulin.
11. Fibronectin and thrombin-stimulated platelets.
12. Growth factors in platelets.
13. 5-Hydroxytryptamine (5-HT, serotonin).

Bone marrow megakaryocytes and platelet formation

Most human nucleated cells have a $2n$ complement of chromosomes. Megakaryocytes are polyploid cells and $4n$, $8n$, $32n$ and up to $64n$ may be found. Thrombopoietin increases the ploidy level. Cells with different ploidy number may form platelets of different sizes. Light platelets (i.e. lower density) have a lower granule content, $32n$ ploidy, greater lipoprotein content in the membranes, more surface canaliculi, higher arachidonic acid content and are more active in particle uptake. Large platelets are denser than small platelets, have $8n$ ploidy and contain more granules and mitochondria. They react more actively with low ADP concentrations. Small platelets are thought to be less active in haemostasis.

In the megakaryocyte, nuclear DNA synthesis stops when cytoplasmic membrane demarcation begins, in which profiles of round, oval or elongated vesicles are apparent when the membrane encloses an empty core or vesicle. These vesicles show budding, coalescing and branching. It appears that the cell membrane invaginates to form this system. Megakaryocytes are located in the subendothelial region of the vascular sinuses. The cytoplasm of the megakaryocytes penetrates the lumen, through and not between endothelial cells. Proplatelets enter the lumen, and each mature megakaryocyte can produce six proplatelets. It is probably outside the marrow that proplatelets each give rise to about 1200 platelets, either in the general circulation, or in the pulmonary circulation (more platelets leaving the lung than entering it). The pulmonary vascular walls produce large amounts of prostacyclin, inhibiting aggregation of the fragmenting megakaryocytes.

Of the platelets in the circulation at any one time, two-thirds are circulating and one third are sequestered in the spleen. The mechanisms for maintenance of steady-state blood platelet count are not known.

Each megakaryocyte in the bone marrow produces 3000–4000 platelets. From stem cell to platelet takes 10 days. Ploidy classes of megakaryocytes include: $8n$ producing dense platelets with increased numbers of granules and mitochondria aggregated selectively by low concentrations of ADP, $16n$ and $32n$ light platelets, with more surface canaliculi, more active particle uptake, and greater surface membrane content of phospholipid, a rich source for prostaglandins and platelet factor 3.

Platelet structure

Each platelet consists of a smooth convex disc with random surface indentations connecting with the open canalicular system inside the platelet. It has a mean diameter of 2–4 μm and a mean cell volume of 8–10 fl (with a right skew distribution). Stained spread blood films show a central granulomere and a surrounding hyalomere, artefactual effects of spreading, concentration organelles and granules centrally.

Detailed structure

Peripheral zone

There is an exterior glycocalyx rich in glycoprotein, providing surface receptors. Beneath this layer are asymmetrically distributed phospholipids providing essential surfaces for interactions with coagulant proteins, rich in substances containing arachidonic acid. Underneath this layer is a third layer which translates surface 'signals' into chemical messages and physical alterations for platelet activation.

Sol–gel layer

This consists of the matrix of the platelet cytoplasm, the fibres supporting the discoid shape of the platelet. They provide a contractile system concerned with

change in shape of the platelet, extrusion of pseudopodia, and internal contraction and secretion. This contractile system comprises 55% of the total platelet protein.

Organelle zone

Dispersed through the cytoplasm are granules, dense bodies, peroxisomes, lysosomes, mitochondria and discrete glycogen particles. There are at least four different types of storage organelles. There is storage for: enzymes including acid hydrolases, adenine nucleotides including ATP, serotonin, proteins, pyrophosphate, fibrinogen, calcium, vascular permeability factor, β-thromboglobulin, platelet factor 4 and growth factor. Calcium and enzymes for prostaglandin synthesis are sequestered in the platelet membrane system. Platelet calcium is 12 ± 3 ng/200 000 platelets (16–53 ng/200 000 platelets in May–Hegglin anomaly).

Examining instantly fixed platelets in whole blood smooth, unactivated disc platelets can be distinguished from platelets with protuberances. There are relatively small differences in such results in individual subjects over time, and it has been suggested that the effects of antithrombotic drugs could be studied.

Reference
Rosenstein, R. (1986) *Am. J. Clin. Pathol.* **85**, 502

Specific binding sites on the platelet surface

The open canalicular system provides access to the platelet interior for plasma-borne substances, and egress for products of the platelet release reaction. The platelet tubules, arranged in concentric rings conforming to the disc shape of the platelet, resemble the transverse tubules and sarcotubules of embryonic muscle cells. There are specific binding sites for the following:

- Thrombin, with neutralization of low concentration of thrombin on glycoprotein GP-I, and binding at higher concentration on glycoprotein GP-V followed by the release reaction.
- Specific binding sites for factor Va, which bind factor Xa and protect it from the actions of AT-III and heparin.
- Binding sites for ADP on GP-II.
- Fibrinogen is essential for platelet aggregation by thrombin or ADP, and fibrinogen binding sites are exposed by adrenaline, fibrinogen binding via its γ-chain. PGI$_2$ binds and inhibits the mobilization of binding sites for fibrinogen.
- Binding sites for adrenaline: these may be affected by oestrogen and progesterone.
- Binding sites for factor vWF on GP-I. Platelets, adhering to collagen in the exposed endothelial wall via factor vWF, adhere at high shear rate.

ADP is released in the immediate vicinity, inducing platelet aggregation.

- Immunoglobulins IgG1 and IgG3 bind more avidly to the platelet surface than IgG2 and IgG4. IgG1 dimers bind more avidly than IgG1 monomers, and less than polymers. They play an important part in immune thrombocytopenia, systemic lupus erythematosus, myeloproliferative disease, pre-eclampsia, septicaemia, Hodgkin's lymphadenoma and malignant tumours.
- Fibronectin binding sites: fibronectin is essential for platelet adhesion and aggregation.
- Thrombospondin in the platelet surface binds heparin.
- Collagen, arachidonic acid, TxA_2 and thrombin all expose factor VIII binding sites.
- Calcium is bound to the protein calmodulin and is in an unionized state. Following the release reaction, free calcium ions reach the platelet surface and bind to it, enhancing coagulation, platelet aggregation and further platelet release reaction.

References
Blumberg, N., Masel, D. and Stoler, M. (1986) *Blood* **67**, 200
Di Minno, G., Shapiro, S. S., Catalano, P. M. *et al.* (1983) *Blood* **62**, 186
Gogstad, G. O., Solum, N. O. and Krutnes, M.-B. (1983) *Br. J. Haematol.* **53**, 563
Jaffe, E. A., Leung, L. L. K., Nachman, R. L. *et al.* (1982) *Nature* **295**, 246
Karas, S. P., Rosse, W. F. and Kurlander, R. J. (1982) *Blood* **60**, 1277
Peerschke, E. I. B., Francis, C. W. and Marder, V. J. (1986) *Blood* **67**, 385

- In the inactive zymogen state, plasma factor XI is not detectable on platelets, but activated factor XII (XIIa) combined with factor XI bind to the platelet surface, and can cause platelet release reaction.

Platelet contents

The *microtubules* which form a ring around the rim of the platelet disc contain the protein tubulin and others. The α-tubulin has a molecular weight of 55 000, and the β-tubulin has a molecular weight of 110 000. The functions of the microtubules include flagellar and ciliary motility, and determination of the cell shape.

Platelet granules

Electron-dense granules (δ-granules)

These contain:

- Metabolically inactive storage form of ADP.
- Serotonin.
- ATP.
- Pyrophosphate.
- Most of the platelet calcium in inert form, bound to the specific calcium-binding protein.

α-Granules

These contain:

- Fibrinogen.
- Factor V.
- Platelet-derived growth factor.
- Platelet-specific proteins.
- Platelet factor 4.
- β-thromboglobulin.
- Albumin.
- Fibronectin.
- Thrombospondin.
- Factors vWF and VIIIR : Ag.

Reference
Wencel-Drake, J. D., Dahlback, B., White, J. G. and Ginsberg, M. H. (1986) *Blood* **68**, 244

Lysosome-like granules

These contain lysosomal enzymes, e.g. acid hydrolase.

Enzymes in platelets

- α_1-Antitrypsin.
- α_2-Macroglobulin.
- Low-molecular-weight antiplasmin.
- Inhibitor of plasminogen activator.
- Vascular permeability factor.
- Bactericidal factor.
- Chemotactic factor.
- Thrombospondin.
- Monoamine oxidase activity (low in migrainous subjects).
- N-Acetylglucosaminidase.
- β-Glucuronidase.
- β-Galactosidase.
- Arylsulphatase.
- Endoglucosidase.
- Neutral protease.
- Cyclic $3' : 5'$-phosphodiesterase.

Reference
Sandler, M., Youdim, M. B. H. and Harington, F. A. (1974) *Nature* **250**, 335

Platelet coagulation factors

In addition to the specific binding sites for circulating plasma coagulation factors, platelets contain coagulation factors in their structure, including the following.

Fibrinogen

Platelet fibrinogen, lacking part of the γ-chain found in plasma fibrinogen, is stored in the α-granules. It is more effective than plasma fibrinogen in supporting ADP- and adrenaline-induced platelet aggregation.

Reference
Peerschke, E. I. B., Francis, C. W. and Marder, V. J. (1987) *Blood* **67**, 385

Factor V (platelet factor 1)

Platelet factor 1, identical with plasma factor V, is stored in the α-granules, and factor V-antigen has been demonstrated in the platelets of patients with congenital plasma factor V deficiency.

References
Bradford, H. N., Annamalai, A., Doshi, K. and Colman, R. W. (1987) *Blood* **71**, 388
Miletich, J. P., Kanes, W. H., Hofmann, S. L. *et al.* (1979) *Blood* **54**, 1013

Factor XIII

Platelet factor XIII contains only the 'a' polypeptide subunit, and not the 'b' subunit found in plasma factor XIII. It accounts for 50% of factor XIII activity in the blood, and there is a linear relationship between factor XIII activity and the platelet count.

High-molecular-weight kininogen (HMWK)

HMWK, a major cofactor substrate of the contact phase of coagulation, is contained within platelets. When platelets are activated, HMWK is expressed on the platelet surface, where platelet enzymes can cleave and increase the coagulant activity of exogenous HMWK.

Reference
Schmaier, A. H., Smith, P. M., Purdon, A. D. *et al.* (1986) *Blood* **67**, 119

α₂-Antiplasmin

Platelets are the only peripheral blood cells carrying significant amounts of α_2-antiplasmin, which is important in the maintenance of the integrity of a thrombus.

Reference
Plow, E. F. and Collen, D. (1981) *Blood* **58**, 1069

Factor XI

Platelet factor XI has a lower molecular weight than plasma factor XI. Both factor XI and factor XIa bind to specific sites on the activated platelet membrane.

Von Willebrand factor

Platelets contain up to 25% of the circulating factor FVIII.RWF, and spreading adhesion of platelets on a subendothelial surface depends on platelet GP-IIb/GP-IIIa, calcium or magnesium ions, fibronectin and/or factor vWF. There is an excellent inverse correlation between the bleeding time and platelet factors vWF and vWFAg.

Reference
Gralnick, H. R., Rick, M. E., McKeown, L. P. *et al.* (1986) *Blood* **68**, 58
Platelet anticoagulation factors

Platelet antithrombin III

Plasma antithrombin III is less important than platelet antithrombin III. Deficiency of platelet antithrombin III has been described in kindred with multiple thrombotic attacks.

Reference
Tullis, J. L. and Watanabe, K. (1978) *Am. J. Med.* **65**, 472

Platelet surface glycoproteins

Glycoprotein I (GP-I)

There are 500 binding sites for thrombin on a platelet. At low thrombin concentration, thrombin is bound to GP-I and inactivated. At higher concentrations, thrombin binds to GP-I, GP-V underneath is uncovered and GP-V is the active substrate for thrombin-induced platelet 'release'.

GP-I contains more sialic acid than the other platelet glycoproteins, and this is lost progressively during storage. GP-Ib releases glycocalicin when exposed to calpain (the cysteine proteinase from the platelet cytosol). Calpain is mostly responsible for cleavage of exogenous HMWK on the platelet surface. Glycocalicin is the binding site for vWF, and is also the target for platelet autoantibodies in idiopathic thrombocytopenic purpura. Plasmin can induce proteolysis of glycocalicin rapidly, and this may be important during endogenous fibrinolysis or fibrinolytic therapy, by interfering with normal platelet function.

References
Michelson, A. D., Loscalzo, J., Melnick, B. *et al.* (1986) *Blood* **67**, 19
Szatkowski, N. S., Kunicki, T. J. and Aster, R. H. (1986) *Blood* **67**, 310

Glycoproteins II and III

These are essential for platelet aggregation by ADP. Glycoprotein III is absent and glycoprotein IIb is markedly reduced in Glanzmann's thrombocytasthenia. GP-IIb-α has a molecular weight of 132 000 and GP-IIb-β has a molecular weight of 23 000 (the two disulphide-linked units). Glycoprotein III consists of a single polypeptide chain with molecular weight of 114 000 and the alloantigen PI[A1] (or Zw[a]) resides in glycoprotein III.

Actin and myosin

Actin and myosin are located on the cytoplasmic face of the platelet membrane. Actin is lost during platelet storage.

Thrombospondin

This multifunctional protein, which has also been called glycoprotein C and thrombin-sensitive protein, and which is involved in platelet adherence and aggregation at sites of vascular injury, is selectively released from α-granules following platelet activation by thrombin. It has a molecular weight of 450 000 and consists of three identical subunits linked by disulphide bonds. Each subunit has a subunit of molecular weight 30 000 which binds heparin. Specific thrombospondin binding sites are elaborated on platelet glycoprotein GP-IIb/GP-IIIa on the platelet surface.

Reduced

Platelet thrombospondin content is reduced in essential thrombocythaemia and the grey platelet syndrome.

References
Jaffe, E. A., Leung, L. L. K., Nachman, R. L. *et al.* (1982) *Nature* **295**, 246
Lawler, J. (1986) *Blood* **67**, 1197

Calcium and calmodulin

Unionized calcium, bound to the protein calmodulin at a concentration of 48–84 nmol/mg protein, is essential for the phosphorylation of the myosin light chain in actinomyosin, and actinomyosin maintains the platelet's shape and helps to keep it intact. The calcium–calmodulin complex, without free calcium ions, inhibits platelet aggregation by ADP, thrombin, adrenaline, collagen and vWF.

Free calcium ions stimulate the activation and disintegration of platelets. Thromboxane A_2 acts as a calcium ionophore, mobilizing free calcium ions during the release reaction. When platelets are stimulated by thrombin, thrombospondin is released from platelet granules, enabling platelets to aggregate if free calcium ions are present.

Adenylate cyclase, which catalyses the formation of cyclic AMP (cAMP) from ATP, inhibiting platelet aggregation, is stimulated by PGI_2 and inhibited by free calcium ions. Free calcium is present in higher concentration in the platelets of hypertensive subjects than normal (168 ± 32 nmol/l compared with 108 ± 16 nmol/l).

Reference
Erne, P., Bolli, P., Bürgisser, E. and Bühler, F. R. (1984) *N. Engl. J. Med.* **310**, 1084

Platelet factor 4 (PF4)

PF4, which neutralizes heparin by forming an inactive complex which is cleared from the circulation, has a molecular weight of about 29 700 and is stored in the α-granules. Structurally it comprises a basic protein combined with a proteoglycan. It is released when platelets undergo activation, and can be used as a marker of platelet activation, as it has a half-life in the plasma of 20 min.

Its function is to help maintain the integrity of a platelet thrombus, by interfering with the action of local heparin which would otherwise act as cofactor to AT-III (neutralizing factor Xa, thrombin, factor IXa etc.). Reduction in the thrombin–heparin clotting time reflects the effects of acute phase proteins rather than any action of PF4. PF4 is heat stable, but is destroyed by plasmin and trypsin.

Increased PF4 activity

This occurs in any condition in which platelets undergo activation, including thrombosis in veins or arteries, atherosclerosis, prosthetic heart valves etc. and also following an injection of heparin. PF4 also increases in patients with cardiac ischaemia following exercise. This increase in plasma PF4 does not occur if aspirin is given beforehand, nor does it occur in normal subjects after exercise.

β-Thromboglobulin (β-TG)

β-TG, stored in the platelet α-granules, has a molecular weight of 30 000–36 000. It is released when platelets are activated, and can be used as a marker of platelet activation, as it has a plasma half-life of 100 min. Its function is to inhibit prostacyclin synthase in the vascular endothelium in the immediate vicinity of a platelet thrombus, reducing PGI_2 production which would othewise inhibit TxA_2 activity released from activated platelets.

Increase

β-TG is increased in any condition in which platelets are activated, including thrombosis in arteries or veins, pre-eclampsia, prosthetic heart valves, renal transplant rejection etc. Increased urine β-TG in diabetic nephropathy correlates with renal damage rather than reflecting platelet activation.

Reference
Hopper, A. H., Tindal, H. and Davies, J. A. (1986) *Thromb. Haemost.* **56**, 229

Plasma assays of PF4 and β-TG are used to detect hyperaggregatable platelet states, and also α-granule deficiency states.

Fibronectin and thrombin-stimulated platelets

Fibronectins are high-molecular-weight glycoproteins, present on many cell surfaces, in extracellular fluids, connective tissues and most basement membranes. Plasma fibronectin, consisting of two subunits linked by two disulphide bonds and with a molecular weight of about 440 000, has specific domains for cell binding. It binds to the α-chain of fibrinogen, vWF, thrombospondin, collagen, platelet GP-IIb/GP-IIIa and fibrin (cross–linked to it by factor XIIIa). Fibronectin is required for platelet adhesion and for thrombus formation on subendothelial and collagen surfaces under flow conditions. It is also concerned with the support of the non-immune defence of the host against foreign protein challenge in infections, burns, surgical trauma and in starvation, and plays a part in the phagocytic function of macrophages in the presence of magnesium ions.

Fibronectin is contained in the platelet α-granules, and is secreted following thrombin stimulation. Both fibronectin and thrombospondin bind to platelet GP-IIb/GP-IIIa. Stimulation by ADP or adrenaline does not release fibronectin, and fibronectin has no effect on either ADP- or thrombin-stimulated platelet aggregation.

References
Moon, D. G., Kaplan, J. E. and Mazukewicz, J. E. (1986) *Blood* **67**, 450
Mosesson, M. W. and Amrani, D. L. (1980) *Blood* **56**, 145
Plow, E. F. and Ginsberg, M. H. (1981) *J. Biol. Chem.* **256**, 9477
Robert, L. (1988) *Rev. Iberoam. Tromb. Hemost.* **1**(S1), 26

Growth factors in platelets

Factor promoting endothelial cell growth

Platelets are essential for the maintenance of the capillary endothelium, because they contain a factor distinct from platelet-derived growth factor (PDGF). In humans with thrombocytopenia, the endothelium of capillaries supplying skin or skeletal muscle has been found to be abnormally thin and fenestrated. Transfusion to normal counts or treatment with steroids restore these vessels towards normal.

References
King, G. L. and Buchwald, S. (1984) *J. Clin. Invest.* **73**, 392
Kitchens, C. S. and Pendergast, J. F. (1986) *Blood* **67**, 203

Platelet-derived growth factor (PDGF)

PDGF is a protein with a molecular weight of 30 000, which is stored in the platelet α-granules. It consists of two polypeptide chains linked by disulphide bonds, and is released locally during platelet activation when the blood vessel endothelium is damaged. The protein is a mitogen for cells of mesenchymal origin, including fibroblasts and human arterial smooth muscle cells. PDGF mediates proliferation of smooth muscle cells in injured artery walls, and excessive activity is thought to play an important part in the development of atherosclerosis. Smooth muscle cells from human atherosclerotic plaque can synthesize and secrete smooth muscle mitogens, some of which resemble PDGF.

PDGF also stimulates direct cell migration of neutrophils, monocytes, fibroblasts and plain muscle cells, and may be important in attracting and activating inflammatory cells to areas surrounding tumours. It is a vasoconstrictor, and contains an amino acid sequence similar to that of transforming protein of the Simian sarcoma virus.

References:
Baglin, T. P., Price, S. P. and Boughton, B. J. (1988) *Br. J. Haematol.* **69**, 483
Libby, P., Warner, S. J. C., Salomon, R. N. and Birinyi, L. K. (1988) *N. Engl. J. Med.* **318**, 1493
Seifert, R. A., Schwartz, S. M. and Bowen-Pope, D. F. (1984) *Nature* **311**, 669
Tzeng, D. Y., Deuel, F. F., Huang, J. S. *et al.* (1984) *Blood* **64**, 1123
Williams, L. T. (1989) *Science* **243**, 1564

5-Hydroxytryptamine (5-HT, serotonin)

Ninety per cent of the total body serotonin in mammals is secreted and stored in the enterochromaffin (argentaffin) cells in the small intestine. The bulk of the remainder is found in the platelets and the central nervous system, normal platelets rapidly taking up 5-HT from the plasma. There is an inverse relationship in healthy women between platelet count and platelet 5-HT, and their platelets are more susceptible to aggregation by ADP and 5-HT than those from men. 5-HT is released during the platelet release reaction; it vasodilates normal coronary arteries, but constricts coronary arteries with damaged endothelium, causing vasospasm. Free plasma 5-HT is catabolized in the liver.

The lung is also an important site of 5-HT metabolism. Massive platelet aggregation in the lungs, with release of platelet 5-HT, plays an important part in the development of pulmonary hypertension in bacterial endotoxaemia.

Platelet uptake of 5-HT is inhibited in both Down's syndrome and during reserpine therapy without causing any haemostatic defect. In storage pool deficiency and the Hermansky–Pudlak syndrome, platelet 5-HT uptake is normal, but its retention is defective.

Reference
Fetkovska, N., Amstein, R., Ferracin, F. *et al.* (1989) *Thromb. Haemost.* **60**, 486
McFadden, E. P., Clarke, J. G., Davies, G. J. *et al. N. Engl. J. Med.* **324**, 648

Platelet function and tests

1. Platelet function
2. Effects of deficient platelet function
3. Excessive platelet activity – blood flow and platelet deposition
4. Bleeding time
5. Platelet adhesion
6. Platelet retention test
7. Platelet aggregation:
   (a) adenosine diphosphate
   (b) platelet aggregation reduced
   (c) platelet cAMP
   (d) collagen
   (e) adrenaline
   (f) thrombin and platelets
   (g) arachidonic acid
   (h) ristocetin
   (i) platelet aggregation in whole blood
8. Platelet release reaction
9. Arachidonate cascade
10. Thromboxane a_2
11. Prostacyclin
12. Platelet factor 3 availability test
13. Platelet survival

Platelet function

Platelets are essential for the maintenance of normal vascular endothelium, with continuous repair of microtears in the endothelial lining of vessels, including the capillaries. They act as mechanical plugs, sealing over breaks in the lining. The pulsatile flow of blood through the vessels, with their expansion and relaxation at each heart beat, the effects of growth and ageing, and the inevitable minor bumps encountered in normal life, all result in minute sites of damage in blood vessels.

Following damage to the vascular endothelium, a layer of platelets is laid down on subendothelial tissue, platelet thrombus forms within 10 min and by the end of 1 h a monomolecular layer of platelets covers the subendothelial surface with a non-thrombogenic covering. Human platelets are the most negatively charged cells circulating in the blood, with a negative resting potential of at least $-60\,mV$. The negative charge on platelets depends in part on N-acetyl-neuraminic acid in the platelet surface, and this negative charge repels them from the normal negative charge on the endothelial surface, whilst coaxial flow in the blood forces platelets into the outer layers of the blood column. Damage to the blood vessel surface results in the loss of its negative charge at the site of damage, which may become positively charged, attracting negatively charged circulating platelets.

The velocity of platelets $1\,\mu m$ from the vessel wall endothelium is about $50\,\mu m/s$ and they would flow past an injury site $100\,\mu m$ long in 2 ms, during which time platelets must adhere to be effective. In a coronary artery with blood flowing at the rate of 40 cm/s, 3×10^8 platelets would flow every second along a small artery of 2-mm internal diameter, when the whole blood platelet count is $250 \times 10^9/l$. If a platelet thrombus forms, and continues to grow, as it would in a coronary artery thrombosis, it can grow very rapidly and block the vessel.

In the protection from blood loss following a macroscopic tear or cut with associated bleeding, platelets provide an essential protection and catalytic surface for the interaction of coagulation factors to produce a clot; they carry coagulation factors which, on release, increase local platelet aggregation, and release reaction, and stimulate thrombosis. Clot retraction depends on platelet action. In addition, bacterial endotoxin can coat platelets, causing their activation, or the endotoxin-coated platelets can be destroyed by reticuloendothelial cells, helping to clear the circulation of endotoxins.

Formation of the haemostatic plug

In a superficial skin wound, firmly interdigitated platelets are seen at the centre of the haemostatic plug. Platelets start to degranulate within 30 s, and most are degranulated by 3 min.

Fibrin deposition begins between the empty platelet vesicles, and is visible by 30 min. The wound is infiltrated with neutrophils which extend up to $200\,\mu m$ from the wound, by 2 h.

The effects of deficient platelet activity

Inadequate numbers of circulating platelets or defective platelets are associated with fenestrations in the skin and muscle capillaries, and probably in other capillaries throughout the body. Platelet lack results in the development of spontaneous petechiae, ecchymoses ('devil's pinches'), bruises, haematomas and frank bleeding either occurring apparently spontaneously or after trivial injury. Bleeding may occur from the nose, gums, in the gastrointestinal tract, the renal tract or in the brain. After tooth extraction or more serious injury, bleeding may be excessive and prolonged.

Excessive platelet activity

Blood flow and platelet deposition

Atherosclerotic plaques are most prominent in the segment of the proximal internal carotid artery segment opposite the branch flow divider, where flow velocity and wall shear stress are low. Flow separation results in vortex formation, recirculation and delayed clearance of circulating particles, the platelets. Plaque formation is accelerated by pulsatile flow, i.e. during forward and reverse flow pattern, and especially during the downstroke of systole. Plaque formation is also prominent in the coronary arteries opposite branch flow dividers; pulsatile flow is marked in the coronary arteries, and flow is subjected to two systolic and one diastolic episodes of flow acceleration and deceleration in each cardiac cycle. Episodic reverse flow occurs during periods of fast heart beat, and slowing of the heart rate by β-blockers is associated with reduction in coronary artery atherosclerosis.

Other arteries affected by plaque formation and platelet deposition include the abdominal segment of the aorta, and the arteries of the lower extremities. Arteries which are almost unaffected include the mesenteric, renal, pulmonary, intercostal and mammary arteries.

Both fibrinogen and platelets 'wear out' in the circulation, following the trauma of passing through branching vessels, and the repeated periods of temporary reversible adhesion to vessel walls.

Reference
Beere, A., Glasgov, S. and Zarins, C. K. (1984) *Science* **226**, 180

There is evidence that platelet deposition occurs preferentially in low shear regions (suggesting that exercise and increased rate of blood flow retard platelet thrombus formation). Irregularities and sharp bends in small vessels are important since platelet adhesiveness is increased in proportion to the velocity of impact on a surface.

Platelet α-granules contain mitogenic growth factor, which is released when platelets undergo the release reaction. This factor causes arterial wall smooth muscle cell proliferation. Within a few days, smooth muscle cells migrate through the lacunae in the internal elastic lamina of the vessel wall. New endothelial cells appear, probably derived from smooth muscle cells, to form a continuous layer of endothelial cells by the sixth day.

Proliferation of arterial wall smooth muscle cells requires endothelial injury, plus plasma von Willebrand factor, obviously the presence of platelets, and is enhanced by increased plasma concentrations of LDL cholesterol. Low concentrations of prostaglandins allow the development of smooth muscle cell proliferation, while adequate concentrations of PGE_1 and PGE_2 inhibit cloning of smooth muscle cell cultures. Platelet-released β-thromboglobulin inhibits the formation of prostaglandins by the vessel endothelial cells.

Collagen and proteoglycans are secreted in the vessel wall beneath the proliferation of muscle cells, and proteoglycans bind cholesterol. Regenerating endothelium avidly binds cholesterol, an essential component of cell walls.

If excessive cell proliferation has occurred, several layers of smooth muscle cells are then present between the endothelium and the internal elastic lamina. The thickness of this layer decreases until the layer is three cells thick by 6 weeks. The remaining healed lesion is morphologically identical with the fibromuscular plaque, a known preatherosclerotic lesion.

Smooth muscle cells can synthesize collagen fibrils, microfibrils and elastin, and smooth muscle cells in the fibromuscular plaque are surrounded by collagen fibres. When platelets adhere to collagen, thrombi containing fibrin develop, and are not removed in the subsequent few hours. There is a progressive increase in smooth muscle cells, and subsequently fatty degeneration of these cells. This cycle is repeated and a complete atherosclerotic plaque is formed, on which large thrombi can form, and from which emboli can separate.

Risk factors for atherosclerosis include diabetes mellitus, hypercholesterolaemia, excessive smoking, high blood pressure and 'stress' (whatever that is).

An alternative mechanism for the development of atherosclerotic lesions, is that with rupture of a vessel wall plaque in a subject eating a Western dairy product diet, palmitic acid is released, which causes instant platelet disintegration, on contact, and the rapid development of a platelet thrombus. If this mechanism plays a part in atherosclerosis, then dietary replacement of palmitate in plaques with ω-series polyunsaturated fatty acids would be therapeutically sensible.

Bleeding time

Normal

Using a 'template' method with a standard depth of cut made vertically in the forearm without venous stasis, the normal bleeding time is about 3 min. The test must be preceded by a platelet count, as a prolonged time is of no significance when there is thrombocytopenia. In the presence of normal platelets in normal numbers, the bleeding time is inversely proportional to the haematocrit, increasing in anaemia. The mean bleeding time is significantly longer in adult females than males (18–45 years).

References
Editorial (1984) *Lancet* **i**, 997
Mielke, C. H. Jr. (1982) *Blood* **60**, 1139
Parkin, J. D. and Smith, I. L. (1985) *Thromb. Haemost.* **54**, 731

Pathological

Shortened bleeding time

Within 12 h after acute myocardial infarction.

Reference
Milner, P. C. and Martin, J. F. (1985) *Br. Med. J.* **290**, 1767

Prolonged bleeding time

- Thrombocytopenia: variable results.
- Primary platelet abnormalities, including thrombasthenia, platelet storage disease.
- Von Willebrand's disease: there is no simple correlation between the bleeding time and plasma vWF:Ag in mild forms, but there is excellent inverse correlation between the bleeding time and platelet vWF activity, as platelet vWF plays an important part in the early stages of haemostasis.

Reference
Gralnick, H. R., Rick, M. C., McKeown, L. P. *et al.* (1986) *Blood* **68**, 58

- 'Template' bleeding time is increased in some haemophilia A patients, but bleeding may well persist. This is not a sensible test in this condition. This also applies to severe deficiency of factors I, II, V, VII, IX or XI.

Reference
Smith, P. S., Baglini, R. and Meissner, G. F. (1985) *Am. J. Clin. Pathol.* **83**, 211

- Hereditary haemorrhagic telangiectasia in affected areas. Bleeding from a cut lesion is difficult to stop.
- Disseminated intravascular coagulopathy.
- Acute fibrinolysis (pathological or therapeutic).
- Dextran infusion, persisting for some hours.
- Cardiac bypass surgery.
- Cyanotic heart disease.
- Severe liver disease, and some cases of obstructive jaundice.
- Uraemia.
- Acute systemic lupus erythematosus.
- Glycogen storage disease type I.
- Aspirin: no longer a sensible test for von Willebrand's disease, and contraindicated in factor VIII or factor IX deficiency. Low-dose aspirin inhibits platelet α-granule release and formation of thrombin at the template bleeding site. Other non-steroidal anti-inflammatory drugs may also prolong the bleeding time.

References
Barber, A., Green, D., Galluzzo, T. *et al.* (1985) *Am. J. Med.* **78**, 761
Kyrle, P. A., Westwick, J., Scully, M. F. *et al.* (1987) *Thromb. Haemost.* **57**, 62

- Ticlopidine after 4 days of treatment.

Platelet adhesion

Following endothelial damage, negatively charged platelets are attracted to the positively charged lesion of exposed subendothelial collagen. During blood flow at low shear rates, platelet spreading adhesion is independent of platelet glycoproteins GP-IIb/GP-IIIa. At higher shear rates, adhesion depends on GP-IIb/GP-IIIa, calcium or magnesium ions, fibronectin and/or von Willebrand factor, with specific binding sites for fibronectin and vWF on the platelets. Fibronectin promotes platelet spreading on collagen, and of adhesion at high shear rates on collagen types I and III. Types I, II and III collagen in the subendothelium stimulate platelet release, which results in increasing aggregation of platelets over the damaged area. Platelet adhesion increases with the platelet count, and with an increasing haematocrit. Red cells displace platelets to the periphery of the flowing blood column, increasing their chances of impact on the damaged site. If the shear rate is increased, a rate is reached when adherence falls away with further rate increase.

Measurement of pure platelet adhesion is impossible, as aggregation occurs as soon as platelets are activated. The platelet retention test depends in part on platelet adhesion to an artificial surface.

Reference
Aarts, P. A. M. M., Bolhuis, P. A., Sakeriassen, K. S. *et al.* (1983) *Blood* **62**, 214

Platelet retention test

Blood is passed through a standard column of beads at a standard speed. If the flow is too rapid, normal platelets do not stick to the beads. If the flow is too slow, defective platelets are able to stick to the beads. The platelet count in the blood after its flow through the bead column is subtracted from the count in untreated blood, and the difference in the two counts is the number of platelets trapped on the beads. This gives a qualitative assessment of platelet adhesiveness, which is similar to that obtained by comparing capillary and venous blood counts in a patient. Unfortunately, too many factors require standardization for this to be a reliably reproducible test. Even the washing, drying and storage of the glass beads affect results. Whether the test measures platelet adhesion and/or aggregation is uncertain. Whilst there is a diurnal normal variation, with greater retention in the afternoon and a seasonal variation, with greater retention in the Spring, this is a qualitative test. It is only useful in the detection of defective platelet function.

Pathological

Reduced retention

- Von Willebrand's disease: restored to normal following infusion of cryoprecipitate.
- Qualitative platelet defects: including Glanzmann's disease, Bernard–Soulier giant platelet syndrome, platelet storage pool disease, glycogen storage disease type 1.
- Uraemia.
- Thrombocytosis in myeloproliferative disease.
- Following aspirin.

Increased retention

This follows injury, surgical operation, and burns, with peak adhesiveness at about the tenth day. It also occurs in acute infections, some cases of carcinoma, diabetes mellitus, atherosclerosis, hyperlipoproteinaemia and homocystinuria. The test cannot be used to detect those patients liable to develop post-operation thromboembolic disease, or patients liable to suffer from myocardial infarction.

Platelet aggregation

Following platelet adhesion to a lesion in the vessel endothelial wall, further circulating platelets stick to the adhering platelets, and more platelets stick to these, forming a platelet aggregate. During aggregation, the discoid platelets become spheroidal and develop pseudopodia, when they become 'sticky'. The initial adhering platelets and the aggregating platelets in their immediate vicinity undergo 'release reaction', when their adhesion and aggregation become irreversible, beginning the repair of the lesion. The surplus aggregating platelets are released back into the circulation – otherwise continuing aggregation would eventually block the vessel. Platelets which have released their ADP, aggregated, disaggregated and subsequently been released back into the circulation, are unreactive for 20–30 min and do not react to further ADP ('tired' platelets).

The initial reversible aggregation depends on local release of ADP, which alters the platelet shape and causes the appearance of binding sites for fibrinogen on the platelet surface. Fibrinogen and fibronectin are essential for platelet aggregation. There are specific binding sites on the platelet surface for ADP; cAMP, which inhibits platelet aggregation, competes for, and binds to these same sites.

Platelet aggregation can be demonstrated in vitro using a platelet aggregometer. Light is passed through a platelet-rich plasma sample, and aggregating agents are added. As the platelets aggregate and clump together, more light passes through the plasma to reach a light meter, which detects these changes. Thrombin, collagen, ADP, adrenaline (in pharmacological doses), thromboxane A_2 and arachidonic acid all cause platelet aggregation and can be used in vitro to test platelet aggregation. These tests are useful in the detection of defective aggregation, but not for the detection of overactive platelets.

Physiological

Platelet aggregability is reduced by physical training in middle-aged men, with increases in plasma HDL_2 cholesterol and the inert metabolite of PGI_2, and decrease in plasma HDL_3 cholesterol.

References
Rauramaa, R., Salonen, J. T., Seppanen, K. *et al.* (1986) *Circulation* **74**, 939
Rauramaa, R., Salonen, J. T., Kukkonen-Harjula, K. *et al.* (1984) *Brit. Med. J.* **288**, 603

Various agents have been used to induce platelet aggregation in vitro in the detection of platelet function disorders:

- Adenosine diphosphate (ADP).
- Collagen.
- Adrenaline.
- Thrombin.
- Arachidonic acid.
- Ristocetin.
- Attempts have been made to measure platelet aggregation in whole blood.

Adenosine diphosphate (ADP)

Platelets contain both ADP and ATP in their dense granules, and some ADP is bound to actin. ADP is released from damaged red cells in the circulation. Platelet ADP reaches the platelet surface during the release reaction, seen in vitro during the secondary wave of irreversible platelet aggregation. ADP binds to the specific receptors in the platelet surface glycoproteins GP-IIb/GP-IIIa, with free calcium ions. Extracellular fibrinogen then binds in reversible fashion to this activated surface membrane complex. Platelets then change from a discoidal to a spherical shape with protruding pseudopodia. Thrombin and collagen also cause this change in shape.

At low concentrations of ADP (0.5–1.0 mmol/l), platelets subsequently disaggregate and bound fibrinogen is also freed. Some minor aggregation defects are detectable at this strength of ADP.

At higher concentrations of ADP (2.5–10 mmol/l), the irreversible secondary wave of platelet aggregation occurs, with release of α-granule and dense granule contents. ADP stimulates release of arachidonic acid from the platelet surface membrane, release of thromboxane A_2, inhibition of adenylate cyclase with immediate reduction in cAMP activity.

ADP exposes secondary binding sites for factor VIII/vWF on GP-IIb/GP-IIIa, and low concentrations of thrombin act with intrinsic platelet ADP to induce binding of factor VIII/vWF. ADP also activates plasma factor XII and stimulates the synthesis of PGE_1, which in turn activates adenylate cyclase, increasing cAMP activity later, to counteract ADP activity at the time of disaggregation.

$$ATP + AMP \xrightleftharpoons[]{} 2ADP$$

adenylate
kinase

$$Adenosine + ATP \longrightarrow AMP + ADP$$

ATP-generating system of cells

$$maintains \quad \frac{(ATP)}{(ADP)\,(Pi)} \quad at\ about\ 500$$

Relationships and interconversions of ATP, ADP and ADP in and on platelets. When the binding sites on platelets are occupied by ADP, the platelets are 'adhesive', and when the sites are occupied by AMP, they are not adhesive. Pi = inorganic phosphate.

Platelet aggregation reduced

Absence of platelet aggregation
- Glanzmann's thrombasthenia.
- Cyclo-oxygenase deficiency.

Abnormality or absence of secondary wave
- Platelet storage disease.
- Thromboxane synthase deficiency.
- Abnormality of thromboxane receptors.
- Aspirin or other NSAIDs which block cyclo-oxygenase activity.
- A variety of diseases including fulminant liver failure, portal cirrhosis, pre-eclampsia, hereditary spherocytosis, heavy alcohol intake. (Platelets in Bernard–Soulier syndrome aggregate in response to ADP, but do not become spherical.)

Platelet cAMP

cAMP competes for binding sites on the platelet surface in glycoprotein IIb and III, and:
- Reduces ADP-induced aggregation of platelets: the so-called 'exhausted' platelets disaggregating after aggregating reversibly with ADP have probably had many of the bound ADP molecules replaced by cAMP.
- Collagen-induced platelet aggregation and adrenaline-induced platelet aggregation are reduced by increasing platelet cAMP content.
- Platelet retention in the Salzman glass bead column is reduced.
- Release of platelet factor 4 into the plasma is reduced.
- Bleeding time, total platelet count and factor 3 availability are not affected by cAMP.

Reference
Mannucci, P. M. and Pareti, F. L. (1970) *J. Lab Clin. Med.* **80**, 828

Intracellular cAMP inhibits hydrolysis of arachidonic acid from platelet membrane phospholipid.

Collagen

Adhesion of platelets to cover exposed subendothelial collagen when the vascular endothelium is exposed, is the first stage in the repair of such minute damage. Excessive deposition of platelets and their subsequent degeneration are thought to be of importance in the development of plaques and atherosclerosis. Platelets adhere to collagen at high shear rates, as are found in arteries and arterioles, in the presence of factor VIII/vWF. This adhesion is not mediated by ADP, but adhering platelets release ADP, which in turn increases local platelet aggregation.

Platelets bind to the glucosyl-galactosyl moiety in collagen, and do not bind to either denatured collagen or tropocollagen. Fibronectin is the collagen receptor on platelets. Platelets probably respond to type III collagen. Collagen can activate both plasma factor XII and platelets, and the development of collagen-induced activity depends on the binding of plasma factor XI to the platelet membrane. The major activation pathway, via platelet prostaglandins, results in the formation of thromboxane A_2 from platelet membrane phospholipids, and the release of platelet granule contents.

In vitro, platelet aggregation by collagen is preceded by a short 'lag phase' lasting 10–60 seconds; the duration of this phase is inversely proportional to the concentration of the reagents used, and also to the responsiveness of the platelets under test. This lag phase is followed by a single irreversible phase of aggregation.

Higher concentrations of collagen in vitro cause the platelet release reaction without the mediation of the prostaglandin pathway. As a result, concentrations of $1\,\mu g/ml$ and $4\,\mu g/ml$ (final) are used. Higher concentrations give non-specific aggregation. The lower concentration is more specific for detection of abnormalities of the arachidonic acid cascade, thromboxane A_2 generation and subsequent platelet granule release. Aggregation of platelets in vitro by active collagen is reproducible down to platelet counts of $50 \times 10^9/l$, and is not affected by plasma or platelet cholesterol concentrations (compare the responses of platelets to ADP and adrenaline).

Aspirin taken in vivo inhibits in vitro platelet aggregation and release reaction, unless unusually high collagen concentrations are used. A collagenase, present in platelets and released during the release reaction, may play a part in limiting thrombus formation.

Pathological

INCREASED PLATELET RESPONSE TO COLLAGEN IN VITRO

Found in 50% of patients with diabetic neuropathy.

DECREASED RESPONSE

Impaired platelet response to collagen is found in a number of 'easy bruisers' with no history of significant bleeding.

DECREASED PLATELET AGGREGATION IN RESPONSE TO COLLAGEN IN VITRO

- Thrombasthenia: no response to collagen.
- Hermansky–Pudlak syndrome.
- Storage pool disease: no TxA_2 or ADP released during platelet aggregation.
- Wiskott–Aldrich syndrome.
- Chédiak–Higashi syndrome.
- Cyclo-oxygenase deficiency.
- Thromboxane synthase deficiency.
- Grey platelet syndrome.
- Aspirin administration: reduction in platelet aggregation following aspirin intake can persist for up to 7 days. The platelet cyclo-oxygenase enzyme is acetylated and inactivated.

Adrenaline

Adrenaline binds to α-adrenergic receptors on the platelet membrane, and fibrinogen receptors are exposed by a mechanism independent of ADP. In vivo, it enhances the reaction between platelets, factor VIII/WF and exposed subendothelium. Adenylate cyclase is inhibited, reducing platelet cAMP (which would otherwise inhibit platelet aggregation). Adrenaline has a biological half-life in the plasma of less than a minute, and its concentration varies diurnally.

It is used in vitro at a final concentration of $1-10\,\mu m$, which is much higher than the levels reached in extreme pathological stress in vivo. In vitro, platelet aggregation studies using adrenaline are of little clinical value, and no specific clinical platelet abnormalities can be detected using adrenaline, which are not observed using the other reagents.

Reference
Keraly, C. L., Kinlough-Rathbone, R. L., Packham, M. A. *et al.* (1989) *Thromb. Haemost.* **60**, 209

Thrombin and platelets

Whilst prothrombin is an anion at blood pH and is not attracted, thrombin is a cation and is attracted to platelets. At low thrombin concentration it binds to platelet glycoprotein GP-I, and is neutralized by GP-I and glycocalcin. At higher concentrations, the discoidal platelet becomes irregularly spheroidal with pseudopodia projecting from the surface, with thrombin binding to GP-V beneath GP-I in the platelet membrane. Secondary binding sites for factor VIII/WF on the GP-IIb/GP-IIIa glycoprotein complex are exposed, and platelet adhesion to collagen is increased. Thrombin-stimulated platelets bind fibrinogen, fibronectin, factor VIII/WF and thrombospondin.

The platelet is irreversibly activated, releasing its granule contents and liberating protein-bound calcium to increase the concentration of free calcium ions inside the platelet. Phosphorylation of platelet protein occurs in less than a second after thrombin activation, and there is a marked increase in phosphatidyl serine formation (a component of factor 3 in the coagulation cascade). The arachidonic acid cascade and platelet granule release contribute to platelet activation, but at higher concentrations of thrombin, platelet activation does not require TxA_2 generation. Platelet aggregation occurs both via the arachidonate cascade and ADP release, but also by an ADP-independent pathway.

Since thrombin converts fibrinogen to fibrin, platelet aggregation studies with thrombin must be carried out with platelets washed free of plasma at a final thrombin concentration of $0.1-0.5$ unit/ml. Washing the platelets free of plasma also removes the antithrombin agents antithrombin III and α_2-macroglobulin. Low concentrations of thrombin test platelet prostaglandin activation, as all the components of the arachidonic acid cascade are required for a normal response.

References
Carty, D. J., Spielberg, F. and Gear, A. R. C. (1986) *Blood* **67**, 1738
Jenkins, C. S. P., Clemetson, K. J. and Ali-Briggs, E. F. (1983) *Br. J. Haematol.* **53**, 491

Arachidonic acid (AA)

This is the most abundant unsaturated fatty acid in

the platelet ($C_{20:4}$, ω-6), and most occurs in phosphatidyl ethanolamine (PE) and phosphatidyl choline (PC), with much smaller amounts in phosphatidylinositol (PI) and phosphatidyl serine (PS). Phospholipase A_2 in the presence of calcium ions splits off arachidonic acid and phosphatidic acids (phospholipids which accelerate plasma clotting). Arachidonic acid is converted to thromboxane A_2 via the arachidonic acid cascade. The aggregation of platelets by arachidonic acid is irreversible and is accompanied by the release of ADP, but ADP does not take part in the reaction. In vitro, arachidonic acid at a final concentration of 1–2 mmol/l induces TxA_2 generation and granule release in normal platelets and, even if a defect exists, in the phospholipase-induced release of endogenous arachidonic acid or defects before this stage. It does not produce platelet aggregation if the defect is lower down the arachidonic acid cascade.

Increased platelet aggregation

Platelets enriched with cholesterol yield more thromboxane A_2 following release. This may partially explain the increased reactions of platelets to aggregating agents in type IIa hyperlipidaemia, which respond to lower concentrations of adrenaline, collagen and ADP than normal.

Decreased platelet aggregation

ABSENCE OF PLATELET AGGREGATION

- Aspirin administration – cyclo-oxygenase inhibition.
- High concentrations of indomethacin inhibit endoperoxide formation.
- Thrombasthenia.
- Strong calcium chelators.

FIRST STAGE AGGREGATION (REVERSIBLE) ONLY

- Bernard–Soulier syndome.
- Hermansky–Pudlak syndrome.
- Storage pool disease.
- Defects of TxA_2 synthesis.
- Cyclo-oxygenase deficiency.

References
Stuart, M. J., Gerrard, J. M. and White, J. G. (1980) *N. Engl. J. Med.* **302**, 6
Vermylen, J., Badenhurst, P. N., Deckmyn, H. *et al.* (1983) In: Harker, L. A. H. and Zimmerman, T. S., Ed. *Clinics in Haematology*, Vol. 12, pp. 107–151. London: W. B. Saunders

Ristocetin

Ristocetin, originally developed as an antituberculous agent, was found to cause severe thrombocytopenia in patients. It is now used as a platelet aggregating agent. Ristocetin reduces the platelet net negative surface charge, binding via diphenolic groups to platelet surface glycoprotein GP-Ib, and binding to plasma von Willebrand factor (factor VIIIRWF), a large molecule which can bridge between platelets, causing platelet aggregation. An irreversible agglutination of platelets forms, independent of thromboxane A_2 generation or granule contents release. The final concentration of ristocetin in vitro should be 1.2 mg/ml. Non-specific platelet clumping due to interaction with fibrinogen occurs at concentrations above 1.5 mg/ml, masking detection of any platelet or plasma defect.

Physiological

Platelets from normal Negroes give a moderately defective response to ristocetin.

Pathological

INCREASED RESPONSE

Platelets from von Willebrand's disease subtype 11b respond to lower concentrations of ristocetin than normal, due to a lack of high-molecular-weight oligomers of factor VIII-related antigen in the plasma. They are detectable when ristocetin is used at a concentration of 0.5–1.2 mg/ml.

DECREASED RESPONSE

- Bernard–Soulier syndrome: these platelets are deficient in surface platelet glycoprotein GP-Ib.
- Von Willebrand's disease Types I, IIA, IIC and III: for any patient suspected of having a factor VIII complex defect, ristocetin cofactor assay should be carried out using washed fixed normal platelets.
- Vancomycin, which has a chemical structure similar to ristocetin, inhibits ristocetin-induced platelet aggregation by competitive binding to the GP-Ib sites on the platelets.
- Aggregates of IgG and the Fc fragment of IgG inhibit platelet aggregation by ristocetin in plasma. Platelet membrane Fc receptor sites are part of GP-I, and are important in immune thrombocytopenia, systemic lupus erythematosus, myeloproliferative disease and pre-eclampsia.
- Glycogen storage disease type 1, with decreased vWF levels and activity.
- Uraemia in chronic renal disease.

References
Castillo, R., Lozano, T., Escolar, G. *et al.* (1986) *Blood* **68**, 337
Gralnick, H. R., Williams, S. B., Shafer, B. C. *et al.* (1982) *Blood* **60**, 328
Triplett, D. A. (1991) *Mayo Clin. Proc.* **66**, 832

Platelet aggregation in whole blood

Platelet aggregation can be measured, using electrical impedance, in both platelet-rich plasma and whole blood. When whole blood is used, centrifugation is unnecessary, reducing the time lag before testing, and allowing the testing of the whole platelet population.

Centrifugation tends to remove the heavier platelets from a sample. Results obtained using impedance on whole blood, and impedance or densitometry on platelet-rich plasma, are similar.

Platelets are more reactive to ristocetin, thrombin, arachidonic acid and prostacyclin in whole blood than in platelet-rich plasma. The platelet count and the haematocrit do not appear to affect results, whereas there is a negative correlation between the white blood cell count and whole blood platelet aggregation induced by collagen. White blood cells can produce anti-aggregating arachidonic acid metabolites, and can degrade ADP.

Using whole bloode platelet aggregation measured by impedance, it has been shown that social drinking resulting in moderate blood alcohol levels inhibits platelet aggregation using collagen and ADP, suggesting a partial explanation for the protection from ischaemic heart disease found in moderate drinkers.

References
Abbate, R., Favilla, S., Boddi, M. *et al.* (1986) *Am. J. Clin. Pathol.* **86**, 91
Mackie, I. J., Jones, R. and Machin, S. J. (1984) *J. Clin. Pathol.* **37**, 874
Mikhailidis, D. P., Barradas, M. A., Epemolu, O. and Dandona, P. (1987) *Am. J. Clin. Pathol.* **88**, 342
Riess, H., Braun, G., Brehm, G. and Hiller, E. (1986) *Am. J. Clin. Pathol.* **85**, 50
Sweeney, J. D., Labuzetta, J. W. and Fitzpatrick, J. E. (1988) *Am. J. Clin. Pathol.* **89**, 655

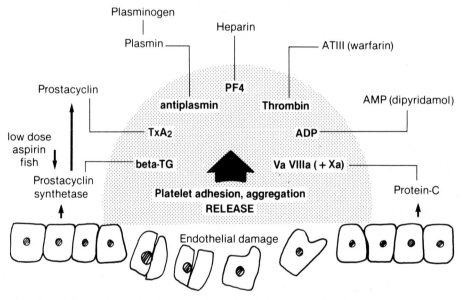

Release reaction of platelets at the site of vascular endothelial damage, with release of platelet contents, and inhibition of active platelet factors at the immediate periphery of the platelet thrombus. In addition to those substances shown, platelets also release a collagenase.

Active factors associated with the releasing platelets	*Neutralized at the periphery of the thrombus by*
Factors Va, Xa and VIIIa ←	Vascular endothelium protein C
ADP (competition for binding sites) ———	Cyclic AMP (protected from conversion to AMP by dipyridamol)
Thrombin ←	Antithrombin III (which also neutralizes factor Xa)
Platelet factor 4 ——→	Heparin
Platelet antiplasmin ——→	Plasmin released from plasminogen by activated factor XII etc.
Thromboxane A$_2$ ←	Prostacyclin from vessel endothelium
β-Thromboglobulin ——→	Prostacyclin synthase
(→ indicates inhibition)	

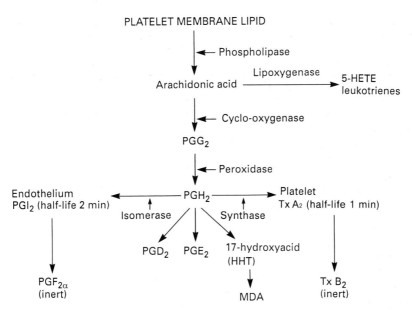

PLATELET MEMBRANE LIPID

Prostacyclin/thromboxane cascade.

Platelet release reaction

During the release reaction, platelets release the contents of their granules, free calcium ions are liberated from protein binding in the platelets, and phospholipids and arachidonic acid in the platelet membranes are split from each other. Phospholipid then takes part in the coagulation cascade with plasma coagulation factors for the production of fibrin. Arachidonic acid is acted on by enzymes in the arachidonic cascade to produce thromboxane A_2 (TxA_2). This series of reactions is autocatalytic, as generated thrombin induces the formation of more thrombin, and TxA_2 causes more platelets to aggregate and undergo release, with formation of more TxA_2.

Platelets release substances which protect the developing platelet thrombus from its neutralization by circulating antithrombotic agents. At the same time, the anti-platelet release substance prostacyclin (PGI_2) is formed from arachidonic acid in the endothelium immediately surrounding the platelet thrombus, and other antithrombotic substances in the circulation help to localize the thrombus. Whilst TxA_2 causes local vessel spasm to protect the thrombus, PGI_2 causes vasodilatation at the periphery.

Evidence of generation of TxA_2 and PGI_2 is shown by raised plasma levels of inert thromboxane B_2(TxB_2) and inert PGF_2, respectively, and of platelet release by raised levels of β-thromboglobulin and platelet factor 4. Platelet release in the circulation is induced by thrombin, ADP and collagen in exposed subendothelium (enhanced by adrenaline).

Arachidonate cascade

Phospholipase A_2, activated by thrombin, collagen and mechanical perturbation, and inhibited by glucocorticoids, dibutryl-cAMP, and some antimalarials, releases arachidonic acid and phosphatidyl choline, phosphatidyl inositols and phosphatidyl ethanolamine from the platelet membrane.

Arachidonic acid is converted to the equally short-lived prostaglandins PGG_2 and PGH_2 by the microsomal enzyme cyclo-oxygenase. This enzyme is irreversibly acetylated and inactivated for the duration of the affected platelet's life by aspirin. Indomethacin and other non-steroidal anti-inflammatory drugs reversibly inhibit this enzyme. Some arachidonic acid is converted by lipoxygenase to HETE and leukotrienes, which stimulate chemotaxis and migration of leucocytes. In the endothelium, prostacyclin synthase converts arachidonic acid to prostacyclin (PGI_2). Other products derived from arachidonic acid include PGD_2, the major prostaglandin produced by mast cells in response to allergic and other stimuli. It is a vasodilator of systemic resistance vessels, and a bronchoconstrictor in the lungs. PGE_2 is the major product from arachidonic acid in the microvascular endothelium, including the kidney and gastrointestinal tract, and is a vasodilator causing diuresis and natriuresis. It inhibits lymphocytes and other cells from participating in inflammatory and allergic responses, and can induce second-wave platelet aggregation.

The platelet microsomal enzyme thromboxane synthase, which acts on PGG_2 and PGH_2 to generate TxA_2, is also inhibited irreversibly by aspirin.

References
Clarke, R. J., Mayo, G., Price, P. and Fitzgerald, G. A. (1991) *N. Engl. J. Med.* **325**, 1137
Oates, J. A., Fitzgerald, G. A., Branch, R. A. *et al.* (1988) *N. Engl. J. Med.* **319**, 689

Thromboxane A_2 (TxA_2)

This extremely active substance with a half-life in the circulation of 30 s, at 37°C, is bound to, and protected by, albumin. It is a potent agent for stimulation of platelet release reaction, aggregation and platelet shape change by contracting thrombasthenin (from discoid to sphere), and a very powerful platelet aggregating agent. It causes centripetal localization of the dense granules, and later releases endogenous materials via the canaliculi. In addition, TxA_2 is a very powerful local vasoconstrictor, up to 100 times more powerful than angiotensin II (molar comparison). Its actions on platelets are mediated by translocation of calcium, after binding to specific sites.

TxA_2 undergoes spontaneous non-enzymatic change to thromboxane B_2 (TxB_2), an inert relatively stable substance. Estimation of circulating TxB_2 is used as a guide to the rate of TxA_2 generation. ?TxB_2 plays some part in chemotaxis. Cholesterol-rich platelets release more TxA_2 than cholesterol-poor platelets.

Reference
Stuart, M. J., Gerrard, J. M. and White, J. G. (1980) *N. Engl. J. Med.* **302**, 6

Prostacyclin (PGI$_2$, epoprostenol)

PGI_2, a metabolite of arachidonic acid, produced by the enzyme prostacyclin synthase in vascular endothelial cells, increases the cAMP content of these cells and of adhering platelets by activating adenylate cyclase. It binds to platelet fibrinogen receptors, preventing fibrinogen binding, and therefore preventing platelet activation and 'release' by thrombin. Platelets cannot synthesize PGI_2.

Transfer of arachidonic acid and its immediate metabolites from adherent collagen-stimulated platelets to endothelial cells is followed by PGI_2 synthesis after minor degrees of endothelial desquamation. PGI_2 inhibits platelet adhesion and aggregation in response to ADP and adrenaline, and free calcium ion mobilization and arachidonic acid is inhibited by both cAMP and non-cAMP mechanisms. Its actions ensure

that the platelet–fibrin plug at the site of vascular endothelial damage does not expand beyond its immediate zone, or block the vessel concerned. It prevents platelet activation and platelet consumption from being excessive and generalized. In addition, it is a vasodilator, relaxing smooth muscle cells in vessel walls, counteracting the vasospastic action of TxA_2 released in a platelet thrombus, and it also stimulates fibrinolytic activity by inducing plasminogen activator. At the edges of a local platelet thrombus β-thromboglobulin inhibits PGI_2 activity, protecting the local repair process.

PGI_2 appears locally within 10 seconds of enzymatic activity, peaking by 90 seconds with a biological half-life of 3.5–10 min (longer than TxA_2). It undergoes rapid non-enzymatic conversion to stable inert $PGF_{2\alpha}$, which can be used to measure PGI_2 production. Red cells bind and inactivate PGI_2. Prostacyclin has been given by local infusion in (1) incipient gangrene due to arterial embolism, (2) Raynaud's phenomenon, (3) severe peripheral vascular disease.

In vitro PGI_2 reduces platelet retention in glass bead columns to a minimum of 15%, and inhibits kaolin-induced platelet factor 3 availability.

Prostacyclin deficiency

- High-dose aspirin therapy inhibits prostacyclin synthase, but for a shorter period than it inhibits platelet cyclo-oxygenase activity. Low-dose aspirin does not inhibit systemic prostacyclin.
- Vascular endothelium in diabetes mellitus, increased by insulin therapy.
- Atherosclerotic vascular tissue.
- The umbilical and placental vessels in pre-eclampsia.
- Systemic lupus erythematosus: circulating 'lupus' anticoagulants inhibits its synthesis.
- Sickle-cell disease.
- Cigarette smokers: urine $PGF_{2\alpha}$ reduced.

References
Chesterman, C. N., Owe-Young, G., Macpherson, J. and Krilis, S. A. (1986) *Blood* **67**, 1744
Schafer, A. I., Zavoico, G. B., Loscalzo, J. and Maas, A. K. (1987) *Blood* **69**, 1504
Stuart, M. J. and Sills, R. H. (1981) *Br. J. Haematol.* **48**, 545
Willems, C., Stel, H. V., Van Aben, W. *et al.* (1983) *Br. J. Haematol.* **53**, 43

Platelet factor 3 availability test

When plasma clotting factor deficiencies have been excluded, faulty release of platelet factor 3, following activation of platelet-rich plasma with kaolin, may be demonstrated if the plasma clotting time is compared with that obtained using platelet-poor plasma from the patient plus patient's platelets which have been lysed by suspension in distilled water, sonicated, or frozen and thawed. Kaolin release of factor 3 is only 15% of that obtained by sonication or repeated freezing and thawing. The test depends on the surface exposure of procoagulant phospholipid in the platelet membrane, platelet aggregation and fibrinogen binding to the platelet membrane. It is only a useful test, if more specific platelet function tests are not available.

Pathological

Increase

Hyperlipoproteinaemia (e.g. type IIa) which returns to normal after successful treatment with clofibrate or nicotinic acid.

Defective release of factor 3

PRIMARY

- Primary platelet disorders, including Glanzmann's disease, Bernard–Soulier giant platelet syndrome, isolated platelet factor 3 deficiency.

Reference
Sultan, Y., Brouet, J. C. and Devergie, A. (1976) *N. Engl. J. Med.* **294**, 1121

- Glycogen storage disease type I – glucose-6-phosphatase deficiency.

SECONDARY

- After 600 mg aspirin factor 3 release is reduced by 50% in 2 hours, returning to normal in 5–8 days.
- Uraemia, improved by dialysis.
- Macroglobulinaemia, lupus erythematosus.
- In some cases of myeloproliferative disease, liver disease, scurvy, sprue and pernicious anaemia, there is also a deficiency of platelet factor 3, and the clotting time is normalized when lysed normal platelets are added.

Platelet survival

Normal platelets survive for 8–10 days in the human circulation. They are removed when senescent, but some undergo 'random' destruction, There is a normal continual loss of surface glycoprotein from platelets, which may occur during reversible aggregation and adhesion, with recirculation, at minute sites of damage in the circulation. Some platelets undergo release reaction to repair minute sites of damage in the vascular endothelium in vessels of all sizes, including especially the capillaries, and are lost from the circulation. A variable proportion of platelets are sequestered in the spleen. About 18% of the platelets are used in the normal circulation each day. The platelet lifespan is only moderately reduced when the whole blood platelet count is $50–100 \times 10^9/l$, but it is markedly reduced when the count falls below $50 \times 10^9/l$.

Reference
Hanson, S. R. and Schlichter, S. J. (1985) *Blood* **66**, 1105

Platelet survival reduced

Antibody action

1. Fetomaternal incompatibility.
2. Post-transfusion.
3. Idiopathic thrombocytopenic purpura.
4. Drug-induced platelet destruction.
5. Secondary to:
   (a) systemic lupus erythematosus;
   (b) lymphoma;
   (c) allergic reactions.

Increased consumption of platelets

- Disseminated intravascular coagulopathy (DIC).
- Microangiopathic haemolytic anaemia.
- Severe infection.
- Postoperation, and post-trauma: platelets utilized at wound sites.
- Venous thrombosis, thromboembolism.
- Cerebrovascular accident.
- Myocardial infarction.
- Myeloma: with increased TxB_2, β-thromboglobulin and PF4 release.

Reference
Fritz, E., Ludwig, H., Scheithauer, W. *et al.* (1986) *Blood* **68**, 514

Inherited platelet abnormalities

Chronic conditions

- Atherosclerosis.
- Venous and arterial thromboembolism.
- Intravascular prosthesis.

Reference
Verstraete, M. (1976) *Am. J. Med.* **61**, 897

- Neoplasia.
- Vasculitis.
- Hypoxia.
- Homocystinuria.
- Hyperlipidaemia.
- Haemorrhagic states.

Platelet disorders

1. Qualitative platelet defects
   (a) defects of platelet membrane
   (b) platelet storage disease
   (c) platelet disorders secondary to disease
   (d) deficiencies of thromboxane synthesis and action
   (e) deficiencies of other enzymes
2. Platelet antibodies
3. Platelet transfusion

Qualitative platelet defects

Defects of platelet membrane

Glanzmann's thrombasthenia [AR]

This condition, due to a deficiency of platelet glyco-proteins GP-IIa/GP-IIIa, is associated with a lifetime of bruising, epistaxis and bleeding from mucous membranes. The platelet count is normal and the platelets appear normal in stained blood films. Homozygotes lack GP-IIb/GP-IIIa and intraplatelet fibrinogen. The bleeding time is prolonged, clot retraction is impaired, as is platelet aggregation in response to ADP, thrombin and adrenaline. Aggregation with collagen is only reversible, but aggregation with ristocetin is normal. Platelet retention is reduced, as is platelet factor 3 availability. ADP induces normal platelet shape change, but TxA_2 production is defective. Thrombin and arachidonic acid both induce normal TxA_2 production.

The reduced amounts of GP-IIb/GP-IIIa in the platelets of heterozygotes are sufficient to make them symptomless, although their clot reaction is impaired.

Bernard–Soulier giant platelet syndrome [AR]

This is a mild bruising and bleeding diathesis, with excessive bleeding after trauma, which may be manifest from the first week of life. The platelet count is normal or moderately reduced, with giant platelets to be seen in stained blood films, although in suspension the platelets are of normal volume. Platelet GP-I, with an abnormally low sialic content, is grossly reduced. The bleeding time is increased, with normal or mildly defective clot retraction. Platelet aggregation in response to ADP, adrenaline, thrombin, collagen and arachidonic acid is normal, but ADP does not induce the normal change in platelet shape from disc to sphere. Aggregation with collagen is faulty, and aggregation with ristocetin is also defective and not corrected by vWF in normal plasma. Platelet retention and factor 3 availability tests are reduced.

Heterozygotes are clinically unaffected.

Primary platelet procoagulant defect [R]

A rare, mild, bleeding diathesis is reported, due to reduced binding sites for factor Va on platelet membrane. The bleeding time is normal and platelet aggregation tests are normal. Platelet factor 3 availability is defective, and is not corrected by lysed normal platelets.

References
Miletich, J. P., Kane, W. H., Hofmann, S. L. et al. (1979) Blood 54, 1015
Weiss, H. J., Vicic, W. J., Lages, B. A. et al. (1979) Am. J. Med. 67, 206

Platelet storage disease

Decrease of substances stored in dense granules

- Chédiak–Higashi syndrome.
- Hermansky–Pudlak syndrome: with oculocutaneous albinism and pigmented ceroid-containing macrophages in the bone marrow. Heterozygotes clinically normal, with platelets normal except for reduced 5-HT content.
- Wiskott–Aldrich syndrome: small platelets.
- Thrombocytopenia with absent radii syndrome.

Decrease of substances stored in α-granules

Grey platelet syndrome: bleeding after tooth extraction, and epistaxes. Platelet aggregation with ADP, adrenaline, collagen and sodium arachidonate normal, but poor reversible aggregation with thrombin. TxB_2 production is normal. Electron microscopy detects reduction in α-granules.

Reference
Srivastava, P. C., Powling, M. J., Nokes, T. J. C et al. (1987) Br. J. Haematol. 65, 441

Decrease in both dense and α-granule contents

This is rare.

Laboratory tests for platelet storage disease

Patients with a mild bleeding diathesis, prolonged bleeding time and decreased total platelet ADP and serotonin are probably suffering from platelet storage disease, and are relatively common. Platelet aggregation tests may be normal.

Reference
Nieuwenhuis, H. K., Akkerman, J-W. N. and Sixma, J. J. (1987) Blood 70, 620

Platelet disorders secondary to disease

Diabetes mellitus

Platelets from diabetics are more reactive, and respond in vitro to lower concentrations of ADP, adrenaline and arachidonic acid than normal. There are also increased numbers of circulating platelet aggregates. Plasma vWF is increased with increasing age of the patient, and also in parallel with increasing severity of peripheral arterial occlusive disease. Plasma fibrinogen is increased and fibrinolytic activity is reduced. These findings help to explain, in part, the increased tendency to premature vascular degeneration and atherosclerosis.

Severe postoperative sepsis with thrombocytopenia

Endotoxins induce platelet release reaction with loss of platelets which, with toxic marrow depression, results in thrombocytopenia. In the absence of DIC, the MPV is low. Cases with increasing MPV and increasing platelet count tend to recover, whilst the MPV remains low in patients who do not recover from sepsis.

References
Bessman, J. D. and Gardner, F. H. (1983) Surg. Gynecol. Obstet. 156, 177
Hawiger, J., Hawiger, A., Steckley, S. et al. (1977) Br. J. Haematol. 35, 285

Thrombotic thrombocytopenic purpura

Degradation of plasma PGI_2 is increased. Treatment with fresh frozen or fresh plasma is more effective than plasmapheresis and albumin replacement, suggesting a plasma factor deficiency.

Reference
Chen, Y-C., McLeod, B., Hall, E. R. et al. (1981) Lancet ii, 267

Idiopathic thrombocytopenic purpura

In this autoimmune disease, there are abnormally large numbers of IgG molecules attached to the Fab factor. The antibody in the IgG3 fraction can cross the placenta to attack fetal platelets.

Reference
McMillan, R., Tani, P. and Mason, D. (1980) Blood 56, 993

Homocystinuria

Platelet adhesiveness is greatly increased in proportion to the increased plasma homocysteine concentration. Premature acute myocardial infarction and pulmonary embolism occur in adolescence.

Deficiencies of thromboxane synthesis and action

Cyclo-oxygenase deficiency [R]

In this rare mild bleeding condition, the bleeding time is abnormally increased. Only the first phase of aggregation of platelets is induced by ADP and thrombin, adrenaline and ristocetin. Neither collagen nor arachidonic acid induce platelet aggregation. Complete platelet aggregation is induced by calcium ionophore. Unlike thromboxane A_2 synthase deficiency, the patient's plasma does not contain malondialdehyde.

References
Legarde, M., Bryon, P. A., Vargaftig, B. B. et al. (1978) Br. J. Haematol. 38, 251
Pareti, F. I., Mannucci, P. M., D'Angelo, A. et al. (1980). Lancet i, 898

Familial thromboxane synthase deficiency [R]

In this rare condition associated with a moderate bleeding tendency, the bleeding time is prolonged. In vitro aggregation of platelets with arachidonic acid is absent, aggregation with 4 mol/l ADP is reversible (irreversible with normal platelets), and adrenaline only induces a single wave aggregation. When platelets are incubated with arachidonic acid, TxB_2 production

is abnormally low, but HETE production is normal. The patient's plasma contains malondialdehyde.

References
Defreyn, G., Machin, S. J., Carreras, L. O. et al. (1981) Br. J. Haematol. 49, 29
Machin, S. J., Carreras, L. O., Chamone, D. A. F. et al. (1980) Acta Therapeut. 6, 34

Defective platelet response to TxA_2 [R]

References
Hardisty, R. M., Keenan, J. P., Machin, S. P. et al. (1982) Br. J. Haematol. 52, 133
Lages, B., Malmsten, C., Weiss, H. J. et al. (1981) Blood 57, 545

Deficiency of other platelet enzymes

Lipoxygenase deficiency [R]

This rare congenital deficiency is associated with spontaneous platelet aggregation and thrombosis. In vitro platelet aggregation in response to arachidonic acid occurs at unusually low concentration.

Platelet antibodies

1. Platelets carry A, B and O antigens, but do not contain Rh antigens.
2. Platelets carry HLA antigens, 70–80% of which are adsorbed. ?Its origin.

Reference
Kao, K. J., Cook, D. J. and Scornik, J. C. (1986) Blood 68, 627

3. Platelet-specific antigens:
   (a) Dazo system;
   (b) Pl^A(Zno) system: population 97% Pl^{A1}-positive, 3% Pl^{A1}-negative;
   (c) Ko system;
   (d) Pl^E system.

Platelet transfusion

Indications

Active bleeding with thrombocytopenia or abnormal platelet function. Transfusion is unlikely to be of benefit if the count with normal platelet function is $> 50 \times 10^9/l$. Platelet transfusion is given to surgical operation when there is thrombocytopenia.

Risks

Risks include alloimmunization, infection and very rarely, graft versus host disease, prevented by irradiation of platelet concentrates before transfusion. Post-transfusion purpura is rare, and occurs most often in patients with Pl^{A1}-negative platelets who develop anti-Pl^{A1}-positive antibodies. These destroy the remaining transfused platelets; these then become adsorbed onto the patient's platelets, which are in turn destroyed.

Reference:
Kickler, T. S., Ness, P. M., Herman, J. H. and Bell, W. R. (1986) *Blood*
68, 347

Compatibility tests

As many as one-third of closely HLA-matched platelet transfusions fail to achieve satisfactory results. An indirect Coombs' test using ^{125}I-labelled goat anti-human IgG has been used where multiple platelet transfusions have been given.

References
Kickler, T. S., Braine, H. G., Ness, P. M. *et al.* (1983) *Blood* **61**, 238
McFarland, J. G. and Aster, R. H. (1987) *Blood* **69**, 1425 (comparison of four methods)
Platelet Transfusion. Concensus Conference (1987) *J. Am. Med. Assoc.* **257**, 1777

Drug actions on platelets

- Aspirin
- Dipyridamol
- ω-3 Fish triglycerides
- Vegetable triglycerides
- Ticlopidine
- Dextran
- Sulphinpyrazone

Aspirin

Oral acetylsalicylic acid (aspirin) acetylates and inactivates platelet cyclo-oxygenase while they are in the gut capillaries during absorption of aspirin. This enzyme inactivation interrupts the arachidonate cascade, and lasts the life of affected platelets. Thromboxane A_2 (TxA_2) synthesis is reduced, as the substrate for TxA_2 synthase is reduced. This is shown by the fall in serum TxB_2, the inert stable metabolite of TxA_2, before aspirin is detected in the systemic circulation.

The effects of aspirin can be demonstrated in vitro, using collagen-induced platelet aggregation as a test, for 4–7 days after a single dose of 300 mg aspirin. Unfortunately a residual 10% capacity in platelets to form TxA_2 in response to stimuli can sustain thromboxane-dependent platelet aggregation.

Aspirin doses of 300 mg per day or more

Aspirin has a plasma half-life of 15 minutes, and salicylate has a plasma half-life of 2–3 h (low dose), or 15–30 h (high dose and poisoning). In high doses, aspirin acts on platelet cyclo-oxygenase in the systemic circulation as well as in the portal circulation, on megakaryocytes in the bone marrow, but also inactivates prostacyclin synthase in the systemic vascular endothelium, reducing protective prostacyclin (PGI_2) generation there for a few hours after each dose.

Secondary aggregation of platelets induced by adrenaline, antigen–antibody complex, γ-globulin-coated surfaces and low concentrations of thrombin is reduced. Platelet collagen glucosal transferase activity is also reduced by acetylation. Given alone in doses of 300 mg/day or more, aspirin reduces reinfarction rates after myocardial infarction by 20%, improves survival after strokes and in transient ischaemia and reduces the risk of death in patients suffering from angina by half. Combining aspirin with dipyridamol has been found to be more effective. The combination reduces the rate of reinfarction after myocardial infarction, maintains the patency of coronary artery grafts and slows the rate of deterioration of renal damage in chronic kidney disease. Unfortunately doses of aspirin 300 mg or more daily over long periods are often associated with gastrointestinal disturbances, and even bleeding into the gut.

Aspirin doses of 80 mg per day or less

Low dose aspirin avoids both gastrointestinal irritation and suppression of PGI_2 synthesis in the systemic circulation. Aspirin 20 mg at midnight for 7 days reduces TxB_2 generation, measured in the morning, by 85–93%, with complete suppression of archidonate-induced platelet aggregation. A daily dose of 40 mg aspirin produces inhibitory effects on platelets indistinguishable from those produced by 325 mg aspirin. Increasing the dose to 80 mg aspirin daily, 40 mg aspirin twice daily or repeated doses of 10 mg aspirin hourly through the day, produces very full suppression of TxA_2 release without gastrointestinal irritation or suppression of PGI_2 synthesis, although PGI_2 production is suppressed in the mesenteric veins.

The degree of suppression of cyclo-oxygenase is not associated with any bleeding tendency as congenital cyclo-oxgenase deficiency is a very mild bleeding diathesis. During low dose aspirin treatment, template bleeding sites show 90% inhibition of TxB_2 formation in both bleeding time blood and clotted blood, with inhibition of thrombin formation.

Low-dose aspirin reduces postoperative thrombosis after total hip joint replacement, and also reduces the incidence of pregnancy-induced hypertension and preeclampsia (associated with TxA_2 generation). The combination of low-dose aspirin with mini-dose warfarin or dipyridamol or both, could have dramatic effects on the treatment of thromboembolic diseases. As plasma aspirin esterase activity is lower in frail hospitalized, elderly patients, they will probably require a lower dose of aspirin.

References
Alfaro, M. J., Paramo, J. A. and Rocha E. (1986) *Thromb. Haemost.* **56**, 53

Cerletti, C., Carriero, M. R. and de Gaetano, G. (1986) *N. Engl. J. Med.* **314**, 316
Di Minno, G., Silver, M. J. and Murphy, S. (1983) *Blood* **61**, 1081
Jakubowski, J. A., Stampfer, M. J., Vaillancourt, R *et al.* (1985) *Br. J. Haematol.* **60**, 635
Kyrle, P. A., Westwick, J., Scully, M. F. *et al.* (1987) *Thromb. Haemost.* **57**, 62
Patrono, C., Ciabattoni, G., Patrignani, P. *et al.* (1985) *Circulation* **72**, 1177
Pedersen, A. K. and Fitzgerald, G. A. (1984) *N. Engl. J. Med.* **311**, 1206
Schwartz, L., Bourassa, M. G., Lesperance, J. *et al.* (1988) *N. Engl. J. Med.* **318**, 1714
Wallenburg, H. C. S., Dekker, G. A., Makovitz, J. W. *et al.* (1986) *Lancet* **i**, 1
Williams, F. M., Wynne, H., Woodhouse, K. W. and Rawlins, M. D. (1989) *Age and Ageing* **18**, 39

Dipyridamol

Dipyridamol, first developed as a coronary artery dilator, acts on platelets in whole blood, but has little effect in platelet-rich plasma. It potentiates and directly stimulates release of prostacyclin (PGI$_2$) from vascular endothelium. It also inhibits cell uptake and metabolism of adenosine, resulting in increased adenosine concentration at the platelet–vascular interface. Platelet survival is prolonged, and abnormally reduced platelet survival in thrombovascular disease is increased towards normal.

Dipyridamol enhances adenylate cyclase activity (potentiated by PGI$_2$) and as a result increases platelet cAMP. cAMP competes for platelet-binding sites with ADP, reducing platelet ADP content and hence platelet adhesiveness. Breakdown of cAMP to AMP by phosphodiesterase is inhibited, prolonging the reduction in platelet adhesiveness. Platelet aggregation by PGE$_1$ is also inhibited. These actions are potentiated by low-dose aspirin. Dipyridamol should be given in combination with aspirin, as there is pharmacokinetic interaction. If low-dose aspirin is used, then warfarin can also be safely given.

Clinical applications

Aspirin and dipyridamol reduce non-fatal myocardial infarction by about 20%. This combination is also useful in maintaining patency in coronary artery grafts. When given with low-dose warfarin, there may be a greater reduction in thromboembolic complications in cardiac valve disease, than when low-dose warfarin is given alone.

Dipyridamol with aspirin slows the deterioration in renal function in patients with type I membranoproliferative glomerulonephritis.

References
Fitzgerald, G. A. (1987) *N. Engl. J. Med.* **316**, 1247
Perez-Requejo, J. L., Aznar, J. and Santos, M. T. (1985) *Thromb. Haemost.* **54**, 799
Weiss, H. J. (1982) *Platelets, Pathophysiology and Antiplatelet Drug Therapy.* New York: Liss

ω-3 Fish triglycerides

This includes eicosapentaenoic acid (C$_{20:5}$, ω-3) and docosahexaenoic acid (C$_{22:6}$, ω-3). Eskimos living on a high fatty fish diet (mackerel, seal blubber etc.) have a very low incidence of coronary heart disease, and almost non-existent atherosclerosis. The incidence of heart disease and atherosclerosis is high in the UK by contrast. When arachidonic acid is added to the Greenland Eskimo fish diet, platelet activity is increased to the western European level of activity.

A high intake of cold water, fatty fish oils, or of fish oil concentrates rich in eicosapentaenoic acid and docosahexaenoic acid, by Europeans results in changes in the blood resembling those found in Eskimos on fish diets. ω-3 Fatty acids replace ω-6 fatty acids in red cells and platelet membranes. There is an increase in platelet survival and a fall in the total platelet count by 15%. Both platelet factor 4 and β-thromboglobulin, markers for platelet destruction in the circulation, are reduced significantly. Platelet aggregation response is reduced within one week, as TxA$_3$ derived from ω-3 fatty acids is much less active than TxA$_2$ (derived from arachidonic acid) in causing platelet aggregation, release and local vasospasm. TxA$_3$ is produced in the prostacyclin–thromboxane cascade at the expense of TxA$_2$. PGI$_3$, derived from ω-3 fatty acids, is as active as PGI$_2$ in inhibiting platelet aggregation and release, and in inhibiting local vasospasm.

The increased bleeding time, found in native Eskimos on high fish diets, does not develop if the diet contains adequate amounts of the essential fatty acid linoleic acid. Red cell deformability is increased, with consequent decrease in whole blood viscosity at constant mean cell volume (MCV) and haematocrit, without change in the plasma viscosity. The maximal incorporation of ω-3 fatty acids in the red cell membrane occurs by 14 weeks.

Blood pressure response to noradrenaline is decreased, and blood vessel wall reactivity to noradrenaline is reduced. It has also been found that plasma fibrinogen falls significantly over a 4-year period on fish oil supplements. Plasma triglyceride levels in hyperlipidaemias fall from abnormally high to high normal values, and from high normal to normal values. Plasma HDL$_2$ is increased as plasma VLDL concentrations fall. When the initial baseline serum cholesterol level is raised, fish oils cause a fall with increase in HDL cholesterol, and fibrinolytic activity is increased.

Eating a fish meal twice weekly results in a significant fall in the incidence of heart attacks. Mackerel contains an inhibitor of platelet aggregation by ADP, which is not eicosapentaenoic acid. Eskimos on high eicosapentaenoic acid intake have higher plasma AT-III levels than Caucasian Danes living in Greenland.

References
Dyerberg, J., Bang, H. O., Stofferson, E. *et al.* (1978) *Lancet* **ii**, 117
Fischer, S. and Weber, P. C. (1984) *Nature* **307**, 165
Hay, C. R. M., Durber, A. P. and Saynor, R. (1982) *Lancet* **i**, 1269
Honda, J., Iwamoto, M., Shichijo, S. *et al.* (1991) *Lancet* **338**, 817
Jorgensen, K. A., Nielsen, A. H. and Dyerberg, J. (1986) *Acta Med. Scand.* **219**, 473
Saynor, R. and Gillott, T. (1988) *Br. Med J.* **297**, 1196
Second MaxEPA Conference (1984) *Br. J. Clin. Pract.* Suppl. 31

Vegetable triglycerides

Dihomo-γ-linolenic acid ($C_{20:3}$, ω-6)

A diet fortified with added dihomo-γ-linolenic acid was thought to result in the generation of TxA_1 by platelets on activation, which was relatively inactive, and PGI_1 by the vessel endothelium, which was active. There was also some decrease in heparin neutralization by plasma, with reduction in ADP-induced platelet aggregation. When this dietary supplement is sustained, there is also in vitro inhibition of ristocetin-induced platelet aggregation. Unfortunately if the daily dose of dihomo-ω-linolenic acid exceeds 2 mg/kg body weight, the substance appears to develop thrombogenic properties.

References
Kernoff, P. B. A., Willis, A. L., Stone, K. J. *et al.* (1977) *Br. Med. J.* **2**, 1441
Sim, A. K. and McCraw, A. P. (1978) *Br. Med. J.* **1**, 236

Ticlopidine

Ticlopidine, a thienopyridine, causes dose-related inhibition of ADP-induced platelet aggregation. It also inhibits platelet aggregation induced by low concentrations of collagen, arachidonic acid, TxA_2 and thrombin. Rapidly absorbed when given orally, with peak plasma values at 2h, full antiplatelet activity does not occur until 2–4 days later, and maximal prolongation of the bleeding time occurs after this. These effects persist for several days after the drug has been discontinued. The inhibitory effects of PGI_2 are enhanced, and arterial production of PGI_2 is increased. Ticlopidine has been used successfully to reduce reocclusion of coronary artery grafts. In doses of 250 mg twice daily ticlopidine reduces the incidence of myocardial infarction, stroke, and death from vascular disorders, in both men and women. Reversible adverse effects include neutropenia, skin rashes and diarrhoea.

References
Ashida, S. and Abiko, Y. (1978) *Thromb. Haemost.* **40**, 542
Ashida, S. and Abiko Y. (1979) *Thromb. Haemost.* **41**, 436
Gent, M., Blakely, J. A. Easton, J. D. *et al.* (1989) *Lancet* **i**, 1215
Johnson, M. and Heywood, J. B. (1979) *Thromb. Haemost.* **42**, 376
Lips J. P. M., Sixma, J. and Schiphorst, M. E. (1980) *Thromb. Res.* **17**, 19

O'Brien, J. R., Etherington, M. D. and Shuttleworth, R. D. (1978) *Thromb. Res.* **13**, 245
Tissinier, A. M. (1988) *Rev. Iberoam. Tromb. Haemost.* **S1**, 59

Dextran

In patients with no haemorrhagic diathesis there is no risk of haemorrhage when doses of less than 1–1.5 g/kg body weight are given. Dextran infusion can cause haemorrhage in haemophilia, von Willebrand's disease, severe uraemia and during heparin therapy. It should therefore only be given under these circumstances with great care.

Dextran causes reduction in ADP-induced platelet aggregation, also a reduction in plasma factor VIIIRAg (von Willebrand factor).

Thrombi formed in blood from patients receiving dextran are more lysable than thrombi formed in blood without dextran.

Reference
Begquist, D. (1982) *Acta Chir. Scand.* **148**, 633

Sulphinpyrazone action on platelets

Sulphinpyrazone is rapidly absorbed, and reaches peak plasma values by 1–2 h. The plasma half-life is about 2–3 h, but action continues for up to 18 h (presumably via metabolites). It is protein-bound in the plasma and, on normal dosage, plasma concentrations are about 80 $\mu mol/l$.

Sulphinpyrazone acts by inhibiting platelet cyclo-oxygenase, and aggregation with collagen, adrenaline and antigen–antibody complexes, but not thrombin, is inhibited. In experiments it has been shown to inhibit the adhesion of platelets to de-endothelialized aorta. In practice, its activity is not great and it is not regularly used as an anti-platelet agent. The whole blood clotting time, prothrombin time and activated partial thromboplastin time are unaffected.

References
Buchanan, M. R., Rosenfeld, J. and Hirsh, J. (1978) *Thromb. Res.* **13**, 883
The Anturane Reinfarction Trial Research Group (1980) *N. Engl. J. Med.* **302**, 250
Wong, L T., Zawidzka, Z. and Thomas, B. F. (1978) *Pharmacol. Res. Commun.* **10**, 939

Fibrinolysis

1. Fibrinolysis
2. Fibrin I and fibrin II
3. Soluble fibrin
4. Fibrinopeptide A
5. Fibrinopeptide B
6. Plasminogen
7. Plasminogen activators
8. Plasminogen activator inhibitor
9. Plasmin

10. Antiplasmins
11. Fibrinolytic activity in the blood
12. Haemorrhage associated with fibrinolytic system activation
13. Tests used in the assessment of fibrinolysis
14. Fibrinogen, fibrin degradation products and cross-linked fibrin degradation products
15. Fibrinolytic therapy
    (a) streptokinase;
    (b) urokinase
16. Thrombolytic therapy
17. Complications of thrombolytic therapy
18. Contraindications to thrombolytic therapy
19. Ancrod – therapeutic defibrination
20. Antifibrinolytic agents

Fibrinolysis

The firm fibrin clot is the end-stage of the acute coagulation cascade, after fibrin monomers have been formed. Fibroblasts move through the fibrin network of the clot during healing, a network of collagen is laid down and fibrin is dissolved by plasmin. Neutrophils play some part in the dissolution of the fibrin. Superfluous fibrin is also dissolved, and clots in the circulation are removed. Fibrin monomer is lysed easily by plasmin, but factor XIII-stabilized fibrin polymer is lysed much more slowly. Ideally, the fibrinolytic system dissolves inappropriate clots as fast as they form, preventing the spread of clotting through the circulation, and also limiting the size of essential clots to their local requirement.

Inadequate fibrinolysis leads to abnormal excessive thrombus formation and embolism, whilst excessive fibrinolysis, with dissolution of essential fibrin clots before healing is complete, can lead to serious bleeding.

A plasminogen activator with enhanced fibrin selectivity cannot differentiate between a thrombus which threatens the heart and one which prevents exsanguination, for example in an artery in an eroded peptic ulcer. On the other hand, streptokinase necessitates production and release of new clotting proteins before normal haemostasis is restored.

Fibrin I and fibrin II

Thrombin cleaves fibrinogen to release first fibrinopeptide A (FPA), and then fibrinopeptide B (FPB), with sequential activation of two sets of polymerization sites. Fibrin I forms as end-to-end polymers, after FPA has been removed, which are rapidly lysed by plasmin. Fibrin I is soluble in monochloroacetic acid, and is rapidly lysed by plasmin.

After release of fibrinopeptide B (FPB), fibrin II is formed, and this has both end-to-end and side-to-side linkages as polymers form. The side-to-side links form following the action of factor XIIIa, which is itself activated by thrombin. Cross-linked fibrin is less susceptible to digestion by plasmin, which is why fibrinolytic therapy is more effective if given soon after a thrombus has formed.

Soluble fibrin

Soluble fibrin is formed when limited action of thrombin releases fibrinopeptide A from fibrinogen. The fibrin complexes with plasma fibrinogen and is kept in solution. It is detected by:

- Protamine sulphate precipitation.
- Ethanol gelation test.
- NH_2-terminal analysis.

Increased
- Early stages of severe disseminated intravascular coagulopathy.
- Low-grade intravascular coagulopathy.
- Myocardial infarction (some cases).
- Normal or complicated pregnancy.

Reference
Mckillop, C., Howie, P. W., Forbes, C. D. et al. (1976) Lancet i, 56
- Therapeutic ancrod defibrination.
- Certain snake bites.

References
van Hulsteijn, H., Fibbe, W., Bertian, R. et al. (1982) Thromb. Haemost. 48, 247
Yudelman, I. (1987) Thromb. Haemost. 57, 11
Yudelman, I. M., Nossel, H. L., Kaplan, K. L. et al. (1978) Blood 51, 1189

Fibrinopeptide A (FPA)

FPA, released when fibrinogen is converted to fibrin I, has a half-life in the circulation of only 3–5 minutes, but can be used as a marker of continuing thrombin activity.

Increase
- Venous thrombosis with or without pulmonary embolism. High plasma levels of FPA occur in patients with impaired resolution, and also possible greater risk of recurrent thromboembolic episodes.
- Malignancy.
- Uraemia.
- Some cases of dysfibrinogenaemia.
- Therapeutic defibrination using ancrod (Arvin). The snake venom releases FPA, but no FPB, so that there is no activation of factor XIII or release of thrombin.

- Severe bacterial infection, including patients with acute myelobastic leukaemia with septicaemia.
- Active lupus erythematosus.

Fibrinopeptide B (FPB)

FPB is released from fibrin I, with the formation of fibrin II, after FPA has been released from fibrinogen by thrombin. It is thought to have chemotactic activity, and may be important in preventing wound infection.

Reference
Nossel, H. L. (1981) *Nature* **291**, 165

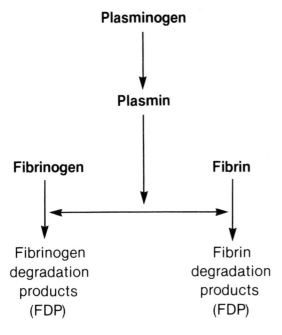

Plasminogen

Plasmin

Fibrinogen   **Fibrin**

Fibrinogen   Fibrin
degradation   degradation
products   products
(FDP)   (FDP)

Action of plasmin on fibrin and/or fibrinogen resulting in the formation of fibrin/fibrinogen degradation products (FDP).

Plasminogen

Plasminogen is a single polypeptide chain, synthesized in the liver, with a molecular weight of 92 000, and is present in the plasma at a concentration of 10–20 mg/100 ml. Part of its molecule contains the active serine esterase of plasmin, with sites homologous in pancreatic serine esterase, prothrombin and factor Xa. The remainder of the molecule contains five 'kringle' structures, comparable in structure with factors X and

II, with three specific binding sites for lysine in fibrin.

Native plasminogen (glutamyl-plasminogen) has a glutamyl residue at its N-terminal, and has a high affinity for fibrinogen and fibrin. On activation, it is converted to two polypeptide chains linked by di-sulphide bridges. Plasminogen, especially Lys-plasminogen, attaches preferentially to fibrin. Plasminogen activators have affinity for fibrin, and their activity is greatly enhanced by contact with fibrin, Therefore plasminogen is converted to plasmin primarily at the surface of fibrin. Free plasmin in the circulation is immediately bound and neutralized by α_2-antiplasmin (or α_2-macroglobulin).

Increase

After strenuous exercise lasting 0–90 min, plasminogen levels increase in the plasma. This increase is no longer apparent after a further 90 min.

Reference
Marsh, N. A. and Gaffney, P. J. (1982) *Thromb. Haemost.* **48**, 201

Decrease

- Plasminogen activity falls after 6 weeks of clofibrate therapy, increasing again after 14 weeks of treatment.
- Liver disease.

Reference
Cederblad, G. and Korsam-Bengsten, K. (1976) *Clin. Chim. Acta* **66**, 9

Abnormal form of plasminogen

Three different abnormalities have been described, associated with recurrent attacks of venous thrombosis:

- Homozygote: defect in the active centre of the molecule.
- K_m activation defect in homozygote.
- Activation defect, impaired activation binding and defective molecular cleavage.

References
Mannucci, P. M., Kluft, C., Traas, D. W. *et al.* (1986) *Br. J. Haematol.* **63**, 753
Wohl, R. C., Summaria L., Chedial, J. *et al.* (1982) *Thromb. Haemost.* **48**, 146

Plasminogen activators

- In plasma Glu-plasminogen is initially converted to Glu-plasmin, which is converted by intrinsic plasminogen activator into active Lys-plasmin.
- In the presence of formed fibrin, Glu-plasminogen is initially converted to Lys-plasminogen, which is converted to active Lys-plasmin by extrinsic plasminogen activator. This reaction is 20 times faster

than the first reaction. Blood is cleared of circulating plasminogen activator by the liver. Native tissue activator binds to fibrin, and activates, fibrin-bound plasminogen.

Intrinsic plasminogen activator

Factor XII-dependent activator, lacking in Hageman factor, is formed by a reaction involving Hageman-factor cofactor, high-molecular-weight kininogen and prekallikrein. Factor XIIa, kallikrein and factor XIa can also activate plasminogen directly. The reaction is weak and slow.

There is also a factor XII-independent activator.

Extrinsic plasminogen activator or tissue plasminogen activator (t-PA)

The more important tissue-type plasminogen activator (t-PA) is a serine protease with a molecular weight of 70 000 and a plasma concentration of about 5 ng/ml, which activates plasminogen to form plasmin. It has a high affinity with the five kringles of plasminogen, and the single kringle of urokinase, and domains responsible for the affinity of fibronectin for fibrin. It is an enzyme with low activity in the absence of fibrin, and is rapidly broken down in the blood. Its activity is greatly increased in the presence of fibrin.

Synthesized by the vascular endothelium, it is more important than the urokinase-type plasminogen activator (u-PA), and increased release follows physical effort, venous occlusion for more than 5 min, catecholamine and DDAVP (vasopressin analogue).

After its release, it is adsorbed onto fibrin, and this renders it relatively inaccessible to t-PA inhibitors. Fibrin-bound t-PA activates fibrin-bound plasminogen to form active plasmin, which degrades fibrin before plasmin inhibitors stop its activity.

Decrease

- Normal pregnancy, with decreased euglobulin lysis.
- Postsurgical operation or injury results in decreased t-PA release or increased neutralization by plasminogen activator inhibitor, with decreased fibrinolytic activity.
- After recovery from a first acute myocardial infarction, it was found that those patients with marked t-PA activity suffered no relapse, whereas patients with little or no detectable t-PA activity reinfarcted within 4 years.
- Some cases of familial venous thrombosis had either low t-PA release, or increased PAI, with resulting low t-PA activity.

References
Gram, J. and Jespersen, J. (1987) *Thromb. Haemost.* **57**, 137
Hamsten, A., Wiman, B., de Faire, U. *et al.* (1985) *N. Engl. J. Med.* **313**, 1557
Paramo, J. A., Colucci, M., Collen, D. *et al.* (1985) *Br. Med. J.* **291**, 573
Verheijen, J. H., Chang, G. T. G. and Kluft, C. (1984) *Thromb Haemost.* **51**, 392
Wan, T-C. and Capuano, A. (1987) *Blood* **69**, 1354

Treatment with recombinant plasminogen activator, in doses which are clot specific and which do not cause general fibrinolysis, has been used to recanalize blocked coronary arteries relatively rapidly.

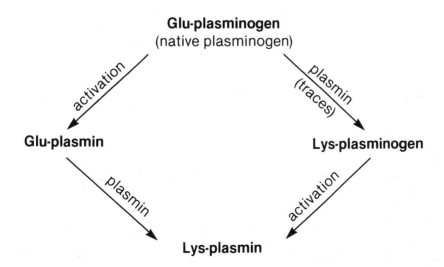

The two routes of plasminogen activation to plasmin.

References
ven de Werf, F. and Arnold, A. E. R. (1988) *Br. Med. J.* **297**, 1374
Verstraete, M. and Collen, D. (1986) *Blood* **67**, 1529

Urinary activator (u-PA, urokinase)

Urokinase is a trypsin-like protein consisting of two polypeptide chains connected by a disulphide link (see p. 185).

Plasminogen activators

Found in human milk, seminal fluid, cerebrospinal fluid, saliva, tears and bile.

Vascular endothelial activator

Released in response to venous occlusion.

White and red cell plasminogen activators

Bacterial activators

Streptokinase (SK) from β-haemolytic stretococci (see p. 185).

SK + Plasminogen →

SK–Plasminogen complex →

SK–Plasmin complex →

Plasmin + SK fragments

Plasminogen activator inhibitor (PAI)

Plasminogen activator inhibitor type 1 (PAI-1) reacts with urokinase-type plasminogen activator (u-PA) and tissue-type plasminogen activator (t-PA). Its activity is reflected by the short half-life of plasminogen activator (100 s). PAI-1 is present in endothelial cells, the liver and the α-granules of platelets. When platelets are stimulated by thrombin, PAI-1 is released on the platelet surface, protecting a blood clot from premature lysis. It is neutralized by activated protein C (APC) from the normal surrounding vascular endothelium, with protein S acting as cofactor.

A second plasminogen activator inhibitor, PAI-II is present in the placenta, and both types I and II are increased in normal pregnancy. Type II is only found during pregnancy.

Increase

- Normal pregnancy.
- Coronary artery disease, including patients with angina and stenosed coronary arteries. It is a risk factor for the recurrence of myocardial infarction.
- One-fifth of a series of 100 patients with 'spontaneous' deep vein thrombosis had increased levels of PAI-1 with normal t-PA, compared with one-tenth with low t-PA and normal levels of PAI-1.

- Triglyceridaemia, insulinaemia, malignancy, sepsis, inflammatory disease, after an operation and excess body weight.

References
Hamsten, A., Wiman, B., de Faire, U. *et al.* (1985) *N. Engl. J. Med.* **313**, 1557
Hamsten, A., de Faire, U., Walldius, G. *et al.* (1987) *Lancet* **ii**, 3
Juhan-Vague, I., Valadier, J., Alessi, M. C. *et al.* (1987) *Thromb. Haemost.* **57**, 67
Nilsson, I. M., Ljungner, H. and Tengborn, L. (1985) *Br. Med. J.* **290**, 1453
Sprengers, E. D. and Kluft, C. (1987) *Blood* **69**, 381

Plasmin

Plasmin has a molecular weight of 80 000, and consists of two polypeptide chains (molecular weights 26 000 and 55 000) linked by disulphide bonds. The light chain contains the active site which binds to fibrinogen and fibrin, attacking susceptible arginine and lysine bonds in the molecules. After 5–7 days, following polymerization and stabilization by factor XIIIa activity, fibrin becomes resistant to lysis by plasmin.

Plasmin activity is controlled by the availability of plasminogen activator, inhibitors competing for lysine-binding sites on plasminogen or plasmin, and inhibitors blocking active sites of the free enzyme. Its activity is continuously required to prevent fibrin deposition in veins.

Plasmin can cause lysis of glycocalicin, a fragment of the α-chain of the platelet membrane GP-Ia, the receptor for factor VIIIvWF, inhibiting platelet adhesion, an important activity in endogenous fibrinolysis or during fibrinolytic treatment, since it limits the extent of platelet adhesion and aggregation around a lesion on a vessel wall. When plasmin levels are excessively high in the circulation, factor V, factor VIII, complement, adenocorticotrophin (ACTH), human growth factor and glucagon can all be attacked, in addition to fibrin and fibrinogen.

Reference
Erickson, L. A., Fici, G. J., Lund, J. E. *et al.* (1990) *Nature* **346**, 74

Antiplasmins

The total antiplasmin activity can probably neutralize 10 times the available total plasmin activity in the plasma, and the main component is α_2-antiplasmin. α_2-Macroglobulin, α-antitrypsin and antithrombin III slowly inhibit plasmin activity, but probably only in pathophysiological circumstances when α_2-antiplasmin is depleted.

α_2-2 Antiplasmin

Free circulating plasmin is bound in a 1:1 complex with α_2-antiplasmin and neutralized. α_2-Antiplasmin is a single-chain glycoprotein with a molecular weight of 65 000–70 000. The normal plasma concentration is 1 μmol/l (60 mg/l). It circulates as a plasminogen-binding form produced by the liver (two-thirds), which inhibits plasmin-activated fibrinolysis, and a non-plasminogen-binding form produced in the circulation (one-third), which reacts more slowly with plasmin. Generalized plasmin activity in the circulation only occurs after all α_2-antitrypsin has been neutralized.

Platelets contain significant amounts of α_2-antiplasmin, which is released along with PF4 (antiheparin) following thrombin stimulation. This release helps to protect the integrity of a small local platelet thrombus. During clotting, 22% of α_2-antiplasmin binds to fibrin in the presence of factor XIII and calcium ions. Detection of plasmin–antiplasmin complexes in plasma is evidence of plasmin formation and fibrinolysis. Plasma α_2-antiplasmin has a biological half-life of about 2.5 days, falling to half a day during thrombolytic therapy. It is essential for factor XIIIa resistance to clot lysis.

Decrease

- Liver disease: reduced synthesis, increased catabolism.
- Disseminated intravascular coagulation.
- Streptokinase and urokinase therapy.
- Congenital deficiency of the plasminogen form [R]: a rare bleeding diathesis with bleeding into the joints in homozygotes, and a mild bleeding diathesis in heterozygotes. This condition demonstrates the importance of α_2-antitrypsin in localizing fibrinolysis.

References
Kluft, C., Los, P., Jie, A. F. et al. (1986) Blood 67, 616
Kluft, C., Vellenga, E., Brommer, E. J. P. et al. (1982) Blood 59, 1169

Fibrinolytic activity in the blood

Physiological

Increased

- After moderate to severe exercise for up to 24 h.
- Hyperventilation.
- Activity is greater during the day than the night, especially with increased physical activity.

Decreased

- Low activity in fetus to maintain a patent fetomaternal circulation.
- Normal newborn infant has lower activity than adult.

- After severe unaccustomed physical exercise, fibrinolytic activity falls during the subsequent day.
- Activity in arterial blood less than in venous blood.
- Normal pregnancy: activity returns to normal levels soon after delivery.
- Postmenopausal females when compared with younger adult females.

Pathological

Increased

- Aspirin.
- ACTH and steroids: after anabolic steriods (e.g. stanozolol) the euglobulin lysis time is restored towards normal if prolonged.
- Fibrinolytic agents – streptokinase, urokinase.
- Therapeutic defibrination with ancrod.
- Cardiopulmonary bypass.
- Secondary to disseminated intravascular coagulopathy (DIC).
- After 48 h following surgical operation, for the next 6–7 days.

Decreased

- Newborn infants with either respiratory distress syndrome, or DIC. There is rapid depletion of the fibrinolytic potential.
- Diabetes mellitus.
- Obesity.
- Pre-term infants.
- During the first 48-h after surgical operation.
- Renal damage: presence of excess fibrinolytic inhibitors in the blood; reduced production of urokinase, in parallel with increasing renal damage.

Haemorrhage associated with fibrinolytic system activation

- Systemic fibrinolysis (hyperplasminaemia).
- Secondary fibrinolysis following DIC.
- Local fibrinolysis: presumed excessive fibrinolytic activity near surgical operation site etc.
- Normal level of fibrinolysis in association with a coagulation defect.

Reference
Prentice, C. R. M. (1975) Thromb. Diath. Haemorrh. 34, 634

Tests used in assessment of fibrinolysis

Whole-blood clot lysis

Whole blood is allowed to clot, and any evidence of lysis is subsequently observed. This test is only useful in the detection of severe fibrinolysis.

Thrombin clotting time

1. If the ratio of the patient's plasma thrombin clotting time to that of a known normal control plasma result exceeds 1.3, repeat the test with equal mixtures of the patient's plasma and the control plasma:

   (a) clotting time approaches normal = deficiency state;

   (b) clotting time approaches patient's clotting time = presence of an inhibitor.

2. Clot serial dilutions of citrated plasma with a standard amount of thrombin, reading at 15 min the highest dilution at which a clot is visible, and reading again at 60 min for evidence of lysis of this clot.

   If addition of ε-aminocaproic acid to the system improves the clot and prevents lysis then this is evidence of the presence of active fibrinolysis.

Euglobulin clot lysis

This tests the ability of dilutions of the patient's plasma to lyse precipitated euglobulin.

Lysis of fibrin plates

Patient's plasma is added to plates of heated fibrin clot (i.e. plasminogen has been destroyed by heat before the test). Lysis of such fibrin by a patient's plasma confirms the presence of free circulating plasmin.

Plasminogen assay

Plasma is treated with streptokinase to convert available plasminogen to plasmin. After acting on casein, the digest is tested for liberation of free amino acid split from the casein by the proteolytic action of active plasmin. The level of plasmin activity indicates the level of available plasminogen. This test is useful during streptokinase therapy in arterial thrombosis.

Fibrinogen and fibrin degradation products (FDP) and cross-linked fibrin degradation products (XL-FDP)

Digestion of fibrinogen and fibrin results in the appearance of fragments of the molecules, with different molecular weights and different physical structures, depending on which lysine and arginine bonds have been attached by the activated enzyme. Platelet aggregation may be enhanced or inhibited. Some fragments are clottable by thrombin, whilst others interfere with coagulation. Increased fibrinopeptide-A (FPA) and β-thromboglobulin (from platelets) in the plasma reflect increased thrombin activity. However, increased cross-linked fibrin-degradation products (XL-FDP) and B_{15-41} (a short-lived product from fibrin with a half-life of 10–12 min) are found when there is increased fibrinolysis, as in DIC or after treatment with t-PA, or to a lesser degree with streptokinase. Normal plasma levels of XL-FDP exclude the presence of active venous thrombosis. The presence of XL-FDP indicates that firm polymerized fibrin has been formed somewhere and has undergone lysis.

References
Eisenberg, P. R., Sherman, L. A., Tiefenbrann, A. J. *et al.* (1987) *Thromb. Haemost.* **57**, 35
Francis, C. W., Alkjsersig, N., Galanakis, D. K. *et al.* (1987) *Thromb. Haemost.* **57**, 110
Rowbotham, B. J., Carroll, P., Whitaker, A. N. *et al.* (1987) *Thromb. Haemost.* **57**, 59
Yudelman, I. (1987) *Thromb. Haemost.* **57**, 11

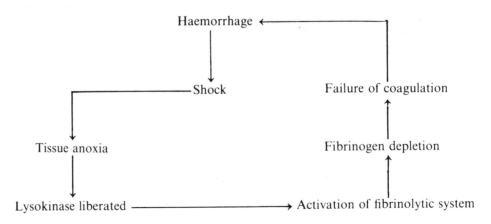

A haemorrhagic state can develop following haemorrhage, which is self-perpetuating.

Cross-linked fibrin and fibrinogen/fibrin degradation products

The normal level is 45 ng/ml. In diseases not associated with haemostatic mechanisms, it is 75 ng/ml. In intravascular activation:

- Treated deep vein thrombosis, uneventful surgical operation, local neoplasia, liver disease, symptomatic arterial disease – 150–400 ng/ml.
- Pulmonary embolism, disseminated carcinoma, severe inflammatory disease, postoperative complications, arterial thromboembolism, disseminated intravascular coagulopathy – 677–6900 ng/ml.

Streptokinase therapy reduces the concentration.

References
Hunt, F. A., Rylatt, D. B., Hart, R. A. *et al.* (1985) *Br. J. Haematol.* **60**, 715
Whitaker, A. N., Elms, M. J., Masci, P. P. *et al.* (1984) *J.Clin. Pathol.* **37**, 882

Fibrinolytic therapy

Streptokinase

Streptokinase is a derivative of β-haemolytic streptococcus group C, and consists of a single-chain α_2-globulin with a molecular weight of 46 000. It has no esterase or protease activity, but forms a complex with plasminogen, activating plasminogen to plasmin.

Treatment

1. Streptokinase 250 000–500 000 units intravenously, followed by 100 000 units hourly. The very large loading dose neutralizes any anti-streptococcal antibodies from previous streptococcal infections.
2. Local infusion of streptokinase onto a local thrombus in a blood vessel.
3. Intermittent therapy: 30-min infusion every 12–24 h, allowing regeneration of plasminogen by the liver.
4. Combination with other drugs has been tried:
   (a) heparin (unsuccessful);
   (b) preceded by ancrod;
   (c) low-dose (5000 units/h) plus systemic heparin.

Streptokinase activity persists for up to 2 h after the therapeutic infusion has been discontinued.

In some books it has been suggested that low-dose streptokinase therapy is dangerous, causing hyperplasminaemia, severe plasminogen and fibrinogen depletion, leading to severe haemorrhage. If this were true, then there would also be a bar on low-dose urokinase therapy for the same reasons, and there is no such bar. Many workers have used local infusions of streptokinase, and since the streptokinase eventually enters the circulation, this also amounts to low-dose streptokinase therapy, without problems. The original authors quoted as authorities for the supposed risk, reported mild ecchymoses and petechiae in the skin in two normal volunteers in whom superficial venous thrombosis had been induced during low-dose streptokinase therapy.

References
Johnson, A. J. and McCarty, W. R. (1959) *J. Clin. Invest.* **38**, 1627
Katzen, B. T. and van Breda, A. (1981) *Am. J. Radiol.* **136**, 1171

Laboratory control of streptokinase therapy

A thrombin time of two to four times the normal control at 3–6-h indicates activity. There are no established tests for the quantitation of therapy.

Following streptokinase infusion, circulating plasminogen, fibrinogen, plasma factors V and VIII, and α_2-antiplasmin levels are all reduced, with increased fibrinogen–fibrin degradation products present.

In some situations, with digestion of fibrin and aggregated platelet thrombi, haemorrhage may develop.

Streptokinase therapy may be associated with complications, including pyrexia, rashes and anaphylactic reactions. After 7–10 days of treatment, antistreptococcal antibodies rapidly increase, and further streptokinase therapy is ineffective. If fibrinolytic therapy is still indicated, urokinase can be used to replace streptokinase, but it is much more expensive.

If severe bleeding occurs during streptokinase treatment, fibrinolysis can be reversed with ε-aminocaproic acid or tranexamic acid plus fibrinogen.

Urokinase

Urokinase is a single-chain β-globulin polypeptide with a large form with a molecular weight of 55 000 and a low-molecular-weight form (mol. wt = 35 000). It is probably formed in the kidney, and the low-molecular-weight form is probably the more active. It converts plasminogen to plasmin.

Urokinase causes leucocyte modulation of plasminogen in tissues to induce fibrinolysis in the tissues. In plasma it is a trypsin-like protease which lyses arginine and lysine bonds, and activates plasminogen to plasmin.

Therapeutic dose

This is 2500–4450 CTA units/kg body weight per hour.

In high dosage, α_2-antitrypsin levels fall, and there is extensive systemic fibrinolysis. In moderate dosage there is only a 50% fall in plasma α_2-antiplasmin and moderate systemic fibrinolysis, with local tissue fibrinolysis at sites of fibrin deposition. Hyperplasminaemia only occurs when plasma α_2-antiplasmin disappears.

Thrombolytic therapy

Various combinations of different thrombolytic agents have been tried in the early stages of acute myocardial infarction. These have been reviewed, and the reviews criticized. These combinations include:

- Aspirin + streptokinase vs placebo + streptokinase vs streptokinase vs nil.
- Aspirin + heparin with, or without recombinant t-PA.
- t-PA vs placebo.
- t-PA + aspirin vs t-PA alone.
- Streptokinase vs t-PA + streptokinase.
- t-PA + heparin vs placebo + heparin.

It is very important that any such treatment be started soon after an acute myocardial infarction. High dosage may be associated both with increased canalization of blocked vessels and an increased incidence of complications. Antibodies and allergic reactions are more likely to occur with streptokinase, but they also occur with recombinant preparations of t-PA. Addition of aspirin reduces mortality, but may slightly increase the risk of intracranial haemorrhage. What should be measured – the rate of survival of patients, the degree of recanalization of blocked vessels? Early treatment can reduce mortality by 25–50%.

References
McNeill, A. J., Flannery, D. J., Wilson, C. M. *et al.* (1991) *Quart. J. Med.* **79**, 487
Marder, V. J. and Sherry, S. (1988) *N. Engl. J. Med.* **318**, 1512, 1585; **319**, 1546
Marx, J. L. (1988) *Science* **242**, 1505

Complications of thrombolytic therapy

- Bleeding.
- Thrombosis.
- Pyrogenic reactions.
- Development of streptokinase inhibitors during the period of use of streptokinase.

Contraindications to thrombolytic therapy

Absolute

- Active internal bleeding.
- Recent cerebrovascular disorder or intracranial procedure within 2 months.

Relative

Contraindicated within 10 days of onset of:

- Major surgery or recent severe trauma.
- Organ biopsy.
- Puncture of non-compressible blood vessel.
- Postpartum (up to 10 days).
- Cardiopulmonary resuscitation in the presence of fractured ribs.

Risk of bleeding

- Uncontrolled haemorrhagic diathesis.
- Pregnancy.
- Severe uncontrolled hypertension.
- Recent streptococcal infection (indication for urokinase rather than streptokinase).
- Previous lytic therapy – change to urokinase from ancrod.

Reference
Sharma, G. V. R. K., Cella, G., Parisi, *et al.* (1982) *N. Engl. J. Med.* **306**, 1268

Ancrod – therapeutic defibrination

Ancrod, the venom from the snake *Agkistrodon rhodostoma*, attacks the fibrinopeptide A portion of the fibrinogen molecule, releasing fibrinopeptide A and progressively shortening the α-chain on the residual soluble fibrin molecule. At the same time, plasminogen is activated to plasmin and neutralized by α_2-antiplasmin. The fibrin molecule is converted to fragments X, Y, D and E with no D-dimer formation. The D and E fragments are not clottable by thrombin. Plasmin fibrinogen levels fall progressively, and α_2-antiplasmin does not bind to the fibrin monomer during ancrod therapy. Thus defibrination proceeds without thromboembolism or renal damage, factor XIII is not activated and therefore no cross-linked insoluble fibrin is formed in vivo (since thrombin is necessary for this, and ancrod does not affect plasma prothrombin). There is no platelet aggregation, in the absence of thrombin, and the soluble fibrin and fragments are rapidly lysed by plasmin. Ancrod reduces the incidence of postoperative thrombosis, and is given by subcutaneous injection twice daily for 4 days after surgical operation.

Antifibrinolytic agents

ε-Aminocaproic acid and *tranexamic acid* act by binding on lysine sites on the plasminogen molecule, preventing fibrinolytic activity developing by inhibiting plasminogen activators competitively. They are used after prostatectomy to prevent bleeding, in menorrhagia and following dental extraction. In mild haemophiliacs, von Willebrand's disease and factor IX deficiency, they can be used to reduce the requirement of cryoprecipitate, factor VIII, or factor IX concentrate, if they are given immediately before dental extraction, and for a week subsequently. They are contraindicated if there is any haematuria or intracranial bleeding. Tranexamic acid (4-aminomethylcyclohexane carboxylic acid) is ten times more potent than ε-aminocaproic acid, and has a half-life in the body of about 80 min.

Aprotinin (Trasylol) is thought to act by inhibiting the formation of contact product, the action of formed contact product, and, in high concentration, the action of factor IX, but in practice it is not very effective.

Bruising and Bleeding Disorders

1. Purpura
2. Purpura in children
3. Ecchymoses due to autoerythrocyte sensitization
4. Spider naevi
5. Acquired increased vascular permeability and fragility
6. Vascular defects:
7. Abnormal menstrual bleeding due to haematological abnormalities
8. Haemorrhage associated with liver disease
9. Circulating anticoagulants
10. Treatment of bleeding disorders:
    (a) congenital coagulation factor deficiencies
    (b) platelet deficiency
    (c) acute fibrinolysis and defibrination syndromes

Purpura

Purpuric lesions are minute haemorrhages in the skin and mucous membranes, about the size of a pinpoint or pinhead. Larger haemorrhages the size of flea bites (petechiae) can occur. Extravasations of blood into subcutaneous or submucous tissue, with visible bruising, may be found in severe cases (ecchymoses).

Thrombocytopenic purpura

See Causes of thrombocytopenia. pp. 158–160

Non-thrombocytopenic purpura

See Vascular defects p. 193.

Purpura in children

Neonatal period

- Thrombocytopenia, transmitted from mother suffering from either primary or secondary thrombocytopenia. Spontaneous recovery occurs in the infant after about 7–10 days.
- Severe asphyxia (e.g. at birth).
- Severe haemolytic disease.
- Purpura neonatorum, often due to non-complement-fixing platelet anti-PL^{A1} antibodies, with marked haemorrhage and a high mortality.

Reference
Duncan, J. R. and Rosse, W. F. (1986) *Br. J. Haematol.* **64**, 331

- Neonatal isoimmune purpura: in up to 1 in 10 000 births maternal alloantibodies react with fetal platelets (directed against paternally derived platelet antigens).

Reference
Moore, S. B. (1982) *Mayo Clin. Proc.* **57**, 778

Childhood

Severe

- Leukaemia.
- Aplastic anaemia.
- Thrombocytopenia (primary).
- Agranulocytosis.
- Severe antemortem marasmus, from any cause.
- Waterhouse–Friderichsen syndrome.

Benign

- Whooping cough.
- Scurvy.
- Salicylate therapy (e.g. in acute rheumatic fever).
- Allergic non-thrombocytopenic purpura (e.g. Schölein–Henoch purpura).

Note: Flea bites and other insect bites may mimic purpura.

Ecchymoses due to autoerythrocyte sensitization

The Gardner–Diamond syndrome [R] occurs predominantly in women. Only seven affected males have been reported. Recurrent painful ecchymoses occur, with normal bleeding and clotting test results. Intradermal autologous blood injection causes immediate burning sensation, followed by an erythematous macular lesion after 2 h with no reaction to intradermal saline. Patients have also suffered from abdominal pain and/or headaches.

Reference
Ingber, A., Alcalay, J. and Feuermen, E. J. (1985) *Postgrad. Med. J.* **61**, 823

'Spider' naevi

'Spiders' are caused by dilatation and branching of terminal arterioles. They are found in the skin, rarely in mucous membranes, and mainly on the upper half of the body. They cannot be demonstrated by infrared photography, unlike telangiectasias, and disappear on death. 'Spiders' occur in the following conditions:

1. Severe and chronic liver disease, especially cirrhosis.
2. Nutritional deficiencies, especially pellagra.
3. Pregnancy: 'spiders' may appear and enlarge from about the third month of pregnancy to full term.
4. Various:
   (a) Cushing's syndrome;
   (b) hyperthyroidism;
   (c) acute rheumatic fever;
   (d) xanthoderma pigmentosa.

'Spiders' due to venous obstruction are rare, and occur in leukaemic infiltration of the skin.

Capillary fragility is reduced by:

- Cortisone.
- Compound F.
- 'Splenin' released by the spleen after ACTH administration.
- Thrombocytosis.

Reference
Stefanini, M. (1953) *Am.J. Med.* **14**, 64

Acquired increased vascular permeability and fragility

Scurvy

Although there may be associated thrombocytopenia in some cases, the fundamental defect is in the synthesis of the cement substance of the capillary wall. Bleeding may occur from almost any capillaries in the body. All tests of haemostasis are normal, except the capillary fragility test, which is strongly positive.

Vitamin K deficiency

Associated with hypoprothrombinaemia and increased vascular fragility.

Senile and cachectic purpura

Infections: capillary damage by toxins

- Smallpox.
- Measles.
- Scarlet fever.
- Diphtheria.
- Typhus.
- Acute glomerulonephritis (related to streptococcal toxin).

Septic emboli

- Subacute bacterial endocarditis.
- Meningococcal septicaemia.
- Pneumococcal septicaemia.

The vessel permeability is increased by the action of hyaluronidase.

Drugs and toxins

- Gold salts.
- Organic arsenicals.
- Sulphonamides.
- Streptomycin.
- Isoniazid.
- Snake venom.
- Copaiba.
- Atropine.
- Quinine.
- Oestrogens.

In these conditions there may be thrombocytopenia and/or capillary damage.

Allergotoxic conditions

Schönlein–Henoch purpura (splenic inhibitor of 'splenin').

Capillary damage associated with thrombocytopenia

- Primary thrombocytopenia.
- Secondary thrombocytopenia.

Purpura simplex

- Hereditary familial purpura simplex.
- Acquired purpura simplex.

In both these conditions all tests of haemostasis are normal.

Various

- Diabetes mellitus⎫ haemorrhages in both sclerae
- Hypertension ⎬ and retina.
- Uraemia: haemorrhages from mucous membranes.
- Hypothyroidism.
- Mechanical constriction.
- Anoxia.
- Convulsions.

Vascular defects

Congenital abnormality of vessel walls

Hereditary haemorrhagic telangiectasia

In this condition there is a hereditary dysplasia of capillaries. The capillaries which are affected occur in non-contractile clusters. The condition is inherited by means of an autosomal dominant gene, transmitted by either sex, affecting both sexes equally.

All tests of haemostasis are normal, except the bleeding time, which is grossly prolonged in the affected areas, and to be avoided.

Pseudohaemophilia (vascular variety)

This rare condition occurs with an increased bleeding time. It is possible that it is inherited as a Mendelian dominant character.

Idiopathic vascular disorders

Pulmonary haemosiderosis

This rare condition occurs most commonly in children and is associated with haemoptysis, pulmonary haemosiderosis, anaemia and reticulocytosis, death usually occurring within 3 years of onset.

Idiopathic haematemesis and melaena

Intermittent severe gastrointestinal bleeding occurs, with no demonstrable bleeding lesion.

Ehlers–Danlos syndrome

This condition is a developmental mesenchymal dysplasia, associated with hyperelasticity of the skin, hyperextensibility of the joints, abnormally friable blood vessels and subcutaneous nodules. Inheritance is by means of a dominant autosomal character.

Abnormal menstrual bleeding (due to haematological abnormalities)

Inherited plasma clotting deficiencies

- Von Willebrand's disease.
- Factor IX deficiency carriers.
- True haemophilia carriers.
- Factor I deficiency ⎫
- Factor II deficiency ⎬ very rare.
- Factor V deficiency ⎪
- Factor VII deficiency ⎪
- Factor X deficiency ⎪
- Dysfibrinogenaemia ⎭

Platelet abnormalities

- Thrombocytopenia (including aplastic anaemia and leukaemia).
- Thrombasthenia (Glanzman's disease).
- Bernard–Soulier syndrome.

(Increased menstrual blood flow is often effectively reduced by antifibrinolytic agents, e.g. ε-aminocaproic acid and tranexamic acid, indicating that active fibrinolysis plays a part in normal menstruation).

Reference
Bonnar, J., Sheppard, B. L. and Dockery, C. J. (1983) *Research Clin. Forum* **5**, 27

Haemorrhage associated with liver damage

The following factors, either singly or in combination, may be depressed. The degree of impairment is roughly proportional to the severity of the liver damage.

- Thrombocytopenia.
- Prothrombin (with no subsequent improvement after treatment with vitamin K).
- Factor V.
- Factor IX (Christmas factor)
- Rarely, fibrinogen is depressed. Abnormal fibrinogen is formed, with increased sialic acid content in the Bβ- and γ-chains. This may result in a prolonged thrombin time.

Reference
Martinez, J., MacDonald, K. A. and Palascak, J. F. (1982) *Blood* **61**, 1196

- Rarely circulating fibrinolysins are present.
- Where there is associated poor fat absorption from the gut, then Factor VII plasma levels may be depressed. Following vitamin K therapy the plasma level of factor VII should improve.
- Plasma antithrombin titre may be increased.
- Vascular resistance is reduced in many cases.

Reference
Finkbiner, R. B., McGovern, J. J., Goldstein R. *et al.* (1959) *Am. J. Med.* **26**, 199

Circulating anticoagulants

- Exogenous heparin during therapy: although endogenous plasma heparin may be increased in anaphylactic shock, after X-ray irradiation or some chemotherapeutic agents, or following amniotic fluid embolism, it is not increased enough to cause bleeding.

- Fibrin degradation products in DIC, or after fibrinolysis may interfere with normal clotting.
- Inhibition of specific coagulation factors (rare except for antibodies against factors VIIIC and IX).
- Circulating anticoagulants may develop in pregnancy or the early puerperium.
- Pemphigus, chronic glomerulonephritis and polyarteritis nodosa, rarely.
- Dysproteinaemias, including myeloma, macroglobulinaemia and cryoglobulinaemia.
- Lupus anticoagulants are often associated with thrombosis – see p. 196.

Detection

When affected plasma is tested using the prothrombin time, partial thromboplastin time and thrombin clotting time, any one or more of these tests may be prolonged. An equal volume of normal plasma added to affected plasma does not return the prolonged clotting time to normal, as would occur with the correction of a simple clotting factor deficiency.

Treatment of bleeding disorders

Congenital coagulation factor deficiencies

More than 19 out of 20 cases suffer from clinical haemophilia, the majority factor VIII deficiency and von Willebrand's disease, the minority factor IX deficiency. The remainder will include deficiencies of factors I, II, V, VII, X, XI XIII, VIII plus V, and α_2-antitrypsin deficiency.

Factor VIII deficiency

Factor VIII concentrate to maintain levels over 50% for 24 hours to cover bleeding episodes. Dental extraction is made safe by raising plasma factor VIII to 50%, and by giving tranexamic acid immediately before extraction. Tranexamic acid is then given three times each day for a further 5 days after tooth extraction. In mild cases no further factor VIII may be needed. Antifibrinolytics should not be given where there is intracranial bleeding or renal bleeding.

Because of AIDS, factor VIII concentrate is now heat treated. It is also wise to vaccinate haemophiliacs against hepatitis B. In the USA, 80% of haemophiliacs requiring transfusion are seropositive for antibody to hepatitis B, and 25% of these have chronic liver dysfunction. Five to ten per cent of such patients are positive for hepatitis B surface antigen. Many haemophiliacs have AIDS acquired from infected plasma. Recently, recombinant DNA techniques have enabled the production of pure uninfected factor VIII.

DDAVP can be used in mild haemophiliacs to produce a two- to four-fold increase in factor VIII and vWF in preparation for minor surgery. Tranexamic acid should also be given, as DDAVP stimulates the release of plasminogen activator.

Reference
White, G. C., McMillan, C. W., Kingdon, H. S. and Shoemaker, C. B. (1989) *N. Engl. J. Med.* **320**, 166

Von Willebrand's disease

Cryoprecipitate and freeze-dried concentrate contain vWF, but cryoprecipitate is preferred as it contains the labile element which enhances platelet adhesiveness. A synthetic analogue of vasopressin (DDVAP) is effective in most mild vWF patients. Bleeding from the uterus, nose or mouth can often be controlled with tranexamic acid or ε-aminocaproic acid, and either agent should be given for 5 days after tooth extraction. (Saliva contains a potent fibrinolytic activator.) DDVAP is contraindicated in type IIB disease, as the large multimers which develop in the plasma cause thrombocytopenia.

Factor IX deficiency

Factor IX concentrate, or fresh frozen plasma for moderate bleeding. Factor IX concentrate also contains factors II, VII and X. Antibodies to factor IX concentrate develop in 5–10% of patients.

Factor I deficiency

Cryoprecipitate or fibrinogen concentrate for afibrinogenaemia to cover bleeding, surgery or injury. Cases of dysfibrinogenaemia (many variants) may suffer from a mild bleeding diathesis or a thrombotic tendency.

Factor II deficiency

Fresh or fresh frozen plasma, or concentrate.

Factor V deficiency

More than 25% of normal is needed to cover injury, surgery or bleeding. Fresh or fresh frozen plasma, or concentrate. Platelets contain 10–20% of the factor V in the blood. Therefore platelet concentrates are useful.

Factor VII deficiency

Plasma every 12 hours, or concentrate to avoid circulatory overload.

Factor X deficiency

Plasma or concentrate for a bleeding episode.

Factor XI deficiency

A level of 30% is required for haemostasis: fresh plasma or fresh frozen plasma.

Factor XIII deficiency

As a level of only 2% of normal is necessary for haemostasis, cryoprecipitate, which in rich in factor XIII, can be used, and can be given weekly as a prophylactic.

Factors V + VIII deficiency

Cryoprecipitate or fresh frozen plasma can be used for the usually mild bleeding in this rare autosomal recessive condition.

Factor XII, prekallikrein and HMWK deficiencies

These have no bleeding tendencies.

α_1-Antitrypsin deficiency

Homozygotes suffer with severe haemophiliac-like bleeding and require treatment with long-term tranexamic acid. In heterozygotes with 50% of normal activity, the mild bleeding tendency, with post-operative bleeding, bleeding after tooth extraction and easy bruising after trauma, can be treated with tranexamic acid or ε-aminocaproic acid.

Platelet deficiency

Transfusion of platelet concentrates may be necessary in severe thrombocytopenia, when dangerous bleeding is possible, during intense chemotherapy, to cover surgery or in severe thrombocytopenia during pregnancy. Ideally platelets should be HLA-compatible; in post-transfusion purpura, PA^A1^-antigen and antibodies should be checked.

Acute fibrinolysis and defibrination syndromes

Obviously the cause should be treated. In addition, blood fresh plasma or fresh frozen plasma, fibrinogen, AT-III concentrate if available, and platelets may be needed. Low-dose heparin has been found to be effective in severe cases.

Thrombosis

1. Increased tendency to thrombosis, both 'spontaneous' and post-trauma
   (a) primary hypercoagulable states
   (b) secondary hypercoagulable states
   (c) lupus anticoagulants
2. Disseminated intravascular coagulation

3. Long-term sequelae to acute venous thrombosis
4. Prediction of thrombosis
5. Detection of venous thrombosis
6. Intravenous saline, the impedance clotting time and hypercoagulability
7. Natural defences against local thrombus extension
8. Prevention of thromboembolic disease following surgery
9. Coronary artery disease
10. Smoking and the circulation
11. Pregnancy and clotting
12. Oral contraceptives and clotting
13. Postmenopausal oestrogen replacement therapy
14. Alcohol and haematology

Increased tendency to thrombosis, both 'spontaneous' and post-trauma

Haemorrhage and/or thrombosis is associated with 40% of newborn deaths.

Reference
Hathaway, W. E. (1970) *Pediatr. Clin. North Am.* **17**, 929

The inherited tendency to thrombosis is more common than inherited bleeding diatheses – 1 in 2500–5000.

Reference
Mannucci, M. and Tripodi, A. (1987) *Thromb. Haemost.* **57**, 247

Primary hypercoagulable states

Coagulant and anticoagulant factors

- Antithrombin III deficiency [AD].
- Protein C deficiency [AD].
- Protein S deficiency [AD].
- Some dysfibrinogenaemias.
- Factor XII deficiency.
- Heparin cofactor II deficiency.

Fibrinolysis disorders

- Reduced plasminogen [AD].
- Abnormal plasminogen – a few families.
- Plasminogen activator – deficiency or defective release of t-PA.
- Plasminogen activator inhibitor (PAI-1) excess.
- Abnormally increased HRGP [AD].

Platelet function abnormalities

Homocystinuria

Homozygotes – premature pulmonary embolism, coronary artery thrombosis, as teenager. Heterozgotes – increased incidence of 'young' early middle-age ischaemic heart disease.

Secondary hypercoagulable states

Abnormalities of coagulation and fibrinolysis

- Normal pregnancy } see pp. 197, 198
- Oral contraceptives }
- Nephrotic syndrome
- Patients with deep vein thrombosis have an increased incidence of carcinoma later – ? already have very early cancer. Mucinous adenocarcinoma of lung and gastrointestinal tract secrete substances which can activate factor X and trigger thrombosis.

Reference
Goldhaber, S. Z., Buring, J. E., Hennekens, C. H., (1987) *Arch. Intern. Med.* **147**, 216

- Rebound on sudden cessation of oral anticoagulant therapy.
- Infusion of some prothrombin concentrates.
- Lupus anticoagulants

Platelet function abnormalities

- Diabetes mellitus.
- Hyperlipidaemias.
- Myeloproliferative disorders.
- Paroxysmal nocturnal haemoglobinuria.

Reference
Schafer, A. I. (1985) *Ann. Intern. Med.* **102**, 814

Abnormalities of blood flow and vessel walls

Venous stasis

During surgical operation under general anaesthesia, the venous tone is reduced to 50% of normal, and this is aggravated by intermittent positive-pressure ventilation. Collapsed veins may be damaged by pressure while the patient is unconscious and flaccid. Further damage to the venous endothelium may occur in the early postoperative period from pressure and anoxia, especially in the less mobile elderly patient. In addition, fibrinolytic activity is markedly reduced during the first 10 days after operation. Immobilization, obesity and congestive cardiac failure, are all causes of peripheral venous stasis.

Blood viscosity

High haematocrit values and, paradoxically, low haematocrit values are both associated with an increased incidence of thrombosis. Whole blood viscosity is greatly increased by increases in the haematocrit and also by rises in plasma viscosity. Plasma viscosity is greatly increased by rises in plasma fibrinogen and, to a lesser extent, increased plasma globulin concentration. Whole blood viscosity is also increased by reduced red cell deformability, as in sickle-cell disease, and rigid red cells can block very small blood vessels,

initiating thrombosis. Increases in plasma fibrinogen and/or globulin cause spontaneous red cell aggregation when the blood flow is slow, another factor promoting thrombosis.

Vessel walls

Atherosclerosis presents an abnormal surface to the blood flowing past a lesion, which can activate plasma clotting factors, and also induce platelet adhesion, aggregation and 'release' reaction, producing local thrombus formation.

Varicose veins are a risk factor in postoperative thrombosis, whilst vasculitis, chronic occlusive vascular disease and artificial surfaces in the circulation (arterial grafts etc.) can all act as foci for thrombosis.

Race, diet, environment and unknown factors

Northern Europeans are at least three times more likely to develop postoperative thromboembolism than Orientals are. Eskimos on their natural high-fat fish diet very rarely suffer from either venous thrombosis or heart attacks.

Lung function

Careful postmortem examination of lungs of patients dying with no history of either pulmonary embolism or lung disease has revealed evidence of numerous small pulmonary emboli of different ages. The lung acts as a normal blood filter, and clinical pulmonary embolism represents emboli large enough to cause circulatory distress.

Lupus anticoagulants

Lupus anticoagulants are circulating immunoglobulins with activities directed against phospholipids in platelets, and also possibly endothelial cell membranes; phospholipids are essential for the effective actions of factors Va, VIIIa and Xa in the coagulation cascade. These antibodies are strongly associated with venous thrombotic attacks, and also with recurrent abortions or unexplained intrauterine deaths, cerebral dysfunction and ischaemic episodes. The majority of patients with the so-called 'lupus anticoagulants' do not suffer from lupus erythematosus.

Tests for detection

- Prolonged APTT or kaolin clotting time (both phospholipid dependent) is not shortened by addition of an equal volume of normal plasma. The clotting time may be shortened if a high concentration of rabbit thromboplastin is used.
- Occasionally the prothrombin time is prolonged.

- There is no specific inhibition of any individual coagulation factor.
- The APTT or kaolin clotting time is prolonged by the addition of an equal volume of patient's plasma to normal plasma.
- Anticardiolipin antibodies may be present in the plasma.
- Thrombocytopenia in some cases.

Reference
Williams, H., Laurent, R. and Gibson, T. (1980) *Clin. Lab. Haematol.* **2**, 139

Occurrence

- Patients with a history of recurrent thrombosis, or thrombosis in sites other than leg veins, in whom no other cause for thrombosis has been found.
- Women with a history of thrombosis and recurrent abortion or unexplained intrauterine deaths.
- Idiopathic or drug-induced lupus erythematosus.

References
Chu. P., Pendry, K. and Blecher, T. E. (1988) *Br. Med. J.* **297**, 1449
Hughes, G. R. V. (1988) *Br. Med. J.* **297**, 700
Rosove, M. H., Ismail, M., Koziol, B. J. *et al.* (1986) *Blood* **68**, 472
Thiagarajan, P., Pengo, V. and Shapiro, S. S. (1986) *Blood* **68**, 869

Disseminated intravascular coagulation

When the mechanisms designed to keep clotting strictly localized and protective fail, and coagulation is activated, then disseminated intravascular coagulation (DIC) may develop.

Triggers

- Entry of foreign material into the circulation, e.g. amniotic fluid.
- Contact of normal blood with extensively damaged tissue surfaces.

Activation occurs

- Plasma clotting factors, with generation of fibrin
- Platelet activation leads to platelet thrombi

  } direct activation of X, tissue factor release, activation of XII etc.

- Later, fibrinolysis is activated.

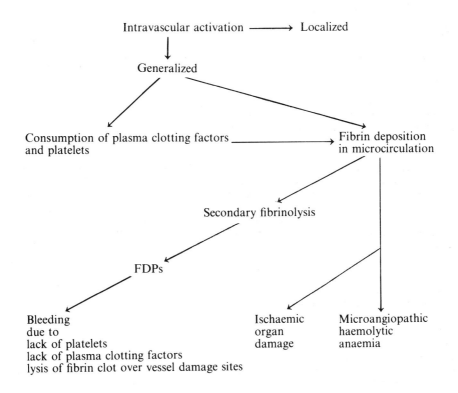

Activating triggers

These include

1. Maternal:
   (a) abruptio placentae;
   (b) amniotic fluid embolism;
   (c) retained dead fetus;
   (d) intrauterine infection;
   (e) eclampsia and pre-eclampsia;
   (f) rupture of uterus;
   (g) severe fetomaternal haemorrhage;
   (h) hydatidiform mole.
2. Newborn infant:
   (a) associated with maternal complications;
   (b) respiratory distress syndrome.
3. Snake venom – snake bite.
4. Acute pancreatitis.
5. Massive injury.
6. Septicaemia.
7. Tumour cell factor release, leukaemia (especially promyelocytic leukaemia).
8. Vessel endothelium damage:
   (a) anoxia;
   (b) acidosis;
   (c) heat stroke;
   (d) virus infections;
   (e) antigen/antibody complex deposition.

Release of thrombin triggers further plasma clotting and also induces platelet activation, aggregation, and release, liberating further stimulus to platelet aggregation and release, and also releasing platelet factor 3 to take part in plasma clotting.

Various factors modify the severity of DIC triggered by the various mechanisms listed:

• Reticuloendothelial blockade – greatly increases severity of attack.
• Activity of secondary fibrinolysis, with release of fibrin degradation products into the circulation.
• Deposition of fibrin, antigen/antibody complexes and platelet thrombi in relation to α-receptors.
• Increased lipids block the reticuloendothelial system (e.g. as in severe diabetic ketoacidosis, which also involves dehydration, anoxia, failing circulation, and variable acidosis).
• Liver disease, with inability to clear circulating partially consumed factors.

Treatment

Treatment consists primarily of treatment of the cause or causes of DIC. Blood, fresh frozen plasma and possibly antithrombin III concentrate (if available) are necessary to replace consumed clotting factors. It has been suggested that low-dose heparin (5000 units 6-hourly intravenously) may be useful in severe cases.

The original idea that active fibrinolysis was a part of DIC has been mostly discarded – fibrinolysis is automatically triggered as soon as fibrin is formed, and also as soon as factor XII is activated.

Local disseminated intravascular coagulation

• Up to 50% of cases of hereditary haemorrhagic telangiectasia suffer from a low-grade continuous DIC, with acute exacerbations on occasion.
• Giant cavernous haemangioma – similarly, these rare cases suffer from chronic DIC.

Both of these conditions are included in the so-called Kasabach–Merritt syndrome.

Classification of disseminated intravascular coagulation

Rate of development

Acute

• Shock.
• Septicaemia.
• Acute intravascular haemolysis.
• Acute pulmonary embolism.
• Cardiac arrest and resuscitation.
• Extensive trauma.
• Snake bite.
• Acute liver disease.
• Major surgery.
• Burns.
• Heat stroke.
• Placental abruption.
• Amniotic fluid embolism.
• Septic abortion.
• Rewarming after hypothermia.

Subacute

• Disseminated malignancy.
• Pancreatic and ovarian carcinoma.
• Promyelocytic leukaemia.
• Aortic aneurysm with clotting.
• Giant haemangioma.
• Retained dead fetus.

Chronic low grade

• Liver disease.
• Myocardial infarction.
• Nephrosis.
• Paroxysmal nocturnal haemoglobinuria.
• Sarcoidosis.
• Eclampsia.
• Systemic lupus erythematosus.
• Allergic vasculitis.
• Ischaemic enterocolitis.
• Renal disease.

Tests useful in disseminated intravascular coagulopathy

- Blood film – fragmented red cells may be seen.
- Platelet count – in active disseminated intravascular coagulopathy, the platelet count falls below $100 \times 10^9/l$.
- One-stage prothrombin time is increased above normal.
- Activated partial thromboplastin time is abnormally prolonged.
- Plasma fibrinogen (measured by clotting assay) is reduced.
- Plasma fibrin/fibrinogen degradation products abnormally increased. (After trauma or major surgery, FDPs are bound to be increased normally – raised FDPs in the presence of low plasma fibrinogen, prolonged prothrombin time, and APTT plus low platelet count justifies presumptive diagnosis of DIC.)
- Thrombin time is prolonged.
- Reptilase or ancrod clotting time is prolonged (not affected by heparin which may have been used during therapy).
- Ethanol gel/protamine sulphate precipitation tests, both detect excess amounts of X–Y complexes following partial fibrinolysis.
- Assays of factors VIII, V and AT-III are all reduced.
- (Fibrinopeptide A only is evidence of initial action of an enzyme such as thrombin on fibrinogen.)

Results of laboratory tests

Decompensated

Thrombocytopenia, fibrinogenopenia, prolonged prothrombin time and APTT, with increased FDPs. Thrombin time prolonged.

Compensated

Platelet count normal or low, plasma fibrinogen low normal, prothrombin time and APTT normal or increased, with thrombin time normal in 50%. Plasma FDPs are increased abnormally.

Hypercompensated

Variable platelet counts, with plasma fibrinogen normal prothrombin time and shortened APTT with increased plasma FDPs.

Pleural fluid

Fibrin/fibrinogen degradation products are increased in the pleural exudate in cases of pulmonary malignancy.

Reference
Astedt, B., Adielsson, G. and Mattson, W (1976) *Lancet* ii, 414

Long-term sequelae to acute venous thrombosis

The status of distal deep veins is very important in the development of sequelae, and the outlook is good if they are patent and competent. The outlook is less favourable if they are occluded or have incompetent valves.

Reference
Strandness, D. E. Jr., Langlois, Y., Cramer, M. *et al.* (1983) *JAMA* **250**, 1289

Prediction of thrombosis

Obviously the demonstration of a specific deficiency known to be associated with thrombosis, e.g. AT-III deficiency or reduced fibrinolytic activity, is clinically valuable, as suitable prophylactic measures can be taken before operation. The preoperative APTT may indicate a thrombotic tendency, if the result is shorter than normal; it normally becomes shorter with increasing age. Patients who are overweight, have varicose veins, atherosclerosis, diabetes mellitus, are old and /or also have a history of previous thrombotic attacks, are known to have a greater risk than normal of developing postoperative thromboembolism. As underlying cancer is known to predispose to venous thrombosis, it has been suggested that patients who develop 'spontaneous' thrombosis should be carefully examined for an unsuspected cancer. It has recently been found that patients with repeated episodes of thromboembolic disease have increased F_{1+2} fragments circulating in their blood while they are symptom free. F_{1+2} fragments are released from the prothrombin molecule when thrombin is formed, indicating in these patients an inappropriate generation of thrombin somewhere in the circulation.

Reference
Bauer, K. A. and Rosenberg, R. D. (1987) *Blood* **70**, 343 (review)

Prediction of liability to postoperation deep vein thrombosis after elective abdominal surgery:

Age > euglobulin lysis > previous abdominal surgery > varicose veins > AT-III level > cigarette smoking > platelet count.

Reference
Sue-Ling, H. M., Johnston, D., McMahon, M. J. *et al.* (1986) *Lancet* i, 1173

Detection of venous thrombosis

Radioactive fibrinogen uptake

A thrombus continues to grow with deposition of fibrin, and shrink with fibrinolysis. This method detects venous thrombosis in the calf veins, but is not useful in the detection of thrombosis in the common femoral and iliac veins, because of the presence of the bladder and large arteries nearby.

Venography

This is invasive and unpleasant for the patient, but it is useful for the detection of femoral vein occlusion. It misses small thrombi.

Ultrasonography

This non-invasive method is quick, but may not detect small thrombi.

Impedance plethysmography

This non-invasive method measures the rate of emptying of the veins in the leg, and can be used to detect major thrombi in the femoral, popliteal and iliac veins. It is not good in the detection of thrombosis in tibial and soleal veins.

Radionuclide venography

This method enables satisfactory visualization of iliac and inferior vena caval thrombosis.

Clinical assessment

Unless the thrombosis is florid, clinical detection can miss thrombi, and misdiagnose local haematomas.

Post mortem

Many unsuspected cases of pulmonary embolism are found. The presence of fibrin degradation products confirms that fibrin has been formed somewhere and that fibrinolysis is in progress (i.e. not diagnostic of either venous thrombosis or DIC).

Intravenous saline, the impedance clotting time and hypercoagulability

When the impedance across a clotting blood sample and the impedance across a heparinized sample of the same blood are measured, the impedance clotting time can be obtained. In vitro addition of physiological saline to blood has been found to increase its coagulability, and a saline test based on this has been used as a preoperative predictor of postoperative venous thrombosis.

Intravenous saline, given during surgical operations, increases the incidence of postoperative thrombosis (a worrying thought, when saline infusion has been used as a negative control procedure in clinical trials of injections of other materials in attempts to reduce thrombosis).

References
Heather, B. P., Jennings, S. A. and Greenhalgh R. M. (1980) *Br. J. Surg.* **67**, 63
Janvrin, S. B., Ur, A. and Greenhalgh, R. M. (1978) *Br. J. Surg.* **65**, 825
Jarvrin, S. B., Davies, G. and Greenhalgh, R. M. (1980) *Br. J. Surg.* **67**, 690

Natural defences against local thrombus extension

Anticoagulant factors in the circulation

- AT-III acting at many levels in the coagulation cascade.
- Heparin cofactor II neutralizing thrombin.
- Plasminogen available for activation to plasmin, when bound to fibrin.
- Plasminogen activator.
- Circulating protein C activated by protein S from endothelial cells, neutralizing factors Va and VIIIa.

Endothelial cell resistance to extending thrombus.

- Endothelial cells are intrinsically non-thrombogenic, and non-stimulated platelets will not adhere to them. Adherence by stimulated platelets is inhibited by secretion of PGI_2 by normal endothelial cells in response to thrombin, bradykinin, ADP and ATP. PGI_2 (prostacyclin) inhibits platelet aggregation and release reaction.
- t-PA is released to activate plasminogen to plasmin.
- Thrombomodulin – activation of protein C, with neutralization of the thrombotic activity of thrombin.
- Heparan sulphate and dermatan sulphate – cofactors for AT-III and heparin cofactor II.
- α_2-Macroglobulin from plasma and heparin from endothelial mast cells neutralize platelet factor 4 (anti-heparin).

Neutralization of factors promoting vessel spasm in vicinity of thrombus

Local removal or degradation of thrombin, bradykinin, complement factor C3, PGD_2, and spontaneous degradation of platelet TxA_2, leukotrienes.

Factors promoting vasodilatation near a thrombus

PGI_2, PGF_1, PGE_1 and PGF_2.

Reference
Petty, R. G. and Pearson, J. D. (1989) *J. R. Coll. Phys.* **23**, 92

Prevention of thromboembolic disease following surgery

Local methods

- Tilting the surgical operating table by 15°, with the patient's head lower, to improve venous return from the lower limbs. Not popular with surgeons.
- Gradient compression stockings applied when patient still conscious, and removed when the patient is awake after the operation or worn for longer.
- Active intermittent compression of the calf muscles, by foot-pedals, pneumatic cuffs, regular galvanic electric shocks applied to the calves, early ambulation. The natural venous pump in the foot helps to return blood up the leg on movement.

General methods

1. Heparin – subcutaneous injection or continuous flow.
2. Low dose warfarin 1 mg/day before and immediately after the operation.
3. Reduction in platelet activity:
   (a) low-dose aspirin – 40–80 mg/day.
   (b) dipyridamol 100 mg three times daily plus low dose aspirin.
4. Perioperative dihydroergotamine tartrate 0.5 mg twice daily to improve venous return.
5. Dextran infusion at the time of operation.

   Note: Intravenous saline at the time of operation may increase the incidence of thromboembolic disease.

6. Ancrod defibrination: very little fibrinogen available to form inappropriate fibrin clots.
7. Long-term preoperative preparation: regular exercise increases plasma HDL and reduces LDL, with also improved fibrinolysis. Increased intake of fish oils for 6 weeks before operation reduces platelet TxA_2 production. Moderate alcohol intake daily increases PGI_2 production and reduces platelet TxA_2 production.

Reference
Colditz, G. A., Tuden, R. L. and Oster, G. (1986) *Lancet* **ii**, 143

Coronary artery disease

Coronary artery endothelium curtails episodes of vasoconstriction elicited by substances released by aggregating platelets. In the presence of normal vascular endothelium, platelets evoke relaxation of the coronary artery, whereas with arteriosclerotic lesions, vasospasm could be induced. See Serotonin p. 162.

Reference
Cohen, R. A., Shepherd, J. T. and Vanhoutte, P. M. (1983) *Science* **221**, 273

Smoking and the circulation

The smoking of tobacco, especially in the form of cigarettes, results in the following.

Increased

- White blood cell count (a risk factor for heart disease).
- Haematocrit.
- Whole blood viscosity (as red cell deformability is reduced).
- Plasma viscosity (as plasma fibrinogen is increased – also a risk factor for heart disease).
- Plasma oncotic pressure.
- Spontaneous red cell aggregation.
- Platelet count.
- Circulating platelet factor 3 in the plasma.

Inhibition

Fibrinolytic activity is reduced. Carbon monoxide in the blood of smokers inhibits arachidonic acid-induced platelet aggregation, and second wave aggregation with adrenaline, but prostacyclin production by the vessel wall endothelium is also inhibited.

Clinical effects

Smokers are less liable than non-smokers to postoperative thrombosis, possibly as a result of the relative venous spasm caused by nicotine, which would cause a faster venous blood flow with less stagnation immediately after surgery. Nicotine also increases both the heart rate and the blood pressure. However, the coronary arteries and aortas from smokers have a higher collagen content, with higher cholesterol concentration in their aortas, when compared with those of non-smokers. The small arteries responsible for penile engorgement during erection are also similarly damaged, and heavy smoking can be associated with impotence.

The effects of smoking, other than those of vessel wall damage, are reversible on abstention.

Reference
Fowkes, F. G. R. (1989) *Br. Med. J.* **298**, 405

Pregnancy and clotting

The woman becomes more liable to thromboembolism during pregnancy. Whilst plasma volume increases more than the red cell mass does, with a normal fall in the haematocrit and haemoglobin concentration, there is significant obstruction to the venous outflow from the legs in later pregnancy. Plasma fibrinogen is increased, with a parallel increase in plasma viscosity, and fibrinogen and fibrin are important in both the implantation and maintenance of the fertilized ovum in the uterine wall. Spontaneous abortion and placental dysruption occur in cases of both hypofibrinogenaemia and dysfibrinogenaemia. Congenital lack of factor XIII results in habitual abortion, and factor XIII cross-links fibrin with fibrin, and fibrin with fibronectin. Plasma factors VIII, IX and X are also all increased. FDP and D-dimers, and evidence of intravascular clotting are frequently detectable in late pregnancy.

Whilst protein C levels remain normal, both total and free protein S levels are reduced significantly during pregnancy, levels falling as low as those found in congenital protein S deficiency (15–37%). $C4_b$-binding protein, which complexes with, and carries, protein S in the plasma, is unchanged or increased during pregnancy.

Fibrinolytic activity decreases during pregnancy, with plasma euglobulin lysis falling from the second trimester onwards, returning rapidly to normal postpartum. Although plasminogen increases throughout pregnancy, t-PA activity falls and PAI activity increases. In addition, the pregnancy-specific inhibitor (PAI-2), undetectable in non-pregnant women, is measurable in the first trimester, and increases in activity throughout pregnancy.

Reference
Wright, J. G., Cooper, P., Astedt, B. *et al.* (1988) *Br. J. Haematol.* **69**, 253

Oral contraceptives and clotting

When combined low-dose oestrogen and progestogen oral contraceptives are taken cyclically by normal women between the ages of 16 and 30 years, the plasma levels of factors I, X and XII increase, and levels of the natural anticoagulants antithrombin III and protein C decrease, increasing the overall tendency to thrombosis. The combined pill should be discontinued at least 4 weeks before operation.

Reference
Cohen, H., Mackie, I. J., Walshe, K. *et al.* (1988) *Br. J. Haematol.* **69**, 259
Robinson, G. E., Burren, T., Mackie, I. J. *et al.* (1991) *Brit. Med. J.* **302**, 789

Postmenopausal oestrogen replacement therapy

Ethinyl oestradiol, a component of some oral contraceptives, is also used for hormone replacement in the climacteric period in women. It has been shown to cause increases in factor VII: Ag, factor VIII: C and

β-thromboglobulin, and falls in both AT-III and the platelet count, resulting in an increased tendency to thrombosis.

Reference
Lindberg, U. B., Crona, N. and Stigendal, L. *et al.* (1989) *Thromb. Haemost.* **61**, 65

Alcohol and haematology

[A] = advantage, if not excessive. [D] = disadvantage.

Moderate intake

(less than 30 ml ethanol/day, and less for women than for men)

- Plasma HDL_2 and HDL_2-cholesterol increased, with decreased plasma LDL-cholesterol [A].
- Plasminogen activator, secreted by vascular endothelial cells, increased in plasma [A].
- Plasma PGI_2 increased in volunteers, with increased inert PGI_2 metabolite in the urine after 1 h. ? Vasodilatory effect of ethanol due to PGI_2 release from vascular endothelium [A].
- PGI_1 release stimulated [A].
- Platelet thromboxane A_2 synthesis inhibited, and platelet response to TxA_2 reduced [A].
- Platelets also less responsive to adrenaline, ADP and collagen [A].
- Inverse relationship between plasma fibrinogen concentration and alcohol intake [A].
- Prolongation of bleeding time by aspirin potentiated [A].
- Negative correlation between fatal ischaemic heart disease and moderate ethanol intake [A].

Excessive intake

1. Sideroblastic anaemia with increased serum iron [D].
2. Direct marrow toxicity with increased MCV [D]. Vacuoles appear in marrow pronormoblasts and, later, in promyelocytes, independently of folate deficiency.
3. Megaloblastic change [D]:
   (a) folate deficiency, effects on cell membrane folate transport;
   (b) decreased efficiency of DNA synthesis;
   (c) malabsorption of vitamin B_{12}.
4. Liver damage – fatty infiltration of liver and eventually alcoholic cirrhosis, with consequent haematological troubles including thrombocytopenia, marrow hypoplasia, bleeding, with inadequate production of vitamin-K-dependent plasma clotting factors, and defective platelets. Suppression of thrombocytopoiesis occurs in the maturing megakaryocyte in chronic ethanol abuse [D].

5. Thrombocytopenia independent of folate deficiency and cirrhosis, with reduced platelet life span occurs after 3–5 weeks of high ethanol intake [D].
6. Iron overload: high iron content of native beer in South Africa and in some red wines in northern Italy [D].
7. Precipitation of attacks in susceptible patients with: (a) acute intermittent porphyria, (b) porphyria cutanea tarda [D].
8. Bleeding time prolonged: this may contribute to the bleeding tendency and increased incidence of gastrointestinal haemorrhage in chronic alcoholics [D].

Withdrawal after prolonged excess alcohol intake

- Platelet count temporarily increased, and bleeding time returns to normal, unless the liver is severely damaged.
- Circulating platelet aggregates temporarily increased [D].
- β-Thromboglobulin in plasma increased, reflecting increased platelet activation and turnover [D].
- Increased platelet sensitivity to ADP [D].
- PGE_1 production reduced: PGE_1 reduces platelet aggregation [D].

References
Deykin, D., Janson, P. and McMahon, L., (1982) *N. Engl. J. Med.* **306**, 852
Fink, R. and Hutton, R. A. (1983) *J. Clin. Pathol.* **36**, 337
Horrobin, D. F. and Manku, M. S. (1980) *Br. Med. J.* **280**, 1363
Landolfi, R. and Steiner, M. (1984) *Blood* **64**, 679
Laug, W. E. (1983) *JAMA* **250**, 772
Levine, R. F., Spivak, J. L., Meagher, R. C. *et al.* (1986) *Br. J. Haematol.* **62**, 345
Mikhailidis, D. P., Jenkins, W. J., Barradas, M. A. *et al.* (1986) *Br. Med. J.* **293**, 715

Anticoagulant Therapy

1. Heparin
2. Vitamin K action
3. Action of warfarin and other related anti-vitamin K anticoagulants
   (a) treatment
   (b) laboratory control
   (c) mechanisms of interference with warfarin
   (d) contraindications
   (e) complications
   (f) low dose and mini-dose warfarin therapy
4. Dextran
5. Dihydroergotamine
6. Multiple therapy for prophylaxis and multifactorial thrombosis
7. Secondary tumour spread, platelets and anticoagulant therapy

Heparin

Heparin is a glycosaminoglycan and consists of alternating copolymers of n-acetylglucosamine and glucuronic acid with postsynthetic modifications. It has a very large negative charge density, and is a natural anticoagulant stored in, and released from, the mast cells lying beneath the vascular endothelium. Commercial heparins are extracted from animal tissues, purified, and concentrated, and have molecular weights from 3000 to 57 000.

Actions

The interaction between activated plasma clotting factors and antithrombin III (AT-III) is slow. Heparin binds to lysine residues in the AT-III molecule, rendering its active site more accessible to thrombin and other serine proteases, including factors Xa, IXa, XIa and XIIa, e.g. the biological half-life of thrombin without heparin of 30–40 seconds, is 0.5 second with therapeutic doses of heparin, and 20 μs with high-dose heparin. The affinity of heparin for AT-III alone is greater than for the (AT-III–thrombin) complex, so heparin is released to combine with more AT-III, whilst the (AT-III – thrombin) complex is cleared from the circulation, with consumption of AT-III.

Heparin cofactor II also neutralizes thrombin, using either heparin or dermatan sulphate as cofactor.

Heparin does not cross the placental barrier to reach the fetus (compare warfarin), and can be used in the treatment of maternal thromboembolic disease during pregnancy, although it may be associated with an increased fetal loss rate. Low-molecular-weight heparin (LMWH) is more active with AT-III in neutralizing factor Xa. As the molecular weight and degree of sulphation increase, the activity against factors IXa, XIa and XIIa increases, with increasing risk of bleeding. Heparin is partially neutralized by PF4 (released by platelets), so that local platelet thrombi are protected. When factor Xa is bound by factor Va to platelet membrane phospholipid, it is protected from the action of heparin – AT-III. Circulating acute phase proteins in the plasma, increased during active thrombosis and in the first few days after acute myocardial infarction, also neutralize heparin activity. It is found that during these first few days a higher dose of heparin may be required to maintain satisfactory anticoagulation.

After bolus heparin injection, the plasma AT-III falls, whereas during subcutaneous low-dose heparin therapy plasma AT-III levels may increase.

Finally, heparin is a component of the lipoprotein lipase which hydrolyses the triacyl glycerol of chylomicrons and other lipoproteins in the circulation.

Modes of administration

Intermittent 6-hourly bolus therapy

This may be convenient, but there is a wide swing in the degree of anticoagulation produced, from over-coagulation with a risk of bleeding to under-coagulation during each 6-hour period.

Continuous infusion

After an initial loading dose this produces a steadier level of anticoagulation with a lower risk of bleeding, and less heparin is used.

Subcutaneous low-dose heparin given 8-hourly to 12-hourly

This must be started before surgical operation to be effective, as its success depends on the neutralization of traces of factor Xa in microthrombi as it is formed. Subcutaneous calcium heparin has been reported as more effective than conventional intravenous sodium heparin in helping to lyse existing thrombi, and in preventing the propagation of thrombi.

Low-molecular-weight heparin (LMWH)

This is prepared by enzymatic depolymerization of conventional porcine heparin, with a mean molecular weight of about 5000 and has been found to be more effective than calcium heparin in the prevention of postoperative deep vein thrombosis following abdominal surgery, with no difference in intra- or postoperative blood loss, wound haematomas or transfusion requirement. LMWH does not prolong the APTT as much as high-molecular-weight heparin, and binds less to platelets. It is effective in preventing thrombosis after hip replacement with less intra and postoperative bleeding.

References
Eriksson, B. I., Zachrisson, B. E., Teger-Nilsson, A.-C. and Risberg, B. (1988) *Br. J. Surg.* **75**, 1053
European Fraxiparin (EFS) Study Group (1988) *Br. J. Surg.* **75**, 1058
Scully, M. F. (1991) *Postgrad. Med. J.* **67**, 848

Heparin biological half-life

Conventional heparin has a half-life of less than 1.5 hours, but LMWH has a half-life of 111 minutes by factor Xa inhibition assay, 76 minutes by thrombin inhibition assay and 40 minutes by APTT assay.

Reference
Matzsch, T., Bergquist, D., Hedner, U. and Ostergaard, P. (1987) *Thromb. Haemost.* **57**, 97

Control of heparin dosage

Various methods are used, each of which measures different characteristics of heparin activity. The various heparins available also vary from species to species of origin, and with molecular size and degree of sulphation.

- Whole blood clotting time – a crude measure.

- APTT – an effective measure for conventional heparin if the APTT is kept at 1.5 –2 times the control APTT. Different platelet substrates or substitutes and different activating agents give different results. LMWH causes only slight prolongation of the APTT.

Reference
Poller, L., Thomson, J. M. and Yee, K. F. (1980) *Br. J. Haematol.* **44**, 161

- Thrombin time – requires careful standardization.
- Anti-Xa potentiation method.
- Chromogenic (amidolytic) assay of heparin. This is not a measure of heparin activity in the circulation.

Complications of heparin therapy

Overdosage

This causes bleeding, bruising and haematuria, and is especially liable to occur in the group of patients at risk with anticoagulant therapy. Since heparin has a relatively short half-life of less than 1.5 hours, simply stopping an infusion results in a rapid fall in circulating heparin. If a very large amount of heparin has been infused by accident, it can be neutralized by careful titration with protamine sulphate. Excess protamine sulphate acts both as a mild anticoagulant, prolonging the APTT and the prothrombin time, but also shortens the thrombin time and precipitates thrombin.

References
Horrow, J. C. (1985) *Anesth. Analg.* **64**, 348 (review of protamine toxicity)
Perkash, A. (1980) *Am. J. Clin. Pathol.* **73**, 676

Thrombocytopenia

Mild thrombocytopenia may occur soon after the onset of heparin therapy, and it usually resolves spontaneously. Delayed and severe thrombocytopenia persists until heparin therapy is stopped. The thrombocytopenia is caused by antibodies which only aggregate platelets in the presence of heparin.

References
Chong, B. H. and Castaldi, P. A. (1986) *Br. J. Haematol.* **64**, 347
Pfueller, S. L. and David, R. (1986) *Br. J. Haematol.* **64**, 149

An in vitro test for the severe type of thrombocytopenia induced by heparin has been devised.

Reference
Sheridon, D., Carter, C. and Kelton, J. G. (1986) *Blood* **67**, 27

Osteopenia

This is caused by high doses of heparin over a prolonged period, during pregnancy.

Reference
Wise, P. H. and Hall, A. J. (1980) *Br. Med. J.* **281**, 110

Alopecia

Reference
Thomas, D. P. (1981) *Clin. Haematol.* **10**, 443

Vitamin K action

Vitamin K action on vitamin K-dependent plasma clotting factors

Vitamin K is a cofactor for post-translational oxidative carboxylation of certain proteins at selected glutamic acid residue sites. Vitamin-K-dependent carboxylation converts 10 glutamate residues (weak chelators of calcium ions) into γ-carboxyglutamate residues. The NH_2-terminal chain of prothrombin contains 10 such residues per molecule. The binding of calcium ions to prothrombin anchors it to phospholipid membranes from the platelets, bringing it into close proximity with factors Va and Xa.

Factor Xa and prothrombin are adsorbed and concentrated on phospholipid-rich surfaces via calcium bridges on γ-carboxyglutamyl residues. Wounds and accompanying cell damage provide adequate phospholipid-rich sites. Similar γ-carboxyglutamyl residues are necessary for the activation of factors VII and IX. (Membrane tissues including bone, tooth dentine and ectopic calcification, are very rich in protein containing glutamyl residues (osteocalcin).) On activation of prothrombin to thrombin, the fragment containing calcium-binding sites is released, and can competitively inhibit further activation of prothrombin by factor Xa. The other portion of the prothrombin molecule is the precursor of thrombin. When anti-vitamin K oral anticoagulants are given (e.g. warfarin), acarboxyprothrombin is formed, with the 10 glutamyl residues not carboxylated, with potential for binding less that 1 calcium ion per molecule. Similar acarboxyderivates of factors VII, IX and X

are formed. Protein C, synthesized by the vascular endothelium, requires vitamin K before it can become active, and neutralize factors Va and VIIIa, as does Protein S.

Reference
Shearer, M. J. (1990) *Br. J. Haematol.* **75**, 156

Action of warfarin and other related anti-vitamin K anticoagulants

Warfarin is rapidly and completely absorbed from the gut, with peak plasma levels within 1 h. Food slows the rate of absorption. The biological half-life of racemic warfarin given intravenously is about 35 h. Therefore a single daily dose is adequate, and multiple doses through the day are not necessary. The separation of racemic warfarin into its two isomers, which have different anticoagulant potencies, has not been commercially viable. The plasma warfarin level cannot be used to control anticoagulant therapy, as a very wide range of plasma values at any given INR (international normalized ratio) is found in a group of patients (e.g. 0.8–4.1 mg/l in 'steady-state' anticoagulation).

Warfarin acts by interfering with the insertion of the calcium-binding site in vitamin-K-dependent plasma procoagulant factors, which include plasma factors II, VII, IX, X, protein C and protein S. The anticoagulant factor antithrombin III is increased by warfarin action, and it is used in the treatment of congenital AT-III deficiency.

The procoagulant factors II, VII, IX and X circulate in PIVKA forms (protein-induced vitamin K absence or antagonist), which have no calcium-binding sites,

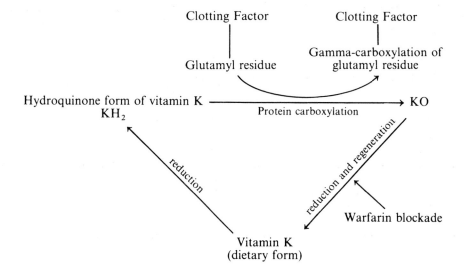

shorter biological half-lives and absence of ability to take part in the coagulation cascade. Long-term therapy with anticonvulsant drugs, including phenytoin, carbamazepine, phenobarbitone and valproate, in the absence of oral anticoagulant therapy produce a small increase in circulating PIVKAs, and PIVKAs are also increased in severe liver disease.

Reference
Davies, V. A., Rothberg, A. D., Argent, A. C. *et al.* (1985) *Lancet* **i**, 126

Start of treatment

Large loading doses during the first few days (15–30 mg/day) should not be used, because protein C has a very much shorter life than factors II, VII, IX and X. When very low levels of protein C are reached before the other vitamin-K-dependent factors have had time to fall, skin necrosis may develop, due to microvascular thrombi. Theoretically, a venous thrombosis could extend, because the surrounding vascular endothelium would not be protected by protein C release.

Warfarin 5–10 mg daily, depending on the patient's weight, should be given with heparin therapy in addition for the first 4–5 days, until adequate anticoagulation has been obtained, when the heparin therapy can be discontinued.

Laboratory control of oral anticoagulant therapy

The most commonly used test is based on the original prothrombin time devised by Armand Quick in the 1930s. This has been standardized as the INR (see p. 212).

Duration of oral anticoagulant therapy

There are no simple laboratory tests which can be used reliably to show whether the underlying thrombotic tendency has decreased or not. Treatment for 3 months is usually adequate for the control of venous thrombosis, with young patients recovering more rapidly than the elderly. Long-term therapy is needed following a second attack. It also prevents reinfarction and reduces cerebrovascular accidents after myocardial infarction.

References
Fennerty, A. G., Dolben, J., Thomas, P. *et al.* (1987) *Clin. Lab. Haematol.* **9**, 17
Lagerstedt, C. I., Olsson, C-G., Fagher, B. V. *et al.* (1985) *Lancet* **ii**, 515
Petitti, D. B., Strom, B. L. and Melmon, K. L. (1986) *Am. J. Med.* **81**, 225
Smith, P., Arnesen, H. F., Holme, I. (1991) *New Engl. J. Med.* **323**, 147

Cessation of oral anticoagulant therapy

Protein C has a very short life, recovering to 50% activity within 16h of stopping warfarin. Because factor VII has a half-life of only 7h, there is a rebound with increased factor VII levels if warfarin therapy is stopped suddenly, with a risk of a further thrombosis if any thrombotic tendency persists. It is therefore recommended that oral anticoagulation should be withdrawn over a period of some days after long-term administration.

Reference
Schofield, K. P., Thomson, J. and Poller, L. (1987) *Clin. Lab. Haematol.* **9**, 255

Mechanisms of interference with warfarin and other oral anticoagulants

Gastrointestinal tract

Vitamin K is present in a normal diet, but is also synthesized by bacteria in the gut, and absorbed. Malabsorption and destruction of vitamin-K-synthesizing bacteria by broad-spectrum antibiotics both increase the effect of oral coumarin-type anticoagulants. If other medicines or tonics contain pharmacological doses of vitamin K, these will depress warfarin activity.

Carriage of warfarin in the plasma

Displacement of warfarin from the albumin-binding sites which normally carry it in the plasma increases the free active circulating warfarin, which acts on the liver cells (e.g. phenylbutazone, clofibrate, indomethacin, sulphonamides etc).

Liver

- Increased affinity for coumarin derivatives, warfarin and other anticoagulants induced by clofibrate, thyroxine, glucagon etc.
- Differing responses of individuals to vitamin K. Genetically inherited varying levels of enzyme activity.
- Rate of synthesis of procoagulant factors II, VII, IX and X increased by anabolic steroids and androgens.
- Induction of enzymes which are responsible for the catabolism of warfarin, by phenobarbitone, chloral hydrate and glutethimide. The activity of these enzymes is reduced by chloramphenicol and by liver damage. Competition for these enzymes by tolbutamide and phenytoin results in increased duration of warfarin activity.

Fibrinolytic activity

Both oxymethalone and phenformin increase fibrinolytic activity, and have been associated with bleeding during oral anticoagulant therapy.

Altered platelet function

Platelet function is depressed by aspirin (acetylsalicylic acid), phenylbutazone and other non-steroidal anti-inflammatory drugs (NSAIDs). Aspirin also displaces warfarin from its binding to albumin.

Increased capillary fragility

In the presence of increased capillary fragility, warfarin may be associated with excessive bruising following trivial injury.

Factors increasing oral anticoagulant activity

- If the agent begins to act during established warfarin therapy, gross over-treatment results, unless the warfarin dosage is reduced.
- If satisfactory anticoagulation was established while the agent was being administered, and the agent is then suddenly discontinued, rapidly developing under-coagulation can occur, with a risk of thrombosis.

These agents include antibiotics, antidiabetic drugs, analgesics and antipyretics.

Factors decreasing oral anticoagulant activity

- If the agent begins to act during warfarin therapy, sudden under-treatment, with risk of thrombosis, may occur unless the warfarin dose is increased.
- If the agent ceases to act during established warfarin therapy, sudden over-treatment with consequent risk of bleeding, may occur.

These agents include vitamin K taken inadvertently, griseofulvin, glutethimide, haloperidol and meprobamate. Anticonvulsants can both impair and enhance warfarin activity, and patients on long-term anticonvulsant therapy are difficult to stabilize.

The Standing Advisory Committee for Haematology of the Royal College of Pathologists classify drug action:

- Drugs expected to potentiate warfarin action.
- Drugs which may potentiate warfarin action.
- Drugs which antagonize or may antagonize warfarin action.
- Drugs potentiated by warfarin.
- Drugs which do not affect anticoagulant therapy.

References
Editiorial (1982) *Br. Med. J.* **285**, 274
Study Advisory Committee for Haematology of the Royal College of Pathologists (1982) Drug interactions with coumarin derivative anticoagulants. *Br. Med. J.* **285**, 274–275

Contraindications or need for careful clinical and laboratory control

Potentially difficult to treat

- Elderly patients may be unreliable, forgetting doses, or taking too many. They require less warfarin than younger patients to achieve anticoagulation.
- Suicidal patients.
- Patients with hazardous occupations.

- Uncooperative patients and patients who lack understanding.
- Difficulty in obtaining laboratory control, with patients living many miles away from control centre.

Clinical conditions

- Gastrointestinal disorders, including diarrhoea, gastrocolic fistula, current or recent gastrointestinal haemorrhage or ulcer.
- Cardiac failure.
- Hypertension, especially in the elderly, with risk of intracranial bleed.
- Suspected cerebral haemorrhage, or recent brain surgery.
- Indwelling catheter, as bleeding occurs at its site.
- Uraemia, with its own bleeding tendency.
- Liver disease and cholestasis.
- Hypoalbuminaemia.
- Thyrotoxicosis.
- Pregnancy, with risk of damage to the fetus, and abortion or miscarriage.
- Lactation: some oral anticoagulants are secreted in breast milk.
- Inherited deficiency of plasma clotting factors, e.g. haemophilia.
- Concurrent heparin therapy for more than a few days.
- Abnormal platelet function – defective platelet function or thrombocytopenia.

Successful long-term oral anticoagulant therapy depends on:

- Vigilant physician.
- Cooperative intelligent patient.
- Reliable laboratory.

When full oral anticoagulant therapy is not possible, it may be useful to consider low-dose aspirin (see p. 176) and /or mini-dose warfarin (see p. 204), with or without added dipyridamol (see p. 177).

Complications of warfarin therapy

- Bleeding and bruising occur with increasing intensity and frequency as the level of anticoagulation is increased. Bleeding may occur at catheter sites, minor muscle damage (e.g. shoulder muscles after throwing a ball in play), gastrointestinal tract and renal tract (haematuria). Cerebral haemorrhage is dangerous. Haemarthrosis is rare. The activated partial thromboplastin time has been used to guard against bleeding during oral anticoagulant therapy.

References
Eastham, R. D. (1968) *Br. Med. J.* **2**, 337

- Skin necrosis is avoided if large loading doses are not used, and the first 4 days include heparin therapy.
- Rethrombosis after cessation of warfarin therapy. It is better to tail off warfarin dosage at the end of a course of treatment. rather than stopping suddenly.
- Fetal damage can occur when oral anticoagulants are given during pregnancy. A proportion of fetuses suffer developmental defects, and life-threatening haemorrhages may occur with abortion or stillbirths. About two-thirds of pregnancies result in normal infants.

References
Hall, J. G., Pauli, R. M. and Wilson, K. M. (1980) *Am. J. Med.* **68**, 122
Stevenson, R. E., Burton, O. M., Ferlauto, G. J. *et al.* (1980) *JAMA* **243**, 1549
Hirsh, J. (1991) *New Engl. J. Med.* **324**, 1865

- Amaurosis fugax: if the sight is threatened in a patient with rheumatic heart valve disease, low-dose aspirin (40 mg/day) and dipyridamol 100 mg three times daily can be safely and effectively combined with routine long-term warfarin therapy without increased risk of bleeding.

Low dose and mini-dose warfarin therapy

Warfarin in low dosage sufficient to increase the prothrombin time by only + 1.5–3 seconds before operation and by 5–8 seconds after operation reduces the incidence of venous thrombosis following hip and knee joint replacement. Warfarin 2 mg daily prevents thrombosis in indwelling central vein catheters. Warfarin 1 mg daily for 20 days before operation and after operation significantly reduces venous thrombosis after gynaecological surgery, and only increases the prothrombin time by 1–2 seconds above the untreated time. This low warfarin dosage was not associated with any excessive bleeding, and the reduction in thrombosis was as great as if full, and therefore potentially dangerous, warfarin anticoagulation had been used. These results strongly suggest that induction of plasma antithrombin III combined with reduced or absent suppression of protein C and protein S (also natural anticoagulants), play some part in the effects of low-dose warfarin, in the absence of marked depression in plasma factors II, VII, IX and X. It remains to be seen if low-dose warfarin can safely replace full-dose warfarin in the long-term treatment of venous thrombosis and pulmonary embolism, reducing the risk of haemorrhage, and eliminating the need for regular monitoring of plasma vitamin K-dependent clotting factors II, VII, IX and X.

References
Bern, M. M., Bothe, A Jr., Bistrian, B. *et al.* (1986) *Surgery* **99**, 216

Francis, C. W., Marder, V. J., McCollister, E. *et al.* (1983) *JAMA* **249**, 374
Poller, L., McKernan, A., Thomson, J. M. *et al.* (1987) *Br. Med. J.* **295**, 1309

Dextran

Dextran produced by a strain of *Leuconostoc mesenteroides* consists of an almost linear chain of glucose molecules linked by their $\alpha 1$–6 bonds, with side chains predominantly consisting of 1–2 glucose units attached by their $\alpha 1$–4 bonds at about every 20 glucose units in the main chain. The fewer and the shorter the side chains, the fewer side-effects are produced in patients. Very large dextran molecules with long side chains are strongly antigenic.

In the preparation of dextran, the high-molecular-weight components are removed, and the most commonly used preparations are Dextran 70 and Dextran 40.

Dextran 70, given at the time of operation, reduces the incidence of fatal pulmonary embolism to one-third of the incidence in untreated patients.

The smaller dextran molecules are eliminated in the urine, whilst the larger molecules diffuse slowly through the capillary walls to be slowly oxidized in the tissues over a period of weeks.

The incidence of dextran-induced anaphylaxis is thought to occur in perhaps 1 in 41 000 patients. Recently hapten inhibition has been tried, 3 g of Dextran 1 being given in 20 ml of solution 1–2 min before the main infusion of Dextran 40 or Dextran 70 is given. Type III anaphylaxis apparently occurs with the formation of large noxious immune complexes (dextran molecules combined with dextran-reacting antibodies of the IgG class), and there is a higher incidence with Dextran 70 than with Dextran 40 (which has a smaller molecular size). Dextran 1, which rapidly combines with, and neutralizes dextran-reacting antibodies, has a molecular weight of only 1000, and is not antigenic.

Complications associated with the use of dextran

- Circulatory overload (as can occur when too much of any plasma expander is given).
- Allergic reaction (perhaps 1 in 41 000 patients): there is cross-reactivity between dextran and a number of capsulated bacteria, including pneumococci.
- ?Haemorrhage, when the patient has thrombocytopenia, as dextran interferes with platelet function.

Haematological actions of dextran

1. Decreases plasma factor VIII activity.
2. Interferes with platelet function.

3. Improves venous blood flow:
   (a) encourages disaggregation of erythrocytes;
   (b) haemodilution with reduction in haematocrit;
   (c) whole blood viscosity reduced.
4. Accelerates factor XII activation by kallikrein and accelerates intrinsic fibrinolysis.
5. Any fibrin formed in the circulation is coarser than normal, and more easily lysed (by fibrinolysis).

Reference
Ljungström, K.-G. (1983) *Acta Chir. Scand. [Suppl.] 54.*

Dihydroergotamine

Prior to hip surgery 0.5 mg dihydroergotamine given subcutaneously twice daily on admission, and continuing for 3–5 postoperative days, combined with Dextran 70 infusion on alternate days, has been found to reduce the incidence of deep vein thrombosis from 31% to 3%. Dihydroergotamine reduces the volume of the capacitance vessels (veins and venules which contain the bulk of the blood volume), and it is thought that the increased rate of blood flow which is the result, reduces the risk of local venous thrombosis.

Dihydroergotamine also causes a temporary reduction in adrenaline-induced platelet aggregation, and has been shown to increase PGI_2 synthesis in vascular samples in vitro. When dihydroergotamine is given with heparin, the blood heparin level is higher than when heparin is given alone, and similar results are found when dihydroergotamine is given with dextran (blood dextran levels are higher than when dextran is given alone). This may be due to reduction of diffusion of either dextran or heparin through the vein walls.

Multiple therapy for prophylaxis and multi-factorial thrombosis

Since many cases of venous thrombosis are multifactorial in origin, it has been proposed that future trials should include combination therapy, for example, with low dose warfarin + low-dose aspirin or ticlopidine + atenolol etc.

Similarly, since platelets respond to, and are activated by, various distinct mechanisms, combination therapy should be considered for the prevention of platelet thrombosis in patients liable to myocardial infarction, stroke etc. with low-dose aspirin + low-dose warfarin + cold water fatty fish triglycerides in the form of regular fish meals or oil concentrates, low-dose alcohol (two glasses of wine daily), inclusion of olive oil in the diet etc.

Reference
O'Brien, J. R. (1987) *Thromb. Haemost.* **57**, 232

Secondary tumour spread, platelets and anticoagulant therapy

A high proportion of patients suffering from cancer die as a result of metastases. Most tumour cells are arrested in the lungs when they circulate from the primary growth, and die within 24 h. It has been suggested that platelets and platelet aggregates help cancer cells to survive, and that therefore antiplatelet drugs could be useful.

Reference
Karpatkin, S. and Pearlstein, E. (1982) *Ann. Intern. Med.* **95**, 636

Individual variation in the ability of platelets to form aggregates with human tumour cells has been found, i.e. there is an explanation for the difference in the spread and growth of secondary tumour deposits.

Reference
Bastida, E., Ordinas, A. and Jamieson, G. A. (1981) *Nature* **291**, 661

It has also been suggested that coagulation facilitates secondary tumour development and a trial with warfarin therapy has been advocated in suitable cases. It is known that tissue factor (factor III) produced by activated monocytes may contribute to the development of disseminated intravascular coagulopathy in cancer patients.

References
Marx, J. L. (1982) *Science* **218**, 145

It is therefore possible that some bland but effective antiplatelet aggregation agent such as eicosapentaenoic acid supplements plus low-dose aspirin and warfarin therapy maintained at the lower end of the therapeutic range might reduce the spread and growth of certain malignant tumour secondaries without harming the patient.

Tests Used in Bleeding and Clotting Studies

Platelet tests

see 'Platelet' section (p. 163).

Bleeding time

see 'Platelet' section (p. 164).

Capillary fragility

The qualitative test of capillary fragility, with its many variations of performance, is of limited clinical value.

It tends to be strongly positive in thrombocytopenia, abnormal platelet function and scurvy. Other conditions in which abnormal numbers of petechiae appear on the arm in response to a restrictive cuff include vascular purpura, liver disease and some diabetics. A few petechiae will develop in 10% of normal subjects.

Reference
Stavem, P. (1969) *Scand. J. Clin. Invest.* **17**, 607

Clot retraction

During the process of clotting, the network of platelets and fibrin retract, and this can be demonstrated in vitro. Various factors affect this test. Clot retraction is directly proportional to the platelet count up to about $126 \times 10^9/l$. Higher counts have no further effect, until very high platelet counts actually impede clot retraction. Defective platelets may also impair clot retraction. Similarly, hypofibrinogenaemia and hyperfibrinogenaemia result in reduced clot retraction. Also, as the packed cell volume is increased, so retraction is reduced, due to the increasing bulk of the cells. The time of onset of clot retraction is inversely proportional to the temperature, and the degree of clot retraction is directly proportional to the temperature. Above 42°C the reaction is inhibited.

Reference
Budtz-Olsen, O. E. (1951) *Clot Retraction.* Oxford: Blackwell

Whole blood clotting time

Both the Lee and White glass tube method (normal range 5–11 min), and the Dale and Laidlaw capillary tube method are insensitive. Five methods, each of which measure different physical characteristics of clot formation, have recently been compared.

Reference
Blair, S. D., Menashi, S., Samson, D. and Greenhalgh, R. M. (1987) *Clin. Lab. Haematol.* **9**, 91

Heparin tolerance test

This is an obsolete test. Heparin is neutralized, locally at sites of thrombi by PF4 released by platelets, and by acute phase proteins in the circulation during thrombosis and after acute myocardial infarction, explaining the varying requirements of conventional heparin to maintain adequate anticoagulation in these, and similar conditions.

Plasma-activated partial thromboplastin clotting time (APTT)

Platelet-poor citrated plasma is activated by diatomaceous earths (kaolin, celite, bentonite), colloidal silica or ellagic acid, in the presence of platelet substrate or platelet substitute. Calcium chloride solution is added after activation, and the time required for clotting to occur is measured. The normal range of clotting times is wide, and varies with the reagents used. There is no standard method. Different reagents are sensitive or insensitive to individual plasma coagulation factor deficiencies. For example, micronized silica and ellagic acid are both more sensitive in the detection of deficiencies of factors VIII, X and XII, than is micronized kaolin. All three reagents detect factors XI deficiency. When factor IX is deficient, ellagic acid is better than micronized silica, which in turn is better than micronized kaolin. All three reagents are insensitive to HMWK deficiency, but will detect moderate prekallikrein deficiency.

Laboratory factors

Overfilling the blood sample tube with blood, with consequent dilution of the citrate in the tube, has little effect on the clotting time, unless the citrate is so dilute that clotting occurs prematurely. Underfilling the blood sample tube, or testing blood from severely polycythaemic patients, artefactually prolongs the APTT, as the citrate concentration in the plasma becomes excessive.

The test should be carried out as soon as possible after sampling, or should be stored without centrifugation at 4°C. If delay before testing is inevitable, the addition of a mixture of theophylline, adenosine and dipyridamol to the citrate (CTAD) allows storage at room temperature for some hours, with prolongation of the APTT by only 0–11%.

References
Turi, D. C. and Peerschke, E. I. (1986) *Am. J. Clin. Pathol.* **85**, 43
van den Besselaar, A. M. H. P., Meeuwisse-Braun, J., Jansen-Grüter, R. *et al.* (1987) *Thromb. Haemost.* **57**, 226

Physiological

Reduced clotting time

- With increasing age.

Reference
Cawkwell, R. D. (1978) *Thromb. Haemost.* **39**, 780

- Following prolonged strenuous exercise.

Reference
Marsh, N. A. and Gaffney, P. J. (1981) *Thromb. Haemost.* **48**, 20

Pathological

Reduced clotting time

- Acute pancreatitis.
- Disseminated malignancy.
- Following acute haemorrhage.
- Following acute thrombosis or myocardial infarction.
- Three to four days after surgical operation or injury. A preoperative shortened APTT may frequently be associated with the development of postoperative thrombosis.

An APTT shorter than normal indicates an associated resistance to heparin.

Prolonged clotting time

- Anticoagulants - including heparin, warfarin and other oral anticoagulants, and some circulating anticoagulants.
- Deficiencies of factors II, V, VIII, IX, X, XI, XII, prekallikrein and/or HMWK – but not factor VII.

The prolonged APTT associated with prekallikrein deficiency is shortened following longer activation with kaolin, or activation with ellagic acid (which activates factor XII in the absence of prekallikrein). The prolonged APTT associated with HMWK deficiency is shortened when the plasma is activated with ellagic acid for a longer period.

Plasma recalcified clotting time (calcium time)

Excess calcium chloride is added to citrated plasma, and the time taken before the appearance of a fibrin clot is measured.

This is now an obsolete test.

Clotting time in siliconized tubes

The normal range of clotting time of whole blood in siliconized tubes is 25–45 min.

The ratio (siliconized glass clotting time/plain glass clotting time) is referred to as the *wettability index* (normal = 2–3).

This is now an obsolete test.

Prothrombin time

Based on the test devised by Quick over 50 years ago, tissue thromboplastin, in the form of rabbit's brain extract or bovine combined thromboplastin, is added

to citrated plasma. Excess calcium chloride solution is added, and the time taken to form a fibrin clot is measured. Human brain thromboplastin is no longer used because of possible health hazards (Jakob–Creutzfeldt disease and AIDS). The test prothrombin time is divided by the control prothrombin time to give the prothrombin ratio – normal ratio = 1.0–1.2.

The international normalized ratio (INR) is based on a comparative standardization of results obtained with pooled plasma from normal subjects, using rabbit brain thromboplastin, bovine combined thromboplastin and human brain thrombopolastin. The sensitivity and precision of thromboplastin at different concentrations and the difficulties in comparing different thromboplastins has been investigated recently.

References
Denson, K. W. F. (1988) *Clin. Lab. Haematol* **10**, 315
Lewis, S. M. (1987) *Br. J. Haematol.* **66**, 1

Therapeutic range for control of anticoagulant therapy

The generally accepted therapeutic range of the INR = 2.0–4.5, although there are no studies which indicate that this is either the ideal or the safest range. Dangerous bleeding occurs with increasing frequency at the upper end of the range, and this should not be exceeded.

Using mini-dose warfarin therapy of 1 mg per day, thrombosis after abdominal surgery has been greatly reduced without side effects, and studies are needed to see whether long-term oral anticoagulation at the lower end of the therapeutic range is effective; it is certainly less likely to cause dangerous bleeding. Oral anticoagulation with warfarin and related drugs not only depresses levels of factors II, VII, IX and X (reducing the tendency to thrombose), but unfortunately also depresses the natural anticoagulants protein C and protein S, while fortunately probably inducing AT-III.

Reference
Davies, J. A. and Tuddenham, E. G. D. (1986) In: Weatherall, D. J., Ed. *Oxford Textbook of Medicine*, 2nd Edn Vol. 2, p 229. Oxford: Oxford University Press.

Shortening of the prothrombin time

Contact with glass when plasma is stored at 4°C before estimation shortens the clotting time by 1–2 s.

Pathological

Deficiency of C1 esterase inhibitor (C1 INH) greatly reduces the prothrombin time

Reference
Palmer, R. N. and Gralnick, H. R. (1982) *Blood* **59**, 38

Increased prothrombin time

Pathological

- Factor VII deficiency: the test is most sensitive to reduced factor VII.
- Factor II deficiency.
- Factor X deficiency.
- Depression of factors II, VII and X during oral anticoagulant therapy, or severe vitamin K deficiency.
- Factor V deficiency.
- Circulating anticoagulants, including high levels of circulating heparin.
- In simple obstructive jaundice, with poor absorption of vitamin K, a small dose of vitamin K (1 mg) will often restore the prothrombin time to normal, whereas in severe liver disease, with failure of synthesis of the vitamin-K-dependent factors and factor V, larger doses of vitamin K may not have much effect on the prothrombin time.
- Paracetamol overdose. Continued increase from day 4 onwards equals poor chance of survival.

Two-stage prothrombin estimation

Now that a specific method for the estimation of factor II is available, this test is obsolete.

Thrombin time

A standard dilution of buffered thrombin is added to the patient's citrated plasma, and the clotting time (reflecting the thrombin–fibrinogen reaction) is compared with that of normal control plasma, using the same dilution of thrombin.

Increase

- Heparin: the thrombin time has been used to control intravenous heparin therapy.
- Other circulating anticoagulants (?).
- Fibrinogen deficiency: the thrombin time is inversely proportional to the plasma fibrinogen concentration, at low plasma fibrinogen concentrations.
- Fibrin – fibrinogen degradation products (FDPs): these impair the thrombin–fibrinogen reaction (e.g. as in DIC).
- Dysfibrinogenaemia: the thrombin time is prolonged in certain varieties of inherited dysfibrinogenaemias.

Heparin–thrombin clotting time

After addition of a standard amount of heparin to citrated plasma (insufficient to prevent clotting by thrombin), 20s later, buffered thrombin is added, and the clotting time is compared with that using control plasma.

Pathological reduction in clotting time

- Acute myocardial infarction.
- Venous thrombosis and/or pulmonary embolism.
- Severe atherosclerosis.

Inhibition of the action of heparin results in the shorter time. It was originally thought that this was due mainly to release of platelet factor 4 (anti-heparin) from disrupting platelets in vivo, but appears to be due mainly to inhibition by non-specific acute phase glycoproteins.

References
Andersen, P. and Godal, H. C. (1977) *Thromb. Haemost.* **38**, 193
Cella, G. and Russo, P. (1977) *Thromb. Haemost.* **38**, 696
O'Brien, J. R., Etherington, M. D. and Jamieson, S. (1976) *Lancet* **i**, 878

Venom 'cephalin' prothrombin assay

Oxalated plasma and 'Stypven' (Russell viper venom) are mixed, and excess calcium chloride is then added. The time after the addition of calcium solution when clotting occurs is measured. The normal plasma clotting time = 15–20 s.

This test does not measure prothrombin activity accurately, and since viper venom has an activity like factor VII, the method cannot safely be used for the control of anticoagulant therapy.

On the other hand, this technique can be used to differentiate between factor VII deficiency, in the one-stage method, and Stuart–Prower factor defect. Venom corrects deficiency in factor VII but not in Stuart–Prower factor, and activates factor X directly. It can be used to assess the degree of factor X deficiency. Cephalin or lecithin is essential for the reaction.

The 'Stypven' time is inversely proportional to the serum triglyceride concentration, i.e. chylomicrons and low-density lipoproteins.

References
Biggs, R. and Macfarlane, R. G. (1949) *J. Clin. Pathol.* **2**, 33
James, G. A. (1949) *J. Clin. Pathol.* **2**, 45
Rifkind, B. M. and Gale M. (1967) *J. Atheroscler. Res.* **7**, 704

Serum prothrombin consumption

During normal clotting thromboplastin converts practically all plasma prothrombin to thrombin, which is then neutralized by serum antithrombin. In those cases in which thromboplastin is generated inadequately during clotting, only part of the prothrombin is converted to thrombin (i.e. consumed). Thus, the test, which measures the residual prothrombin in serum after clotting has occurred, can be used as a simple screening test before the performance of a full thromboplastin generation test. It has the advantage that it can be performed on citrated plasma, but it suffers from wide variations in the values obtained from normal cases unless the conditions of the test are strictly observed.

Normal range

Prothrombin consumption index $= 0–40\%$ (usually less than 20%). Serum prothrombin time, measured 1 h after clotting has occurred, is normally more than 30 s.

Pathological

This test is used, if at all, for the detection of abnormal platelet function. More specific tests of platelet function are available.

One 4 year-old boy with a bleeding disorder has been described, and the only abnormal test found was the prothrombin consumption test. It was assumed that he had an abnormal form of factor II, with slow conversion to thrombin.

References
Rocha, E., Paramo, J. A., Cuesta, B. *et al.* (1985) *Br. J. Haematol.* **61**, 177

Thromboplastin generation

With the availability of estimation of the individual plasma clotting factors (and especially factor VIII and factor IX) this test is obsolete.

Thromboelastography

This apparatus is used in research and is not in general use. A torsion steel wire is inserted into a cuvette containing whole blood or recalcified plasma. A small mirror is mounted on the wire and the cuvette is rotated.

Whilst the blood or plasma remains fluid, the wire remains motionless, but as fibrin appears, adhering both to the cuvette walls and the wire, the pin is rotated. The movements of the wire are observed by means of the mirror.

Deficiencies of coagulation factors show variations in the thromboelastogram and some cases of thrombasthenia are only demonstratable by this technique. Reaction time during surgical operation is shortened in proportion to: (1) depth of narcosis; (2) duration of operation; this is possibly evidence of hypercoagulability.

References
de Nicola, P. (1956) *The Laboratory Diagnosis of Coagulation Defects.* Springfield, IL; Thomas
Wille, P (1959) *Folia Haematol. (Leipz.)* **3**, 339

Anticoagulants (in vitro)

Oxalate

Potassium oxalate 4 mg, plus ammonium oxalate 6 mg prevents 5 ml blood from clotting.

Oxalate acts by removing calcium from plasma, as the insoluble calcium oxalate. Recalcification with excess calcium chloride solution annuls this effect.

Note: Factor V deteriorates more rapidly in oxalated blood than in citrated blood.

Sodium citrate

Citrate ions form a non-ionized complex with plasma calcium, thus preventing clotting until excess calcium salt is added. Commonly 1 part of 3.8% sodium citrate solution is mixed with 9 parts of blood. Although this is satisfactory for prothrombin estimations, the final citrate concentration prolongs the activated partial thromboplastin time if the haematocrit value exceeds 45%, having a marked effect if the haematocrit value exceeds 50%. This effect can be avoided by reducing the volume of citrate to 8 parts citrate to 92 parts blood. This is very important in anticoagulant therapy in polycythaemic patients.

Reference
Koepke, J., Rodgers, J. L. and Ollivier, M. J. (1985) *Am. J. Clin. Pathol.* **64**, 591

EDTA

This chelating agent binds calcium and prevents clotting until excess calcium chloride is added. Also it inhibits the conversion of fibrinogen to fibrin.

Complement, Circulating Immune Complexes, Properdin

Complement

The complement system includes an interrelated, interacting group of serum proteins, which together are responsible for the biological activity of complement-fixing antibodies. It is the prime mediator of cytotoxic injury to antibody-sensitized cells, an important part in the inflammatory response. Antibodies may become attached to corresponding antigens in particular cells, and these cells become engulfed by macrophages and destroyed. If complement is involved, the rate of phagocytosis is increased.

Complement includes a number of components C1, C2, C3 etc. and may become activated rapidly and systematically by sequential enzymatic cleavage of each complement component to $\overline{C1}$, $\overline{C2}$ etc. the bar signifying activation, or may become fragmented, e.g. 3a, 3b, 3c etc. Complement is activated by a wide range of antibody molecules after they have reacted with antigen, and it therefore assists in the destruction of substances foreign to the body.

Sequential activation of components of complement

- C1 is a macromolecule consisting of three subcomponents held together in the presence of calcium ions: C1q which carries binding site for antibody; C1r: C1s which is pro-esterase, after activation it becomes esterase.

  A site on the Fc fragment of certain immunoglobulins becomes capable of binding with C1 when antibody combines with antigen. A single IgM molecule attached to a cell may activate complement. Two adjacent IgG molecules attached to a cell can activate complement, and non-specific activation of complement occurs in the presence of aggregated IgG molecules.

  Of the components of IgG, IgG3 is very active, IgG1 is moderately active, IgG2 is slightly active, and IgG4 has no activity, in the activation of complement. Antibody molecules must be bound to more than one antigen site before complement fixation occurs.
- Activated C1 is designated as $\overline{C1}$, and $\overline{C1}$ acts on C4 which attaches to cell membrane, other C4 molecules, and antibody molecules.
- $\overline{C14}$ activates C2 in the presence of magnesium ions.
- The complex $\overline{C42}$ then acts on C3, a proportion of which binds to the cell surface, and some binds with antibody. C3 is split into smaller fragments: C3a which has anaphylotoxic activity; C3b which binds to the cell surface. Generation of C3b results in opsonization of red cells.
- Activation of C5 requires the presence of both $\overline{C42}$ and C3b; C3b on the cell surface is converted to two further fragments C3c and C3d, and red cells in vitro with complement-binding antibody can be shown to have C3c and C3d on their surfaces.
- C5 activated by $\overline{C423}$, and the complex C567 is activated to produce $\overline{C567}$ attached to the cell surface, binding C8.

- C8 alone can slowly lyse red cells, but the reaction is accelerated by C9. Generation of C8 and C9 results in destruction of red cells in the circulation.
- Lesions in the cell membrane are produced, leading to increasing osmotic damage. All cells lysed by the action of complement have holes in their membranes, 10 nm in diameter, which can be demonstrated by electron microscopy. The final destruction of the cell is by osmotic imbalance resulting from the presence of these holes. Red cell-bound complement components increase red cell membrane rigidity. This is important in complement-mediated red cell destruction.

Reference:
Sung, K-L. P., Freedman, J., Chabanel, A. *et al.* (1986). *Br. J. Haematol.* **61**, 455

'Alternate' mechanism of complement activation

C3 can also be activated by 'C3 activator', bypassing the C142 step. Normal serum contains 'C3 proactivator' (? factor B of the properdin system), which can be converted to C3 activator by aggregated IgG, IgA, zymosan and inulin. C3 activator can cause C3 attachment to the cell surface, leading to eventual cell lysis. This alternative pathway is important in hypocomplementaemia in association with:

- Cirrhosis of the liver.
- Systemic lupus erythematosus.
- Glomerulonephritis.

Reference:
Perrin, L. H., Lambert, P. H., Nydegger, U. *et al.* (1972) *Schweiz. Med. Wochenschr.* **102**, 1604

Complement activation

Moderate

Extracorporeal perfusion: (1) haemodialysis; (2) cardiopulmonary bypass.

Massive and prolonged

Resulting in severe pulmonary damage progressing to shock lung (adult respiratory distress syndrome)

- Severe sepsis.
- Trauma.
- Acute pancreatitis.

Reference:
Jacob, H. S. (1983) *Quart. J. Med.* **52**, 289

Activation of C1 by plasmin

Plasmin can activate C1. In other words, there is an interrelationship between:

- Coagulation.
- Kinin generation.
- Fibrinolysis.
- Complement activation.

Anticomplementary activity

Calcium ions are required for C1 integrity, and magnesium ions are needed for C42 activation. Both these ions are chelated by anticoagulants. Large doses of heparin also interfere with complement integrity. Heating serum to 56°C for 30 min inactivates C1 and C2 activities, and partially destroys C4 activity.

Inhibitors of complement

Serum normally contains an inhibitor of C$\bar{1}$, which does not interfere with the conversion of C1 to C$\bar{1}$. Stored serum is anticomplementary.

Congenital deficiency of inhibitor of C$\bar{1}$

- Type A: total amount of inhibitor low.
- Type B: normal amounts of inhibitor protein antigen but biological activity low.

Attacks associated with laryngeal oedema and intestinal colic.

Normal newborn

Fifty per cent of normal adult levels.

Abnormalities of complementary components

Congenital

Inheritance of these conditions autosomal recessive, except for properdin deficiency which is X-linked recessive, and C1 inhibitor which is autosomal dominant.

- Syndromes resembling systemic lupus erythematosus: C1r, C1s, C4, C2, C5 and CR1 deficiencies.
- Recurrent pyogenic infections: C3, C5, properdin, factor $\bar{D}$, factor I, CR3 deficiencies.
- Recurrent disseminated neisseria infections: C6, C7, C8-β-chain and C8-α-γ-chain deficiencies.
- Glomerulonephritis: C3, factor H deficiencies.
- Hereditary angioneurotic oedema plus increased incidence of autoimmune disease: C$\bar{1}$ inhibitor deficiency.
- The most common inherited complement deficiency in western Europe, frequently associated with autoimmune disease, but subjects may be clinically well: C2 deficiency.

References
Cole, F. S., Whitehead, A. S., Auerbach, H. S. *et al.* (1985) *N. Engl. J. Med.* **313**, 11
Frank, M. M. (1987) *N. Engl. J. Med.* **316**, 1525

Acquired

Increase

Total complement activity is increased in various infectious diseases.

Reduced

- Bacterial endocarditis complicated by glomerulonephritis.
- Prodromal acute viral hepatitis.
- Systemic lupus erythematosus, especially with renal involvement. Serial measurements of C3, C4 and CH$_{50}$ are useful in clinical assessment.
- Decreases liver synthesis of C3 and C4: alcoholic cirrhosis; congestive cardiac failure with liver anoxia; chronic active hepatitis; schistosomiasis.
- Rheumatoid arthritis: complement levels are reduced in the synovial fluid.
- Autoimmune haemolytic anaemia: complement binds to red cells.

Complement activity plays a part

- Paroxysmal nocturnal haemoglobinuria: there is a population of cells which are extremely susceptible to complement lysis.
- Allograft rejection.
- Activation of alternate pathway in glomerulonephritis.

Cases in which the total haemolytic complement activity is increased have a worse prognosis than cases in which complement activity is reduced.

Reference:
Gabriel, R., Glynn, A. A. and Joekes, A. M. (1972) *Lancet* **ii**, 55

- DIC appears to follow intravascular lysis, and is usually associated with complement-activating antibodies, particularly anti-A and anti-B.
- In human haemostasis, C6 component is not significantly involved. In other animal species, platelets are susceptible to complement activation.

Urine C3 excretion in glomerulonephritis is an indicator of continuing disease activity with deposition of C3 by immune complexes in the glomerular capillary wall.

Reference:
Cumming, A. D., Thomson, D., Davison, A. M. *et al.* (1976) *J. Clin. Pathol.* **29**, 601

Species differences

These are present in complement.

References
Bruninga, G. L. (1971) *Am. J. Clin. Pathol.* **55**, 273
Mollison, P. L. (1970) *Br. J. Haematol.* **18**, 249
Ruddy, S., Gigli, I. and Austen, K. F. (1972) *N. Engl. J. Med.* **287**, 489, 545, 592, 642

Circulating immune complexes

Immune complexes can be estimated in the circulation by measurement of the C1q binding activity. Platelets appear to play an important part in clearing immune complexes, and in protecting the vascular endothelium from damage. Although demonstration of immune complexes is of no value in clinical diagnosis, their estimation may be useful in monitoring the progress of lupus nephritis. In idiopathic thrombocytopenic purpura (ITP), the level of immune complexes appears to be inversely related to the platelet count. Antigen-specific immune complexes increase in the plasma after the ingestion of challenge foods.

References
Levinsky, R. J. (1981) *J. Clin. Pathol.* **34**, 1214
Paganelli, R., Levinsky, R., Brostoff, J. *et al.* (1979) *Lancet* **i**, 1270
Trent, R. J., Clancy, R. L. Danis, V. *et al.* (1980) *Br. J. Haematol.* **44**, 645
Walker, S. M. and Khateeb, S. F. Al. (1981) *J. Clin. Pathol.* **34**, 400

Plasmapheresis

It is possible to remove a patient's plasma and replace it with albumin solution, plasma, and/or plasma expanders, removing at the same time, antigen–antibody complexes, poisons etc. originally in the patient's plasma. The procedure, using a cell separator, gives the clinician the opportunity to treat the underlying condition by chemotherapy, radiotherapy, transfusion etc. while the noxious effects of the circulating substances are reduced. The procedure has been used effectively in:

- Hyperviscosity syndrome, removing monoclonal immunoglobulins and relieving hyperviscosity syndrome.
- Poisoning, including parathion, methyl alcohol, digoxin overdose and alpha-amanatin from poisonous fungi.
- Antibodies, including high-titre Factor VIII antibodies in severe haemophilia when Factor VIII infusion is essential to control severe bleeding; severe post-transfusion purpura developing 1 week after transfusion in a P1^{A1}-ve patient; myasthenia gravis with circulating anti-acetylcholine receptors; autoimmune haemolytic anaemia; Goodpasture's syndrome to remove antiglomerular basement membrane antibodies; cold agglutinin haemolytic anaemia; immune complex vasculitis in some cases of lupus erythematosus and rheumatoid arthritis; bullous pemphigus to remove antibody complex; cryoglobulinaemia; some cases of severe idiopathic thrombocytopenic purpura; Guillain-Barré syndrome to remove circulating antibodies.
- While plasmapheresis may be of benefit in thrombotic thrombocytopenic purpura, infusion of fresh plasma is effective, suggesting an underlying acute deficiency state.

- Plasmapheresis has been used in Refsum's disease to remove phytanic acid; familial hypercholesterolaemia to remove cholesterol; severe Rhesus haemolytic disease.

Complications which may occur – allergic reactions, electrolyte disturbances, circulatory disturbances including fluid overload, hypotension, cardiac arrhythmias, and possible infections from contaminated donor plasma.

Serum properdin

Note: Properdere: to prepare to destroy.

This substance, which is present in all mammals, is a β-globulin, and makes up 0.03% of the total serum protein. Its molecular weight is approximately 1 000 000, and it acts with the third component of complement in the presence of magnesium ions to combine selectively with polysaccharides of high molecular weight. This property accounts for its antibody-like action and its haemolytic action.

During the first 6 months of a normal infant's life there is no fall in the serum properdin level (compare serum complement level which falls in the normal infant after birth). Also, properdin from an animal of one species interacts with polysaccharides derived from its own tissues equally as well as with polysaccharides derived from tissues of other species, or even bacteria (i.e. very non-specific).

It is worth noting that patients suffering from congenital agammaglobulinaemia in the absence of infection have normal serum properdin levels.

The known constituents of the properdin system have been designated:

- Factor A: ?derived from the C3 component of complement.
- Factor B: this has been identified with C3 proactivator, part of the alternative mechanism for indicating complement dependent tissue injury. The properdin system appears to function by initiating complement action rather than through the generation of active products from components of the properdin system itself.

Reference:
Naff, G. B. (1972) *N. J. Med.* **287**, 716

Decreased serum properdin levels
- Dextran transfusion: it is possible to ameliorate an acute attack of haemolysis with dextran transfusion in paroxysmal nocturnal haemoglobinuria.
- Acute leukaemia.
- Haemolytic anaemia during crisis.
- Aplastic anaemia.
- Some carcinoma cases.

- Hodgkin's disease and some cases of lymphosarcoma, in which the serum complement is increased.
- Von Gierke's glycogen storage disease: the properdin is bound to the glycogen.
- Experimentally after zymosan injection (polysaccharide in yeast cell capsules) the properdin level falls, but rises to about three times normal after 2–3 days.

References:
Hunter, W. De. and Hill, J. M. (1958) *Am. J. Clin. Pathol.* **29**, 128
Rottino, A. and Levy, A. L. (1959) *Blood* **14**, 246
Wedgwood, R. J. (1958) *Pediatrics* **22**, 991 (review)

Blood Transfusion

Only in the last 50 years have the full therapeutic potentials of blood and blood products begun to be properly utilized.

The first well-documented transfusions were carried out by Richard Lower of Oxford, England and Jean Baptiste Denise in France, in 1667. These were sheep-to-human transfusions, and whilst Lower's patient apparently had little in the way of side effects, several of the patients treated by Denise reported passing 'dark' or 'black' urine' – certainly due to intravascular haemolysis!

Following these reports blood transfusions were banned and those still carried out were for treating insanity, or mood changes! It was not until 1824, when James Blundell, a physiologist and obstetrician at Guy's Hospital, London showed that blood could be used to treat haemorrhagic shock, that transfusion came to the fore again. Blundell treated 10 women with severe post-partum haemorrhage; remarkably 5 survived.

During the remainder of the nineteenth century the following problems arose:

- Local infection.
- Unknown incompatibilities.
- Clotting.

The first step towards modern, safe blood transfusion came between 1901 and 1902, when Karl Landsteiner and associates discovered isoagglutinins, and hence the ABO blood groups. Subsequently, ABO grouping meant major incompatibilities were avoided.

The next steps towards modern blood banking came very quickly during World War I. In 1914, Hustin in Belgium reported the use of sodium citrate and glucose to anticoagulate, and then transfuse blood.

In 1915, Weil, in the USA, stored citrated blood in an ice box for several days before transfusion.

Blood banking and the use of blood on a large scale was pioneered by O. H. Robertson (a Canadian army medical officer) who by the end of the war had shown that blood could be stored for as long as 21 days! Regular blood donation sessions and blood banks were gradually developed.

In the UK, with the help of the British Red Cross Society, a voluntary blood donor service was well established by 1939. In the USA, the service unfortunately tended to develop around paid donors.

In 1943, Loutit and Mollinson introduced acid–citrate–dextrose (ACD) as an anticoagulant and storage medium. This used 70 ml ACD to 450 ml collected blood and gave a less dilute infusion. The blood could be stored for 21–28 days.

In 1951, Gibson used citrate–phosphate–dextrose (CPD) which generally gave better results than ACD and allowed blood to be stored for 28 days.

Initially blood was collected and stored using glass bottles and rubber tubing: from 1952 onwards, however, these were gradually replaced by plastic tubing and plastic bags. This gave much greater flexibility in preparing blood products.

Most blood banks now collect blood into citrate–phosphate–dextrose–adenine (CPD-A), which gives a shelf life of 35 days. Some will separate off all the plasma and resuspend the red cells in saline–adenine–glucose–mannitol (SAG-M) which will happily support red cells for 40 days.

The modern blood transfusion service has changed dramatically since the 1950s, when it was really only expected to produce whole blood and plasma (from outdated blood). Today, with modern storage methods, plastic bags, accurate centrifugation, differential pheresis and plasma fractionation, a whole host of different products are available for the eager clinician to use. The important ones are listed over.

The blood transfusion service has had to adapt to advances in clinical medicine more recently; for instance, it has had to support the development of bone marrow transplantation with large numbers of platelets and CMV negative blood products.

Blood transfusion hazards

Red cell incompatibility

ABO incompatibilities may be fatal, e.g. transfusing group A blood into group O patient, and are due to

Whole blood	For treatment of severe blood loss or in some heart surgery

Red cell concentrates
  Plasma reduced
  SAG-M red cells
	For treating anaemia due to marrow failure
	Not responsive to haemotinics

Washed or filtered red cells	For patients requiring transfusion support who have had transfusion reactions due to white cell orplatelet antibodies
Frozen red cells	Patients with very rare blood groups or where compatible blood may be very difficult to find
Platelets	To treat thrombocytopenia, particularly in aplastic anaemia and leukaemia, but increasingly to support bone marrow transplantation
CMV negative red cells CMV negative platelets	In immunosuppressed patients or in bone marrow transplantation
Albumin 4.5% 20%	As a plasma expander or for more specific treatment in liver failure or renal disease with proteinuria
Fresh frozen plasma (FFP)	To replace depleted clotting factors in hypertransfused patients or consumption of clotting factors in, for example, DIC
Cryoprecipitate	Contains high concentration of factor VIII and was previously used to treat heamophilia. Now also used to replace fibrinogen in DIC
Factor VIII Factor IX	Pure freeze-dried factor VIII is now used to treat haemophilia Freeze-dried factor IX is used to treat Christmas disease (haemophilia B)
Immunoglobulin	To treat hypogammaglobulinaemia or to treat autoimmune thrombocytopenia
Rhesus anti-D	To prevent rhesus haemolytic disease
γ-Globulin	From high-titre donors to treat specific diseases, e.g. measles, herpes zoster

the naturally occurring isoagglutinins anti-A and anti-B. Such serious problems can be avoided by accurate ABO grouping of blood; unfortunately, most mistakes are clerical and not technical.

Acquired antibodies due to previous transfusion or pregnancy may also cause serious problems but can be screened out by cross-matching.

In serious red cell incompatibility, the patient will become very unwell soon after the start of transfusion, due to intravascular haemolysis. The patient may complain of nausea or loin pain. There may also be the following:

- Tachycardia.
- Fall in blood pressure.
- Sweating.
- Fever.
- Passing of dark urine.
- Ultimately anuria!

The transfusion must be stopped and physiological saline given to maintain a good urine flow. If urine flow falls, frusemide or mannitol may be required. DIC might complicate severe reaction and will require platelet and cryoprecipitate support.

Bacterial infection of blood or blood products

Bacteria may contaminate the blood at the time of

collection. Some are capable of surviving or even growing at 4°C.

Diseases transmitted from the donor

Viral hepatitis

Hepatitis A

The carrier state is rare and transfusion risk very small.

Hepatitis B

This used to be a major problem in blood transfusion but screening of donors for hepatitis B surface antigen (HBsAg) has considerably reduced the risk.

Non-A, non-B hepatitis (now called hepatitis C).

This remains a real problem because serological tests have only just become available to detect the non-A, non-B form. The true incidence of post-transfusion non-A, non-B hepatitis is very difficult to establish, but may be as high as 2.5%. It seems likely that two separate viruses are involved. Some transfusion centres check the liver enzymes of donors in an attempt to screen out non-A, non-B hepatitis (e.g. alanine transaminase levels). Infected recipients can go on to develop chronic liver disease and cirrhosis.

HIV-1

This virus was first discovered and described by French workers in 1983. HIV-1 antibody detection, by an ELISA (enzyme-linked immunosorbent assay) technique, has been available since 1985. All blood donations are now tested for HIV-1 antibody; unfortunately, prior to 1985 the virus was transmitted to many patients in blood and blood products, the most unfortunate group being severe haemophiliacs – 75% of whom were infected by contaminated factor VIII. Transfusion centres have made tremendous efforts to reduce the risk of HIV-1 and hence of AIDS.

- Donor selection (discouraging donors from high-risk groups).
- Screening all donors for antibody.
- Inactivation of virus during production (e.g. heat inactivation of virus in factor VIII).

The risk of HIV-1 infection from blood and blood products is currently estimated at 1 : 3 000 000.

HIV-2

This virus has been described in Africa, and also in Europe and the USA. It is not detected by tests for HIV-1.

HTLV-1

This virus, from the same group as HIV, causes a malignancy of T4 lympocytes called adult leukaemia lymphoma. It was first described in Japan, but has

now been found in the Caribbean, USA and UK. It is associated with a bad prognosis and, interestingly, hypercalcaemia.

CMV

Cytomegalovirus transmission is important in immunocompromised patients.

Malaria

In the UK and USA, donor selections should eliminate the danger of transmission. Prophylactic administration of antimalarial drugs should be given in countries where selection of non-infected donors is not possible.

American trypanosomiasis (Chagas' disease)

This is prevalent in South America from Mexico to northern Argentina. Millions of people are infected and can transmit the disease by blood donation.

Syphilis

Transmission could occur if fresh blood from a donor in the secondary stage were given. The spirochaete dies after a few days at 4°C in stored blood. All donated blood is serologically tested.

Trypanosomiasis and kala-azar

In Africa these could be transmitted.

Toxoplasmosis

Infection is dangerous in immunosuppressed patients.

Microfilaria

The worms survive for up to 2 weeks in refrigerated citrated blood.

Relapsing fever

Transmission has been reported, but the spirochaete dies within 24 hours at 4°C.

Fluid overload

This is particularly a problem in the elderly or in patients with cardiac and renal disease. Transfusions should be slowed and small doses of frusemide used. Red cell concentrates reduce the risk of overload.

Potassium loading

The longer blood is stored, the more potassium leaks out of the red cells. This is potentially dangerous, particularly if large amounts of blood are transfused quickly, or if 'old' blood is given to small babies.

Citrate toxicity

This may develop when large volumes of citrated blood are transfused in a short period. This applies especially in neonates and patients with liver disease, where citrate is not metabolized as rapidly as normal. Citrate toxicity can be treated using 10% calcium gluconate, 10 ml i.v. for every 5 units of blood transfused.

Iron overload

Iron overload can occur in any patient receiving long-term blood transfusion support, provided they are not also bleeding, e.g. thalassaemia, aplastic anaemia (with a haemostatic platelet count), myelodysplastic syndromes.

Significant iron overload will occur after 100 units of blood have been transfused. Iron chelation with desferrioxamine can be used to reduce iron overload.

Blood transfusion therapy has made a significant contribution to the advancement of modern medicine. Many people are alive today who would not be, but for good transfusion practice. The advent of HIV was a shattering experience and reminds us all that blood transfusion should not be taken lightly, but that we have to maintain high standards to keep it as safe as possible.

Blood has for centuries been known to be 'the giver of life'; it is mentioned over 500 times in the Bible. Leviticus (7:26) forbids the 'eating' (drinking) of blood, but nowhere of course does it say blood cannot be transfused for the benefit of mankind.

References:
Handbook of Transfusion Medicine (1989) London: HMSO
Thomas, D. P. (1988) *Br. J. Haematol.* **70**, 393
Wintrobe, M. (Ed.) (1980) *Blood Pure and Eloquent.* New York: McGraw Hill

Appendix: SI units in Haematology

A coherent metric system is now used in Britain. This system, called the Système International d'Unités (SI), is the approved method of expressing information in all branches of science and medicine.

SI has six basic units: metre, kilogram, second, ampere, kelvin and candela, with the addition of mole for substance concentration. All other units are derived from these bases.

The preferred unit of volume is litre (l).

The following list shows the usual haematological parameters in conventional units and SI units with conversion factor. In every component the figures are the same in both units but there is a shift of decimal point in some cases. The WBC and platelets may appear unfamiliar but as the integers are unchanged there should be no confusion.

Component	Current use*	SI units*	Conversion factor	Notes
Haemoglobin	14.4 g/100 ml(g%)	14.4 g ml	No change	(1) (2)
RBC	$4.5 \times 10^6/(/mm^3)$	$4.5 \times 10^{12}/l$	10^6	(1)
PVC	41%	0.41	0.01	(1) (3)
MCV	$75–95 \; \mu^3$	75–95 fl	No change	(4)
MCH	27–32 pg	27–32 pg	No change	(6)
MCHC	30–35%	30–35 g/dl	No change	(2)
WBC	4000–11000 (/mm³)	$4.0–11.0 \times 10^9/l$	10^6	
Platelets	150 000–400 000 (/mm³)	$150–400 \times 10^9/l$	10^6	
Serum B_{12} (as cyanocobalamin)	160–925 pg/ml	160–925 ng/l	1	(5)
Serum folate	3–20 ng/ml	3–20 μg/l	1	

Notes:
* Figures in these columns are examples within the normal range.

(1) As the normal range varies with age and sex, only one measurement in the normal range has been given as an example.

(2) dl = decilitre, i.e. 10^{-1} litre.

(3) No unit necessary. l/l is implied.

(4) fl = femtolitre, i.e. 10^{-15} litre.

(5) ng = nanogram (10^{-9} g).

(6) pg = picogram (10^{-2} g).

INDEX